Sleep in Medical and Neurologic Disorders

Editor

FLAVIA B. CONSENS

SLEEP MEDICINE CLINICS

www.sleep.theclinics.com

Consulting Editor
TEOFILO LEE-CHIONG Jr

March 2016 • Volume 11 • Number 1

ELSEVIER

1600 John F. Kennedy Boulevard • Suite 1800 • Philadelphia, Pennsylvania, 19103-2899

http://www.theclinics.com

SLEEP MEDICINE CLINICS Volume 11, Number 1
March 2016, ISSN 1556-407X, ISBN-13: 978-0-323-41665-8

Editor: Patrick Manley
Developmental Editor: Donald Mumford

Sleep Medicine Clinics (ISSN 1556-407X) is published quarterly by Elsevier Inc., 360 Park Avenue South, New York, NY 10010-1710. Months of issue are March, June, September and December. Business and Editorial Offices: 1600 John F. Kennedy Blvd., Ste. 1800, Philadelphia, PA 19103-2899. Customer Service Office: 3251 Riverport Lane, Maryland Heights, MO 63043. Periodicals postage paid at New York, NY and additional mailing offices. Subscription prices are $195.00 per year (US individuals), $100.00 (US students), $458.00 (US institutions), $235.00 (Canadian and international individuals), $135.00 (Canadian and international students), $519.00 (Canadian institutions) and $509.00 (International institutions). Foreign air speed delivery is included in all *Clinics* subscription prices. All prices are subject to change without notice. **POSTMASTER:** Send change of address to *Sleep Medicine Clinics*, Elsevier Health Sciences Division, Subscription Customer Service, 3251 Riverport Lane, Maryland Heights, MO 63043. Customer Service: **Tel: 1-800-654-2452 (U.S. and Canada); 314-447-8871 (outside U.S. and Canada). Fax: 314-447-8029. E-mail: journalscustomerservice-usa@elsevier.com (for print support); journalsonline support-usa@elsevier.com (for online support).**

Reprints. For copies of 100 or more of articles in this publication, please contact the Commercial Reprints Department, Elsevier Inc., 360 Park Avenue South, New York, NY 10010-1710. Tel.: 212-633-3874; Fax: 212-633-3820; E-mail: reprints@elsevier.com.

Sleep Medicine Clinics is covered in *MEDLINE/PubMed (Index Medicus)*.

Printed in the United States of America.

PROGRAM OBJECTIVE

The goal of *Sleep Clinics of North America* is to keep practicing physicians up to date with current clinical practice by providing timely articles reviewing the state of the art in patient care.

TARGET AUDIENCE

All practicing physicians and other healthcare professionals.

LEARNING OBJECTIVES

Upon completion of this activity, participants will be able to:
1. Review cardiovascular disorders associated with low sleep duration, such as cardiovascular disease and congestive heart failure.
2. Discuss the effects of sleep on the incidence of stroke and epilepsy.
3. Recognize how sleep affects neuromuscular and neurodegenerative disorders.

ACCREDITATION

The Elsevier Office of Continuing Medical Education (EOCME) is accredited by the Accreditation Council for Continuing Medical Education (ACCME) to provide continuing medical education for physicians.

The EOCME designates this enduring material for a maximum of 15 *AMA PRA Category 1 Credit*(s)™. Physicians should claim only the credit commensurate with the extent of their participation in the activity.

All other health care professionals requesting continuing education credit for this enduring material will be issued a certificate of participation.

DISCLOSURE OF CONFLICTS OF INTEREST

The EOCME assesses conflict of interest with its instructors, faculty, planners, and other individuals who are in a position to control the content of CME activities. All relevant conflicts of interest that are identified are thoroughly vetted by EOCME for fair balance, scientific objectivity, and patient care recommendations. EOCME is committed to providing its learners with CME activities that promote improvements or quality in healthcare and not a specific proprietary business or a commercial interest.

The planning committee, staff, authors and editors listed below have identified no financial relationships or relationships to products or devices they or their spouse/life partner have with commercial interest related to the content of this CME activity:

Umair Afzal, MBBS; Christian R. Baumann, MD; Philip Cheng, PhD; Flavia B. Consens, MD; Naima Covassin, PhD; Antonio Culebras, MD; Xavier Drouot, MD, PhD; Anna Monica Fermin, MD; Anjali Fortna; Jonathan P. Hintze, MD; Alex Iranzo, MD; Lynn Kataria, MD; Douglas Kirsch, MD, FAAN, FAASM; Patrick Manley; Kimberly Nicole Mims, MD; Dionne Morgan, MBBS; Mahalakshmi Narayanan; Robert L. Owens, MD; Shalini Paruthi, MD; Solene Quentin, MD; Scott A. Sands, PhD; Erin Scheckenbach; Prachi Singh, PhD; Sheila C. Tsai, MD; Bradley V. Vaughn, MD.

The planning committee, staff, authors and editors listed below have identified financial relationships or relationships to products or devices they or their spouse/life partner have with commercial interest related to the content of this CME activity:

Christopher Drake, PhD is on the speakers' bureau for Teva Pharmaceutical Industries Ltd. and Merck Sharp & Dohme Corp., is a consultant/advisor for Merck Sharp & Dohme Corp., and has research support from Teva Pharmaceutical Industries Ltd.; Merck Sharp & Dohme Corp.; PERNIX Therapeutics; Aladdin Dreamer, Inc.; Inteliclinic; Jazz Pharmaceuticals plc.

Teofilo Lee-Chiong Jr, MD has stock ownership, a research grant from, and an employment affiliation with Koninklijke Philips N.V., is a consultant/advisor for CareCore National and Elsevier B.V.; and has royalties/patents with Elsevier B.V.; Lippincott; John Wiley & Sons, Inc.; Oxford University Press; and CreateSpace, a DBA of On-Demand Publishing, LLC.

UNAPPROVED/OFF-LABEL USE DISCLOSURE

The EOCME requires CME faculty to disclose to the participants:
1. When products or procedures being discussed are off-label, unlabelled, experimental, and/or investigational (not US Food and Drug Administration [FDA] approved); and
2. Any limitations on the information presented, such as data that are preliminary or that represent ongoing research, interim analyses, and/or unsupported opinions. Faculty may discuss information about pharmaceutical agents that is outside of FDA-approved labelling. This information is intended solely for CME and is not intended to promote off-label use of these medications. If you have any questions, contact the medical affairs department of the manufacturer for the most recent prescribing information.

TO ENROLL

To enroll in the Sleep Medicines Clinic Continuing Medical Education program, call customer service at 1-800-654-2452 or sign up online at http://www.theclinics.com/home/cme. The CME program is available to subscribers for an additional annual fee of USD $140.

METHOD OF PARTICIPATION

In order to claim credit, participants must complete the following:

1. Complete enrolment as indicated above.
2. Read the activity.
3. Complete the CME Test and Evaluation. Participants must achieve a score of 70% on the test. All CME Tests and Evaluations must be completed online.

CME INQUIRIES/SPECIAL NEEDS

For all CME inquiries or special needs, please contact elsevierCME@elsevier.com.

SLEEP MEDICINE CLINICS

THE CLINICS ARE AVAILABLE ONLINE!
Access your subscription at:
www.theclinics.com

Contributors

CONSULTING EDITOR

TEOFILO LEE-CHIONG Jr, MD
Professor of Medicine, National Jewish Health;
Professor of Medicine, School of Medicine,
University of Colorado Denver, Denver,
Colorado; Chief Medical Liaison, Philips
Respironics, Pennsylvania

EDITOR

FLAVIA B. CONSENS, MD
Associate Professor of Neurology, Adjunct
Associate Professor of Anesthesiology and
Pain Medicine, University of Washington Sleep
Center, Harborview Medical Center, University
of Washington, Seattle, Washington

AUTHORS

UMAIR AFZAL, MBBS
Upstate Medical University, Syracuse,
New York

CHRISTIAN R. BAUMANN, MD
Leading Senior Physician, Department of
Neurology, University Hospital Zurich,
University of Zurich, Zurich, Switzerland

PHILIP CHENG, PhD
Research Scientist, Sleep Disorders and
Research Center, Henry Ford Health System,
Detroit, Michigan

NAIMA COVASSIN, PhD
Assistant Professor of Medicine, Division of
Cardiovascular Diseases, Mayo Clinic,
Rochester, Minnesota

ANTONIO CULEBRAS, MD
Department of Neurology, Upstate Medical
University, Syracuse, New York

CHRISTOPHER DRAKE, PhD
Director of Sleep Research, Sleep Disorders
and Research Center, Henry Ford Health
System, Detroit, Michigan

XAVIER DROUOT, MD, PhD
CHU de Poitiers, Department of Clinical
Neurophysiology, Hôpital Jean Bernard; Univ
Poitiers, University of Medicine and Pharmacy;
INSERM, CIC 1402, Equip Alive, CHU
dePoitiers, Poitiers, France

ANNA MONICA FERMIN, MD
Upstate Medical University, Syracuse,
New York

JONATHAN P. HINTZE, MD
Pediatrics House Officer, Saint Louis
University School of Medicine, St Louis,
Missouri

ALEX IRANZO, MD
Neurology Service, Hospital Clínic de
Barcelona, IDIBAPS, CIBERNED, Barcelona,
Spain

LYNN KATARIA, MD
Sleep Medicine Section, Department of
Neurology, Washington DC Veterans
Affairs Medical Center; Assistant Professor
of Neurology, George Washington University
School of Medicine, Washington, DC

DOUGLAS KIRSCH, MD, FAAN, FAASM
Medical Director, CHS Sleep Medicine, Carolinas HealthCare System; Clinical Associate Professor, University of North Carolina School of Medicine, Charlotte, North Carolina

KIMBERLY NICOLE MIMS, MD
Sleep Physician, Charlotte Medical Clinic, Carolinas HealthCare System, Charlotte, North Carolina

DIONNE MORGAN, MBBS
Instructor, Department of Medicine, National Jewish Health, Denver, Colorado

ROBERT L. OWENS, MD
Assistant Professor of Medicine, Division of Pulmonary and Critical Care Medicine, University of California, San Diego, La Jolla, California

SHALINI PARUTHI, MD
Associate Professor of Pediatrics and Internal Medicine, Saint Louis University School of Medicine, St Louis, Missouri

SOLENE QUENTIN, MD
CHU de Poitiers, Department of Clinical Neurophysiology, Hôpital Jean Bernard; Univ Poitiers, University of Medicine and Pharmacy; INSERM, CIC 1402, Equip Alive, CHU de Poitiers, Poitiers, France

SCOTT A. SANDS, PhD
Instructor in Medicine, Division of Sleep Medicine, Brigham and Women's Hospital, Harvard Medical School, Boston, Massachusetts; Department of Allergy, Immunology and Respiratory Medicine, Central Clinical School, Alfred Hospital, Monash University, Melbourne, Australia

PRACHI SINGH, PhD
Assistant Professor of Medicine, Division of Cardiovascular Diseases, Mayo Clinic, Rochester, Minnesota

SHEILA C. TSAI, MD
Associate Professor, Department of Medicine, National Jewish Health, Denver, Colorado; Associate Professor, Department of Medicine, University of Colorado Denver, Aurora, Colorado

BRADLEY V. VAUGHN, MD
Professor of Neurology, Biomedical Engineering and Allied Health Sciences, Department of Neurology, University of North Carolina School of Medicine, Chapel Hill, North Carolina

Contents

Sleep disorders in neuromuscular disorders are generally caused by respiratory dysfunction associated with these diseases. Hypoventilation in neuromuscular diseases results from both respiratory muscle weakness and reduced chemoreceptor sensitivity, which is required for ventilatory drive. This condition results in repeated arousals, sleep fragmentation, and nocturnal hypoxemia, manifesting most commonly as excessive daytime somnolence. Polysomnography can identify sleep disordered breathing in patients with neuromuscular disorders and treatment with noninvasive ventilation may improve quality of life.

Sleep and circadian rhythms significantly impact almost all aspects of human behavior and are therefore relevant to occupational sleep medicine, which is focused predominantly around workplace productivity, safety, and health. In this article, 5 main factors that influence occupational functioning are reviewed: (1) sleep deprivation, (2) disordered sleep, (3) circadian rhythms, (4) common medical illnesses that affect sleep and sleepiness, and (5) medications that affect sleep and sleepiness. Consequences of disturbed sleep and sleepiness are also reviewed, including cognitive, emotional, and psychomotor functioning and drowsy driving.

Inadequate sleep is increasingly pervasive, and the impact on health remains to be fully understood. The cardiovascular consequences alone appear to be substantial. This review summarizes epidemiologic evidence regarding the association between extremes of sleep duration and the prevalence and incidence of cardiovascular diseases. The adverse effects of experimental sleep loss on physiological functions are discussed, along with cardiovascular risk factors that may underlie the association with increased morbidity and mortality. Current data support the concept that inadequate sleep duration confers heightened cardiovascular risk. Thus implementation of preventative strategies may reduce the potential disease burden associated with this high-risk behavior.

This article provides an overview of common pediatric sleep disorders encountered in the neurology clinic, including restless legs syndrome, narcolepsy, parasomnias, sleep-related epilepsy, and sleep and headaches. An overview of each is provided, with an emphasis on accurate diagnosis and treatment. It is important in comprehensive neurologic care to also obtain a sleep history, because treating the underlying sleep condition may improve the neurologic disorder.

Special Articles

The intensive care unit (ICU) environment is not propitious for restoring sleep and many studies have reported that critically ill patients have severe sleep disruptions. However, sleep alterations in critically ill patients are specific and differ significantly from those in ambulatory patients. Polysomnographic patterns of normal sleep are frequently lacking in critically ill patients and the neurobiology of sleep is important to consider regarding alternative methods to quantify sleep in the ICU. This article discusses elements of sleep neurobiology affecting the specificity of sleep patterns and sleep alterations in patients admitted to the ICU.

In this article, the effect of sleep and sleep disorders on endocrine function and the influence of endocrine abnormalities on sleep are discussed. Sleep disruption and its associated endocrine consequences in the critically ill patient are also reviewed.

Congestive heart failure (CHF) is among the most common causes of admission to hospitals in the United States, especially in those over age 65. Few data exist regarding the prevalence CHF of Cheyne–Stokes respiration (CSR) owing to congestive heart failure in the intensive care unit (ICU). Nevertheless, CSR is expected to be highly prevalent among those with CHF. Treatment should focus on the underlying mechanisms by which CHF increases loop gain and promotes unstable breathing. Few data are available to determine prevalence of CSR in the ICU, or how CSR might affect clinical management and weaning from mechanical ventilation.

Sleep in Neurodegenerative Diseases

Alex Iranzo, MD

KEYWORDS

- Parkinson disease • Insomnia • Excessive daytime sleepiness • Obstructive sleep apnea
- Nocturnal stridor • Restless legs syndrome • Periodic leg movements in sleep
- REM sleep behavior disorder

KEY POINTS

- Sleep disorders are common in patients with neurodegenerative diseases.
- Their origin is multifactorial.
- Insomnia, circadian changes, hypersomnia, REM sleep behavior disorder, sleep-disordered breathing, and restless legs syndrome are sleep disorders commonly found in neurodegenerative diseases.
- Some sleep disorders are red flags of some neurodegenerative diseases: stridor indicates the occurrence of multiple system atrophy; in the setting of dementia, REM sleep behavior disorder indicates dementia with Lewy bodies and not Alzheimer disease; the absence of REM sleep behavior in a patient with parkinsonism points toward Parkinson disease and not to multiple system atrophy.
- Therapy of sleep disorders should be individualized.

INTRODUCTION

Neurodegenerative diseases are characterized by neuronal loss in the nervous system and abnormal deposition of proteins (eg, phosphorylated α-synuclein, tau, β-amyloid, ataxins) in surviving cells. Common neurodegenerative diseases are Alzheimer disease, Parkinson disease (PD), dementia with Lewy bodies, multiple system atrophy, spinocerebellar ataxias, progressive supranuclear palsy, Huntington disease, and amyotrophic lateral sclerosis. Some diseases are idiopathic and sporadic (dementia with Lewy bodies, multiple system atrophy, progressive supranuclear palsy) and others are hereditary carrying genetic abnormalities (spinocerebellar ataxias, Huntington disease). In some diseases, the idiopathic presentation is the most common but genetic forms have also been reported (Alzheimer disease, PD, amyotrophic lateral sclerosis).

The origin of most of the neurodegenerative diseases is uncertain. They are manifested by an insidious onset and a progressive course of a variety of disabling neurologic symptoms and signs, such as dementia, parkinsonism (tremor, bradykinesia, rigidity, postural and gait imbalance), motor weakness, ataxia, cerebellar syndrome, dysautonomia, oculomotor abnormalities, bulbar symptoms, and chorea. In addition, sleep disorders are common, may be the first manifestation of the disease, and may impact on the quality of life. Sleep disorders occurring in neurodegenerative diseases are insomnia (difficulty in falling sleep, sleep fragmentation, early morning awakening), excessive daytime sleepiness (EDS), circadian rhythm changes, rapid eye movement (REM) sleep behavior disorder (RBD), periodic leg movements in sleep (PLMS), restless legs syndrome (RLS), central or obstructive sleep apnea (OSA), and nocturnal stridor. Some of these sleep

Neurology Service, Hospital Clínic de Barcelona, IDIBAPS, CIBERNED, C/Villarroel 170, Barcelona 08036, Spain
E-mail address: airanzo@clinic.ub.es

Sleep Med Clin 11 (2016) 1–18
http://dx.doi.org/10.1016/j.jsmc.2015.10.011

sleep.theclinics.com

disorders may occur during the prodromal stage of the disease, years before the emergence of the cardinal symptoms that define the diagnosis of the disease. This finding indicates that identification of such individuals will be of great interest when neuroprotective agents become available. Awareness of sleep disorders by neurologists and sleep specialists is important because correct counseling, management, and therapy may improve patients' quality of life. This article reviews the sleep disorders occurring in PD, as a prototypical disorder of the neurodegenerative diseases,

because most of the sleep disturbances are present. Sleep disorders occurring in other neurodegenerative diseases are summarized in **Boxes 1–7**.

PARKINSON DISEASE

PD is clinically characterized by parkinsonism caused by neurodegeneration of the substantia nigra. Surviving neurons show cytoplasmatic inclusions, called Lewy bodies and Lewy neurites, where abnormal deposits of α-synuclein are the

---

Box 1
Sleep disorders in Alzheimer disease

- Alzheimer disease (AD) is the most common neurodegenerative disease and is characterized by neuronal loss and deposition of β-amyloid and neurofibrillary tangles in the hippocampus and cortex resulting in cognitive impairment.
- It is under debate if reduced sleep duration and OSA in the general population are risk factors for AD. The APOE-4 allele is a risk factor for AD and OSA.
- The link between AD and sleep disorders is bidirectional. Although degeneration of the suprachiasmatic and cholinergic nuclei by the disease produce severe sleep loss and disruption, these abnormalities may have a negative effect in cognition, perhaps by decreasing β-amyloid clearance in the brain.
- Sleep disorders are common, affecting up to 45% of patients having an important impact on patients and caregivers.
- Sleep disorders may be an early manifestation but their frequency and intensity usually progress with disease severity.
- The most common sleep problem is an exaggerated tendency to phase advancing characterized by frequent daytime napping, difficulties in falling asleep at night, nocturnal sleep fragmentation, and early morning awakening. This pattern is similar but more severe than that seen in the elderly and may be related, in part, to degeneration of the suprachiasmatic nucleus resulting in alterations in melatonin secretion rhythm.
- In extreme cases, patients present the sundowing syndrome, which is characterized by agitation, confusion, and aggressiveness in the dark hours of the evening and in the night.
- In the middle of the night patients may experience confusional awakenings with nocturnal wandering and agitation.
- Polysomnography shows reduced total sleep time and sleep efficiency, increased sleep-onset latency and wake time after sleep onset, reduced deep sleep and REM sleep amounts, and increased light sleep amount. In advanced cases sleep scoring is difficult because of the absence of alpha rhythm during wakefulness and loss of sleep spindles and K complexes.
- RBD is very rare.
- RLS seems to be not prominent, although its frequency may be underestimated because diagnosis requires patients describing their sensations in the legs. Specific RLS criteria for dementia have been developed.
- The frequency of OSA is high affecting between 40% and 70% and may aggravate cognitive dysfunction in AD.
- Management of sleep disorders is based in cognitive-behavioral strategies, sleep hygiene, and bright light therapy. In early stages acetylcholinesterase inhibitors may ameliorate the sleep pattern and cognition. Continuous airway pressure therapy is indicated in OSA. Although robust scientific evidence is lacking, several medications are commonly used to enhance sleep, such as melatonin, benzodiazepines, sedating antidepressants, and atypical neuroleptics (eg, quetiapine).

Adapted from Peter-Derex L, Yammine P, Bastuji H, et al. Sleep and Alzheimer's disease. Sleep Med Rev 2015;19: 29–38.

Box 2
Sleep disorders in dementia with Lewy bodies

- Dementia with Lewy bodies (DLB) is the most common cause of dementia after AD and is characterized by dementia, parkinsonism, fluctuations, and visual hallucinations. Neuropathologic changes are the presence of Lewy bodies in the brainstem, limbic system, and cortical areas.
- Sleep disorders affect about 80% of the patients and are more frequent than in AD.
- Insomnia, circadian rhythm disorder with early awakening, EDS caused by frequent napping, nocturnal hallucinations, and confusional nocturnal wandering are frequent.
- Confusional nocturnal awakenings usually arise from non-REM sleep stages.
- OSA, PLMS, and RLS are no more common than in the general population of similar age.
- Patients with idiopathic RBD may develop mild cognitive impairment characterized by executive, visuospatial, and memory dysfunction. The interval between mild cognitive onset and dementia onset is about 2 years.
- RBD occurs in about 80% of the patients and may antedate the onset of dementia in approximately 70%.
- Detection of RBD in a patient with dementia points toward DLB because this parasomnia is rare in other forms of dementia including AD, frontotemporal dementia, and progressive supranuclear palsy. Current diagnostic criteria of DLB consider RBD as a suggestive feature of the disease.
- In the setting of DLB, RBD occurs predominantly in men, has short duration of dementia, early onset of parkinsonism and visual hallucinations, and little AD-related pathology on autopsy.
- Confusional awakenings and nocturnal visual hallucinations are difficult to distinguish from RBD only using clinical history.
- Patients with severe dementia polysomnography may show ambiguous sleep caused by neurodegeneration of the structures that modulate sleep.

From Iranzo A. Sleep disorders in atypical parkinsonisms. In: Videnovic A, Högl B, editors. Disorders of sleep and circadian rhythms in Parkinson's disease. Springer Wien Heidelberg New York Dordercht London; 2015. p. 209–21; with permission.

---

major component. Patients with PD also present nonmotor manifestations, such as depression, dementia, and sleep disorders, which are the result of the neurodegenerative process occurring in neuronal structures and networks outside the substantia nigra.[1] The origins of sleep disorders in PD are multifactorial and include neurodegeneration of regions that regulate sleep, aging, the presence of certain symptoms and signs of the disease that may affect sleep onset and continuity (eg, parkinsonism leading to difficulty in turning, nocturia, pain, depression, dementia, nocturnal hallucinations), and the effect of some medications (eg, dopaminergic agents, antidepressants, antipsychotics).

SLEEP DISORDERS IN THE PRODROMAL STAGE OF PARKINSON DISEASE

Patients with PD may present a prodromal time period of several years before parkinsonism emerges, which is manifested by hyposmia, depression, constipation, and sleep disorders, namely RBD and possibly EDS. This is in line with a proposed staging model of pathology in PD where α-synuclein aggregates are first present in the peripheral autonomic nervous system and in the lower brainstem before advancing to the midbrain and reaching the substantia nigra.[2]

Rapid Eye Movement Sleep Behavior Disorder

RBD is a parasomnia characterized by abnormal motor and vocal behaviors (eg, jerking, kicking, shouting, crying, laughing) and unpleasant dreams (eg, being attacked or chased by people) occurring during REM sleep without atonia. The diagnosis of RBD is made by clinical and polysomnography. RBD is the result of the dysfunction of the lower brainstem structures that regulate muscle atonia during REM sleep, namely the magnocellularis nucleus in the medulla and the locus subcoeruleus in the pons.[3] There are three lines of evidence indicating that RBD represent the prodromal stage of PD.

Longitudinal studies

Longitudinal studies conducted in sleep centers have shown that most subjects with the idiopathic form of RBD (IRBD) eventually develop the cardinal symptoms of PD and two other

---

Box 3
Sleep disorders in multiple system atrophy

- Multiple system atrophy (MSA) is characterized by a combination of parkinsonism, cerebellar syndrome, and autonomic failure in any combination where the pathologic hallmark is α-synuclein-positive cytoplasmic inclusions in the glia of many brain structures.
- About 70% of patients with MSA report sleep problems.
- Sleep-onset insomnia and fragmented sleep occur in about 50%. Many causes may contribute to sleep fragmentation and include urinary incontinence, anxiety, depression, inability to change body position in the bed because of parkinsonism, and the use of several medications.
- EDS occurs in 28% but in most is not a major complaint. In a few patients sleep attacks may occur after the intake of levodopa.
- It is not clear if RLS and PLMS are more frequent than in the general population of similar age.
- MSA is eventually diagnosed in only a few subjects with the initial diagnosis of idiopathic RBD (most of them are diagnosed with PD and dementia with Lewy bodies), probably because in the general population MSA is much less common than PD and dementia with Lewy bodies.
- RBD occurs in 80% to 100%. In a patient with suspected MSA, the absence of RBD should seriously question the diagnosis of this disease. RBD is currently considered a red flag for the diagnosis of MSA.
- In about half of the patients, RBD precedes the cardinal symptomatology of the disease.
- Breathing problems may be of central and peripheral (obstructive) origin.
- Central respiratory disturbances are caused by degeneration of the bulbar respiratory centers leading to abnormal hypoxic ventilatory responses, Cheyne-Stokes respiration, irregular breathing, and central sleep apnea.
- Nocturnal stridor occurs in about 20% of the patients. It is considered one of the red flags that should raise suspicion of MSA in a patient with parkinsonism. Stridor occurs in all stages of the disease and indicates obstruction of the airway at the level of the vocal cords in the larynx. As the disease advances, nocturnal stridor progresses into wakefulness because of an increasing reduction in the glottic aperture.
- Patients with MSA, particularly those with stridor, may present typical OSA episodes with oxyhemoglobin desaturations and in some cases subacute episodes of respiratory failure.
- In most patients with nocturnal stridor the clinical examination of the vocal cords during wakefulness with laryngoscopy shows vocal cord paralysis.
- The presence of stridor in MSA has been linked to decreased survival and sudden death during sleep.
- Nasal continuous positive airway pressure and tracheostomy eliminate stridor and obstructive apneas in MSA.

From Iranzo A. Sleep disorders in atypical parkinsonisms. In: Videnovic A, Högl B, editors. Disorders of sleep and circadian rhythms in Parkinson's disease. Springer Wien Heidelberg New York Dorderclt London; 2015. p. 209–21; with permission.

---

synucleinopathies, dementia with Lewy bodies and multiple system atrophy (**Table 1**).[4–13] The risk for conversion from IRBD diagnosis increases with the duration of follow-up. In one study, the risk of a defined neurodegenerative syndrome from IRBD diagnosis was 35% at 5 years, 73% at 10 years, and 92% at 14 years.[7]

Idiopathic rapid eye movement sleep behavior disorder abnormalities characteristic of Parkinson disease

Patients with IRBD present abnormalities that are characteristic features of PD, such as olfactory deficit, color vision impairment, cognitive abnormalities, subtle cortical electroencephalographic slowing, dysautonomic abnormalities, reduced cardiac ^{123}I-MBIG scintigraphy, decreased dopamine transporter in the striatum, and increased substantia nigra echogenicity (**Box 8**).[14] Longitudinal studies in IRBD have shown that neuropsychological testing and dopamine transporter binding in the putamen decline over time, whereas olfactory dysfunction, color vision impairment, echogenicity of the substantia nigra, and autonomic functions remain stable.[3]

Box 4
Sleep disorders in progressive supranuclear palsy

- Progressive supranuclear palsy (PSP) is clinically manifested by dementia, parkinsonism, falls, and vertical gaze palsy. PSP is a taupathy involving the brainstem, basal ganglia, frontal lobe, and many other brain areas.
- Polysomnographic studies show reduced total sleep time, decreased REM sleep percentage, and reduction in sleep spindles and K complexes. In severe cases the alpha rhythm is absent and wakefulness and sleep stages are difficult to differentiate.
- The most frequent sleep complaint is insomnia with difficulty in falling sleep and maintenance of sleep, and sometimes symptoms suggestive of RBD. In some patients, RBD-like symptoms may reflect true nocturnal wandering and confusional awakenings, which are frequent in patients with any type of dementia.
- EDS, OSA, PLMS, and RLS are not major complications in PSP.
- RBD occurs in about 10% to 20% and is usually of mild severity and frequently develops after dementia onset.
- The subclinical form of RBD (asymptomatic REM sleep without atonia) occurs in about 20%.

From Iranzo A. Sleep disorders in atypical parkinsonisms. In: Videnovic A, Högl B, editors. Disorders of sleep and circadian rhythms in Parkinson's disease. Springer Wien Heidelberg New York Dorderoht London; 2015. p. 209–21; with permission.

Rapid eye movement sleep behavior disorder and Parkinson disease pathology

Deposits of α-synuclein are detected in living subjects with IRBD in the autonomic nerves innervating peripheral organs. The two subjects with IRBD examined neuropathologically to date without clinical evidence of parkinsonism had predominant brainstem Lewy bodies with minimal damage in the substantia nigra.[15,16] One multicenter postmortem study examined the brain of 80 polysomnography-confirmed subjects with RBD who had comorbid parkinsonism or dementia and found α-synuclein pathology in 78 (98%) of the subjects.[17]

The previously mentioned features indicate that IRBD is an adequate population to test neuroprotective agents destined to stop or slow down the underlying degenerative process.

Box 5
Sleep disorders in Huntington disease

- Huntington disease (HD) is a genetic autosomal-dominant condition characterized by dementia, chorea, and psychiatric disturbances linked to expanded CAG repeats in the Huntington gene. Pathologic studies demonstrate severe atrophy of the putamen and caudate, and, to a lesser extent, of the cortex.
- Sleep disorders affect up to 87% of the cases, particularly in advanced stages. Sleep complaints increase with disease severity and duration.
- Patients usually report poor sleep quality, insomnia, sleep fragmentation with frequent awakenings at night, EDS, and the circadian rhythm sleep disorder of the advanced phase type resulting in early morning awakening.
- Polysomnographic studies show reduced sleep efficiency, increased wake time after sleep onset, increased percentage of light sleep, increased REM sleep latency, and reduced percentage of deep sleep and REM sleep.
- RBD, OSA, and RLS may occur but they are not frequent or a major problem.
- Compared with control subjects, premanifest gene carriers had more disrupted sleep, which is characterized by a fragmented sleep profile.

From Iranzo A, Santamaria J. Sleep in neurodegenerative diseases. In: Chokroverty S, Billiard M, editors. Sleep medicine. New York: Springer; 2015. p. 271–84; with permission.

Box 6
Sleep in hereditary spinocerebellar ataxias

- Hereditary ataxias are inherited neurodegenerative disorders that in most cases result from mutations in genes. These diseases affect the spinocerebellar tracts, cerebellum, brainstem, and many other structures in the brain. They are clinically characterized by progressive ataxia and a wide variety of other neurologic symptoms and signs, such as polyneuropathy and parkinsonism.
- OSA and EDS are not common.
- Nocturnal stridor caused by vocal cord abnormalities has been described in spinocerebellar ataxias (SCA) 1 and SCA3.
- RBD occurs in up to 50% of patients with SCA3 (Machado-Joseph disease) and in patients with SCA2 but with mild clinical severity. RBD has not been found in SCA2.
- RLS has been described in SCA1, SCA2, SCA3, and SCA6.

From Iranzo A, Santamaria J. Sleep in neurodegenerative diseases. In: Chokroverty S, Billiard M, editors. Sleep medicine. New York: Springer; 2015. p. 271–84; with permission.

Excessive Daytime Sleepiness

Whether EDS antedates PD is not clarified. Most studies have demonstrated that EDS is not more common in de novo PD than in control subjects.[18–21] In fact, EDS in PD is associated with parkinsonism duration and the use of dopaminergic therapy. In contrast, two population-based studies in the elderly showed that subjects who reported "being sleepy most of the day"[22] and "napping more than 1 hour per day"[23] had increased risk of developing PD with time. Based on this finding, it was speculated that damage of the brainstem structures that modulate the sleep-wake cycle may have contributed to the development of EDS before the appearance of parkinsonism. Limitations of these two population-based studies are that definitions of EDS were unconventional, EDS was not measured objectively, and that most common causes of EDS in the general population (OSA, insufficient sleep syndrome, and depression) were not ruled out. It has been pointed out that OSA may be a risk factor for the future development of PD.[24] More investigations are needed to clarify if EDS is a risk factor for the development of PD.

Box 7
Sleep disorders in amyotrophic lateral sclerosis

- Amyotrophic lateral sclerosis (ALS) is characterized by degeneration of neurons located in the cortex, brainstem nuclei, and ventral horn of the spinal cord. The disorder is characterized by rapidly progressive weakness, muscle atrophy, fasciculations, spasticity, dysarthria, dysphagia, and respiratory compromise.
- Loss of motor neurons in the brainstem and spinal cord results in pharyngeal, laryngeal, diaphragmatic, and intercostal muscle weakness that predispose to respiratory dysfunction.
- The most common sleep abnormality is respiratory dysfunction.
- Sleep-disordered breathing occurs in 17% to 76%, and includes nocturnal alveolar hypoventilation, OSA, laryngeal stridor, and central sleep apnea. The most common form is nocturnal hypoventilation caused by palsy of the diaphragmatic, intercostal, and accessory respiratory muscles.
- Sleep apnea occurs less frequently than hypoventilation. Most apneic events are central because diaphragmatic weakness and palsy of respiratory accessory muscles predispose to this form of sleep apnea.
- Nocturia, muscle cramps, sleep-onset insomnia, reduced sleep amount, and EDS are the main sleep complaints.
- RBD and RLS are not frequent but they may occur.

From Gaig C, Iranzo A. Sleep-disordered breathing in neurodegenerative diseases. Curr Neurol Neurosci Rep 2012;12:205–17; with permission.

SLEEP DISORDERS IN PATIENTS DIAGNOSED WITH PARKINSON DISEASE

Sleep disorders may occur in subjects with idiopathic and hereditary forms of the disease.

Sleep Disorders in Idiopathic Parkinson Disease

In PD, sleep disorders are one of the most common nonmotor features of the disease affecting 60% to 90% of the patients. In one study evaluating 1072 subjects with PD from 55 centers, sleep disorders were the most common nonmotor feature (64%) and its frequency increased with disease severity. In this study the most common reported sleep disorders were insomnia (37%), abnormal sleep behaviors suggesting RBD (30%), EDS (21%), and restless legs (15%).[25] Nocturnal polysomnography in PD discloses reduced total sleep time and sleep efficiency, increased latency to sleep onset, decreased percentages of slow wave sleep and REM sleep stages, reduction or loss of spindles and K complexes, OSA, PLMS, and RBD.[26,27]

Insomnia, sleep fragmentation, nocturia, stiffness, difficulties in turning over in bed, akathisia, nocturnal restless legs, cramps, nightmares, vigorous motor and vocal dream-enacting behaviors, visual hallucinations, confusional awakenings, snoring, witnessed apneas, painful early morning dystonia, and EDS are sleep problems described in PD. Sleep complaints in PD are multifactorial. They are related to damage and functional dysregulation of the brain structures and mechanisms involved in sleep onset and maintenance; the effects of antiparkinsonian drugs on sleep; parkinsonism severity; comorbid conditions, such as anxiety, depression, and dementia; and genetic-individual susceptibility. In general, sleep disturbances gradually worsen with the progression of the disease.

Insomnia

This is the most common sleep complaint in idiopathic PD. In one study involving 689 patients with PD, disrupted sleep was reported by 81%, early morning awakenings by 40%, nonrestorative sleep by 38%, nocturnal awakenings by 31%, and difficulty of initiating sleep by 18%.[28] Insomnia is uncommon in newly diagnosed patients with PD and its prevalence increases with parkinsonism severity and duration. As noted in primary insomnia, poor quality and reduced duration of nocturnal sleep in PD is related to diurnal fatigue but not to EDS.[29,30] Surprisingly, a more robust and continuous sleep architecture has been associated with more severe EDS.[29] This is in agreement with the finding that sleep benefit

(improvement of parkinsonism on awakening in the morning before dopaminergic drug intake) is associated with shorter total sleep time and longer sleep latency at night.[31]

The main cause of reduced and fragmented sleep in patients with PD is the severity of parkinsonian symptoms at night. Akinesia and stiffness cause poor nocturnal mobility that manifests as difficulties turning in bed or getting out of bed. This situation can be extremely distressing to patients with nocturia who need to go to the toilet several times at night. Constant and stable plasma concentration of a dopaminergic drug during the night, such as the rotigotine patch, improves sleep quality in PD because of a better nocturnal mobility and more continuous sleep.[32] A similar benefit in sleep quality and quantity is found with other strategies to improve parkinsonism at night, such as treatment with ropinirole prolonged release,[33] levodopa/carbidopa intestinal gel infusion,[34] and deep brain stimulation of the subthalamic nucleus.[35]

The main contributors to sleep-onset insomnia in PD are anxiety, depression, RLS, severe parkinsonism, and dyskinesia. Patients with PD who also have dementia may exhibit confusional awakenings and visual hallucinations leading to sleep fragmentation and nonrestorative sleep. RBD does not fragment nocturnal sleep. Depression and early morning trunk and foot dystonia can cause early awakening.

Circadian sleep-wake cycle disruption

Patients with this abnormality have an exaggerated tendency toward an advancement of phase, thereby developing an irregular sleep-wake pattern characterized by EDS in the evening and early awakening at night. In PD, this pattern may be related with the coexistence of depression, dementia, reduction in the amplitude of melatonin secretion, reduced circulating melatonin levels, hypercortisolemia, and altered peripheral clock gene expression.[36,37]

Excessive daytime sleepiness

In PD, EDS is a common complex phenomenon that may lead to social problems, automobile accidents, and a negative impact on quality of life. EDS in PD is manifested either as a state of continuous and persistent hypersomnolence or as episodes of sudden onset of sleep ("sleep attacks").

The prevalence of persistent subjective EDS in patients with PD ranges from 16% to 74% and is higher than in control subjects.[38–45] However, studies evaluating EDS by an objective method, such as the Multiple Sleep Latency Test, show that the mean sleep latency is similar between

Table 1
Longitudinal studies in idiopathic RBD showing conversion to a defined neurodegenerative syndrome

Author	Number	Male (%)	Age at Estimated IRBD Onset (y)	Age at IRBD Diagnosis (y)	Follow-Up from IRBD Diagnosis (y)	Conversion Rate (%)	Estimated Risk for Conversion from IRBD Diagnosis	Emerging Disorders (N)	Interval Between Estimated RBD Onset and Disease Diagnosis (y)	Interval Between RBD Diagnosis and Disease Diagnosis (y)	Age at Disease Diagnosis (y)
Schenck et al,[4] 1996	29	100	55.4 ± 8.7	64.4 ± 5.8	6.1 ± 2.4	41	NR	PD = 11 Dementia = 1	12.7 ± 3.3	3.7 ± 1.4	68.1 ± 6.0
Schenck et al,[5] 2013	26	100	57.7 ± 7.7	NR	16	81	NR	PD = 13 DLB = 5 Dementia = 3[a] MSA = 2	14.2 ± 6.2	NR	71.9 ± 6.6
Iranzo et al,[6] 2006[b]	44	89	62.6 ± 7.3	68.9 ± 6.3	5.1 ± 2.7	45	NR	PD = 9 DLB = 6 MSA = 1 MCI = 4	10.7 ± 5.2	3.8 ± 1.9	71.6 ± 6.6
Iranzo et al,[7] 2013[b]	44	89	62.6 ± 7.3	68.9 ± 6.3	10.5	82	35% at 5 y 73% at 10 y 92% at 14 y	PD = 16 DLB = 14 MSA = 1 MCI = 5	12	6	74
Iranzo et al,[8] 2014[b]	174	78	62.4 ± 7.8	68.7 ± 6.4	5.1 ± 3.9	37	33% at 5 y 76% at 10 y 91% at 14 y	PD = 22 DLB = 29 MSA = 2 MCI = 12	11.5 ± 5.1	4.8 ± 3.4	74.5 ± 5.0

Postuma et al,[9] 2009	93	80	NR	65.4 ± 9.3	5.2	28	18% at 5 y 41% at 10 y 52% at 12 y	PD = 14 DLB = 7 Dementia = 4 MSA = 1	11.5 ± 6.8	5.5 ± 3.9	NR
Postuma et al,[10] 2015c	89	73	NR	66.9 ± 9.3	5.4 ± 2.9	46	30% at 3 y 66% at 7 y	PD = 17 DLB = 18 Dementia = 3 MSA = 3	NR	NR	NR
Wing et al,[11] 2012d	91	82	60.0 ± 12.7	65.5 ± 9.9	5.6 ± 3.3	16	5% at 3 y 8% at 5 y 21% at 7 y 38% at 9 y	PD = 8 DLB = 1 AD = 8	NR	NR	NR
Youn et al,[12] 2015e	84	69	60	65.5 ± 6.7	4.1 ± 2.1	21	9% at 3 y 18% at 5 y 35% at 6 y	PD = 9 DLB = 4 AD = 3 MSA = 1 SCA = 1	NR	NR	NR
Postuma et al,[13] 2015e	279	80	NR	NR	NR	33	25% at 3 y 41% at 5 y	PD = 39 DLB = 28 Dementia = 19 MSA = 7	NR	NR	NR

Abbreviations: AD, Alzheimer disease; DLB, dementia with Lewy bodies; MCI, mild cognitive impairment; MSA, multiple system atrophy; NR, not reported; SCA, spinocerebellar ataxia.

[a] In two patients postmortem examination showed Lewy bodies in the brainstem plus AD pathology.
[b] Development of mild cognitive impairment was a disease outcome.
[c] 59% of patients diagnosed with iRBD had concomitant mild cognitive impairment at baseline.
[d] Development of mild cognitive impairment was not defined as disease outcome but it was found to evolve in 25 patients.
[e] Mild cognitive impairment was not considered a disease outcome and was present in some patients when the diagnosis of RBD was made.

Box 8
Clinical and subclinical abnormalities in idiopathic REM sleep behavior disorder

- Reduced arm swinging
- Face akinesia
- Depression
- Impaired olfaction
- Color vision impairment
- Asymptomatic cognitive abnormalities on cognitive tests, especially in the executive, memory, and visuospatial domains
- Subtle electroencephalographic slowing
- Orthostatic hypotension
- Systolic blood pressure drop
- Decreased beat-to-beat variability in the cardiac rhythm
- Constipation
- Reduced postprandial ghrelin response
- Erectile symptoms
- Episodes of acute psychosis after minor or major surgery
- Reduced cardiac scintigraphy 123I-MBIG
- Decreased dopamine transporter in the striatum, particularly in the left putamen
- Substantia nigra hyperechogenicity
- Hypoechogenicity of the brainstem raphe
- Brainstem changes in diffusion tensor imaging
- Decreased cortical and increased pontine perfusion

Adapted from Iranzo A, Santamaria J, Tolosa E. Idiopathic rapid eye movement sleep behavior disorder. Lancet Neurol, in press; and Boeve B. REM sleep behaviour disorder. Updated review of the core features, the REM sleep behavior disorder- neurodegenerative disease association, evolving concepts, controversies, and future directions. Ann N Y Acad Sci 2010;1184:15–54.

---

patients with PD and control subjects.[46] In one study involving 134 patients with PD, 46% reported subjective EDS, whereas only 13% had short sleep latencies in the Multiple Sleep Latency Test.[47] The frequency of EDS increases with disease duration in PD. In one study with 153 drug-naive patients the frequency of EDS increased from 12% at baseline to 23% after 5 years of follow-up.[48]

The main factors contributing to persistent EDS are the intrinsic pathology of PD and the sedative effects of the dopaminergic drugs used for parkinsonism. In patients with PD, development of persistent EDS may be related to progressive cell loss in the mesolimbic dopaminergic and nondopaminergic brain circuits that modulate sleep mechanisms. This is in line with the finding of the association between EDS and advanced stage of parkinsonism and longer duration of the disease suggesting that more severe and widespread brain damage leads to the development or worsening of EDS.

The sedative effect of all classes of dopaminergic medications is independent of the disease duration and severity. EDS is associated with low doses of levodopa and high doses of dopamine agonists.[49] Other possible causes of persistent EDS should be considered before determining whether EDS is caused by the disease itself or by the effects of dopaminomimetics. Circadian dysrhythmia, high body mass index, OSA, pain, depression, dementia, and the concomitant use of other sedative drugs, such as hypnotics, can also cause persistent EDS in PD.[47]

There is a subgroup of sleepy patients with PD with short mean sleep latency and the presence of REM sleep periods in the Multiple Sleep Latency Test that resembles what is seen in narcolepsy.[29,30] In unselected patients with PD, autopsies show a loss of 23% to 62% of hypocretin cells in the hypothalamus, which is the pathologic hallmark of narcolepsy.[50,51] In PD, however, hypocretin levels in the cerebrospinal fluid are normal[52] and cataplexy, a patognomonic symptom of narcolepsy, does not occur (**Table 2**).

Table 2
Comparison between Parkinson disease and narcolepsy with cataplexy

	Narcolepsy with Cataplexy	Parkinson Disease
Excessive daytime sleepiness	+	+
Sleep attacks	+	+
Cataplexy	+	−
Hallucinations	+	+
Sleep paralysis	+	−
REM sleep behavior disorder	+	+
HLA DQB1*0602	>90%	30%
Sleep-onset REM periods in the Multiple Sleep Latency Test	+	+/−
Absent hypocretin in cerebrospinal fluid	+	−
Loss of hypocretinergic cells in the hypothalamus	90%	23%–62%

Sleep attacks are less common than persistent EDS in patients with PD and may cause automobile crashes.[53,54] Among patients with PD treated with dopaminergic drugs, the prevalence of sleep attacks ranges from 0% to 32%.[38–41] Sleep attacks are considered the result of a dopaminergic class effect because they are associated with the use of virtually all dopaminergic drugs (levodopa plus dopaminergic agonists); occur several days or weeks after the introduction of the offending drug; and usually resolve or improve after its withdrawal, reduction, or replacement. The most common variables associated with sleep attacks are therapy with dopamine agonists, duration of parkinsonism, elevated Epworth Sleepiness Scale score, high age, and male gender.[55–57]

Obstructive sleep apnea

In PD, the frequency of an apnea-hypopnea index greater than five is 27% to 54%, and the frequency of greater than 30 is 2% to 15% (**Table 3**). Most studies have shown that these figures are not more prevalent than matched control subjects.[20,27,45,46,58–62] In fact, in some studies the prevalence of OSA is lower in PD than in control subjects probably because of a lower body mass index of the patients.[62] Therefore, it seems that PD itself does not confer an increased risk of OSA and that the frequent presence of this condition in PD is a reflection of aging or reduction of the upper airway space. Nevertheless, patients with PD who experience EDS may undergo routine polysomnography to identify the presence of OSA. Interestingly, some subjects with PD with increased apnea-hypopnea index may not experience symptoms typical of OSA, such as EDS, tiredness, and feeling not refreshed on awakening in the morning. The clinical relevance of an increased apnea-hypopnea index in asymptomatic PD is uncertain. In PD, attributing EDS to an abnormal apnea hypopnea-index found in polysomnography can be misleading because EDS in this population may also be caused by many other factors, such depression and the use of dopaminergic drugs.

Rapid eye movement sleep behavior disorder

This parasomnia occurs in approximately 40% to 50% of patients.[63,64] In patients newly diagnosed RBD occurs in 30%[19] and this figure increases with time.[65] In about 20% of cases RBD occurs before the onset of parkinsonism.[66] Types of RBD-related unpleasant dreams, dream-enacting behaviors, and polysomnographic abnormalities are similar among sporadic PD and IRBD.[66] About 65% of the patients with PD with RBD are unaware of their nighttime behaviors and 20% do not recall unpleasant dreams.[66] In patients with IRBD that develop parkinsonism, voice changes and face akinesia appear earliest followed by rigidity, gait abnormalities, and limb bradykinesia.[67] RBD in PD is associated with a subtype of PD characterized by old age,[64,68] male gender,[68] long parkinsonism duration,[69,70] akinetic-rigid subtype,[71,72] freezing,[68] falls,[64] impulse control disorders,[73] and cognitive impairment.[74]

Restless legs syndrome

RLS is a sensorimotor disorder characterized by an urge to move the legs caused by unpleasant sensations that begin during periods of inactivity at night and is relieved by movement. Patients with idiopathic RLS dramatically respond to dopaminergic drugs, a feature that suggests the possible relationship between RLS and PD. It is controversial, however, and still under debate if

Table 3
Obstructive sleep apnea in Parkinson disease

Author, Year	Country	Patients (N)	Mean Age (y)	Mean AHI (N)	AHI >5 (%)	AHI >10 (%)	AHI = 5–15 (%)	AHI >15 (%)	AHI = 15–30 (%)	AHI >30 (%)
Rye et al,[29] 2000	USA	27	68	11	—	—	—	—	—	—
Arnulf et al,[30] 2002	France	54	68	10	47	14	28	20	11	9
Stevens et al,[43] 2004	USA	19	60	9	—	—	—	—	—	—
Iranzo et al,[66] 2005	Spain	45	65	16	—	—	—	—	—	—
Diederich et al,[58] 2005	Luxemburg	49	65	8	43	—	20	22	8	15
Baumann et al,[59] 2005	Switzerland	10	69	11	—	—	—	—	—	—
Trotti & Bliwise,[60] 2010	USA	55	64	7	44	—	29	15	11	4
Noradina et al,[61] 2010	Malaysia	46	64	7	54	—	27	27	18	9
Cochen De Cock et al,[47] 2010	France	100	62	10	27	—	6	21	11	10
Yong et al,[46] 2011	Singapore	56	59	12	49	—	15	24	19	15
Alatriste et al,[27] 2014	Mexico	120	60	16	51	—	26	25	11	14
Prudon et al,[20] 2014	UK	106	66	—	37	—	23	11	9	2
Valko et al,[45] 2014	Switzerland	119	65	—	48	—	23	12	—	13

Abbreviation: AHI, apnea-hypopnea index (number of apneas and hypopneas per hour of sleep).

RLS is associated with PD. There are arguments for and against and more research is needed.[75]

Studies evaluating if idiopathic RLS predisposes to PD have shown conflicting results. An epidemiologic study showed that male subjects from the population who had RLS symptoms more than 15 times per month had a higher risk for PD within a 4 (but not 8)-year period of follow-up.[76] Based on this finding, the authors speculated that RLS was an early feature of PD and not a risk factor. In contrast, patients with idiopathic RLS followed at sleep clinics do not progress to PD. In about 20% of cases RBD occurs before the onset of parkinsonism[77] and postmortem brain examination in idiopathic RLS does not show PD pathology.

It is not yet clarified if RLS is a specific component of subjects already diagnosed with PD. The prevalence of RLS is similar between de novo untreated subjects with PD and matched control subjects.[78,79] When the presence of RLS is evaluated in patients with PD with relatively advanced forms of the disease and treated with dopaminergic drugs (which may mask the presence of RLS) the evidence is limited to studies with methodological problems that have reported conflicting results[80–93] (Table 4). In most of the PD cases with comorbid RLS, parkinsonism precedes the onset of RLS, age of RLS onset is advanced, severity of RLS is mild, and family history of RLS is uncommon. It should be noted that RLS must be carefully distinguished by clinical history from other uncomfortable sensations that are commonly experienced in subjects with PD (stiffness, pain, tingling, heat, numbness, cramps) that may be related to parkinsonian features and not to RLS (rigidity, inner tremor, central pain, off periods, dystonia, and dyskinesias). Thus the prevalence of RLS in PD may be overestimated by these sensations and motor features of PD that may mimic RLS (false positives). Alternatively, it has been speculated that the presence of RLS in subjects with PD treated with dopaminergic medications could be a result of overstimulation by these agents of the dopamine receptors in the spinal cord (a phenomenon similar to augmentation in idiopathic RLS where patients treated chronically with dopaminergic agents experience a worsening of their symptoms).[75]

Periodic leg movements during sleep

PLMS are repetitive, stereotyped leg movements that are 0.5 to 5 seconds in duration and are separated by an interval of more than 5 seconds but less than 90 seconds. The occurrence of PLMS is thought to be related to impairment of central dopaminergic function because PLMS decrease in frequency with the use of dopaminergic medications. Moreover, PLMS in PD increase after chronic

Table 4
Restless legs syndrome in Parkinson disease

Author, Year	Country	Patients (N)	Mean Age (y)	RLS in PD (%)	RLS in Control Subjects (%)
Lang & Johnson,[80] 1987	Canada	100	62	0	NE
Ondo et al,[81] 2002	USA	303	67	21	NE
Kahn & Sahota,[82] 2002	USA	26	NE	38	NE
Tan et al,[83] 2002	Singapore	125	65	0	NE
Krishnan et al,[84] 2004	India	126	57	8	1
Braga-Neto et al,[85] 2004	Brazil	86	65	52	NE
Nomura et al,[86] 2006	Japan	165	68	12	2
Loo & Tan,[87] 2008	Singapore	200	65	3	0.5
Lee et al,[88] 2009	Korea	447	64	16	NE
Calzetti et al,[89] 2009	Italy	118	69	13	6
Peralta et al,[90] 2009	Austria	113	67	24	NE
Verbaan et al,[91] 2010	Holland	269	61	11	NE
Angelini et al,[78] 2011	Italy	109	67	6	4
Gjerstad et al,[79] 2011	Norway	200	65	12	7
Bhalsing et al,[92] 2013	India	134	57	10	3
Ylikoski et al,[93] 2015	Finland	577	67	20	NE

Abbreviation: NE, not evaluated.

treatment with bilateral subthalamic stimulation probably because this type of surgery facilitates the reduction or withdrawal of dopaminergic drug treatment.[35] Most studies have shown that PLMS occur in PD, but they are not more frequent than in control subjects.[94] Most patients with PD who experience PLMS are unaware of these leg movements because PLMS are generally not associated with arousals. Therefore, PLMS in PD may be not considered a main contributing factor for developing insomnia, sleep fragmentation, or EDS.

Sleep Disorders in Hereditary Forms of Parkinson Disease

Mutations in the leucine-rich repeat kinase 2 gene (LRRK2-PD) and in the *Parkin* gene are the most frequent forms of hereditary PD. Patients with *Parkin* mutations may present RBD and RLS both of mild intensity.[95,96] In LRRK2-patients with PD, sleep complaints are more frequent than in subjects with *Parkin* gene mutations. In a recent study sleep complaints were frequent in 18 LRRK2-patients with PD evaluated; 78% reported poor sleep quality, 33% sleep onset insomnia, 56% sleep fragmentation, and 39% early awakening.[97] Sleep-onset insomnia correlated with depressive symptoms and poor sleep quality. EDS was a complaint in 33% and short sleep latencies on the Multiple Sleep Latency Tests, which indicate objective EDS, were found in 71%. Sleep attacks occurred in three patients and the narcoleptic phenotype was not observed. RBD was diagnosed in three individuals. EDS and RBD were always reported to start after the onset of parkinsonism. When compared with idiopathic PD, sleep-onset insomnia was more significantly frequent, EDS was similar, and RBD was less significantly frequent and less severe in LRRK2-PD.

MANAGEMENT OF SLEEP DISORDERS IN PARKINSON DISEASE

Treatment of sleep disorders in PD is challenging, because it is a multifactorial and complex phenomenon.[98] Treatment should be individualized. Cognitive-behavioral therapy, bright light therapy, and several drugs at bed time (eszoplicone, doxepin, trazodone, melatonin, and quetiapine) may be effective in patients with PD with sleep onset insomnia. Rotigotine patch and ropinirole prolonged release may improve sleep quality by decreasing sleep-onset insomnia and fragmentation in subjects with severe parkinsonism at night.[32,33] Rotigotine patch also improves mood and early morning motor function. In patients with advanced PD, chronic treatment with bilateral subthalamic stimulation improves subjective sleep

quality, probably because of increased nocturnal mobility secondary to an improvement in rigidity and bradykinesia.[35] In patients with insomnia, the coexistence of severe nocturia, depression, anxiety, and dystonia should be ruled out and appropriately treated.

Subjects with circadian rhythm disturbance may receive melatonin at bed time and advice on sleep hygiene measures. These measures include scheduling regular times to go to bed and wake up, consolidation of sleep during the night, eliminating time spent in bed awake, avoiding long daytime naps, and promoting daytime activities.

If persistent EDS and sleep attacks are thought to be related to the introduction or increase in dose of a dopaminergic medication, it may be useful to reduce the dose, discontinue the drug, or switch to another dopaminergic agent. Treatment of EDS also includes the administration of waking-promoting medications, such as modafinil and sodium oxybate. In patients with PD with comorbid OSA causing EDS, continuous positive airway pressure is indicated because it improves EDS and restores the sleep architecture.[99]

For unknown reasons, RBD responds to clonazepam (0.5–2 mg) and possibly to melatonin (3–12 mg) at bedtime. However, clonazepam does not diminish the risk for developing PD in IRBD. Pramipexole does not improve RBD symptoms in PD.[100]

If RLS is bothersome or prevents the patient with PD from sleeping, the evening dose of dopaminergic agents can be increased or a long-acting release formulation can be prescribed. Alternatively, other nondopaminergic drugs that are effective for RLS, such as gabapentin, gabapentin enacarbil, pregabalin, and oxycodone/naloxone, can be used.

SUMMARY

Sleep disorders are common among subjects with neurodegenerative diseases and may interfere with the patient's quality of life. Sleep specialists and neurologists should be aware of those disorders affecting individuals diagnosed with a neurodegenerative disease. Correct identification of the problem and its severity are key features for the correct management of these disorders.

REFERENCES

1. Jellinger KA. Neuropathology of non-motor symptoms in Parkinson disease. J Neural Transm (Vienna) 2015;122:1429–40.
2. Braak H, Del Tredici K, Rüb U, et al. Staging of brain pathology related to sporadic Parkinson's disease. Neurobiol Aging 2003;24:197–211.

3. Iranzo A, Santamaria J, Tolosa E. Idiopathic rapid eye movement sleep behavior disorder. Lancet Neurol, in press.

4. Schenck CH, Bundlie SR, Mahowald MW. Delayed emergence of a parkinsonian disorder in 38% of 29 older men initially diagnosed with idiopathic rapid eye movement sleep behavior disorder. Neurology 1996;46:388–93.

5. Schenck C, Boeve B, Mahowald M. Delayed emergence of a parkinsonian disorder or dementia in 81% of older men initially diagnosed with idiopathic rapid eye movement sleep behaviour disorder: a 16-year update on a previously reported series. Sleep Med 2013;14:744–8.

6. Iranzo A, Molinuevo JL, Santamaria J, et al. Rapid-eye-movement sleep behaviour disorder as an early marker for a neurodegenerative disease: a descriptive study. Lancet Neurol 2006;5:572–7.

7. Iranzo A, Tolosa E, Gelpi E. Neurodegenerative disease status and post-mortem pathology in idiopathic rapid-eye-movement sleep behavior disorder: an observational cohort study. Lancet Neurol 2013;12:443–53.

8. Iranzo A, Fernández-Arcos A, Tolosa E, et al. Neurodegenerative disorder risk in idiopathic REM sleep behavior disorder: study in 174 patients. PLoS One 2014;9(2):e89741.

9. Postuma RB, Gagnon JF, Vendette M, et al. Quantifying the risk of neurodegenerative disease in idiopathic REM sleep behavior disorder. Neurology 2009;72:1296–300.

10. Postuma RB, Gagnon JF, Bertrand JA, et al. Parkinson risk in idiopathic REM sleep behavior disorder: preparing for neuroprotective trials. Neurology 2015;17(84):1104–13.

11. Wing YK, Li SX, Mok V, et al. Prospective outcome of rapid eye movement sleep behaviour disorder: psychiatric disorders as a potential early marker of Parkinson's disease. J Neurol Neurosurg Psychiatry 2012;83:470–2.

12. Youn S, Kim T, Yoon IY, et al. Progression of cognitive impairments in idiopathic REM sleep behavior disorder. J Neurol Neurosurg Psychiatry 2015. http://dx.doi.org/10.1136/jnnp-2015-311437.

13. Postuma RB, Iranzo A, Hogl B, et al. Risk factors for neurodegeneration in idiopathic rapid eye movement sleep behavior disorder: a multicenter study. Ann Neurol 2015;77:830–9.

14. Boeve B. REM sleep behaviour disorder. Updated review of the core features, the REM sleep behavior disorder-neurodegenerative disease association, evolving concepts, controversies, and future directions. Ann N Y Acad Sci 2010;1184: 15–54.

15. Uchiyama M, Isse K, Tanaka K, et al. Incidental Lewy body disease in a patient with REM sleep behaviour disorder. Neurology 1999;45:709–12.

16. Boeve BF, Dickson DW, Olson EJ, et al. Insights into REM sleep behaviour disorder pathophysiology in brainstem-predominant Lewy body disease. Sleep Med 2007;8:60–4.

17. Boeve BF, Silber MH, Ferman TJ, et al. Clinicopathologic correlations in 172 cases of rapid eye movement sleep behavior disorder with or without a coexisting neurologic disorder. Sleep Med 2013; 14:754–62.

18. Buskova J, Klempir J, Majerova V, et al. Sleep disturbances in untreated Parkinson's disease. J Neurol 2011;258:2254–9.

19. Plomhause L, Dujardin K, Duhamel A, et al. Rapid eye movement sleep behavior disorder in treatment-naïve Parkinson disease patients. Sleep Med 2013;14:1035–7.

20. Prudon B, Duncan GW, Khoo TK, et al. Primary sleep disorder prevalence in patients with newly diagnosed Parkinson's disease. Mov Disord 2014; 29:259–62.

21. Simuni T, Caspell-Garcia C, Coffey C, et al. Correlates of excessive daytime sleepiness in de novo Parkinson's disease. Mov Disord 2015;30:1371–81.

22. Abbott RD, Ross GW, White LR, et al. Excessive daytime sleepiness and subsequent development of Parkinson disease. Neurology 2005;65:1442–6.

23. Gao J, Huang X, Park Y, et al. Daytime napping, nighttime sleeping, and Parkinson disease. Am J Epidemiol 2011;173:1032–8.

24. Chen JC, Tsai TY, Li CY, et al. OSA and risk of Parkinson disease: a population-based cohort study. J Sleep Res 2015;24:432–7.

25. Barone P, Antonini A, Colosimo C, et al. The PRIAMO study: a multicenter assessment of non-motor symptoms and their impact on quality of life in Parkinson's disease. Mov Disord 2009;24: 1641–9.

26. Joy SP, Sinha S, Pal PK, et al. Alterations in polysomnographic (PSG) profile in drug-naïve Parkinson's disease. Ann Indian Acad Neurol 2014;17: 287–91.

27. Alatriste-Booth V, Rodríguez-Violante M, Camacho-Ordoñez A, et al. Prevalence and correlates of sleep disorders in Parkinson's disease: a polysomnographic study. Arq Neuropsiquiatr 2014;73:241–5.

28. Ylikoski A, Martikainen K, Sieminski M, et al. Parkinson's disease and insomnia. Neurol Sci 2015; 36(11):2003–10.

29. Rye DB, Bliwise DL, Dihenia B, et al. FAST TRACK. Daytime sleepiness in Parkinson's disease. J Sleep Res 2000;9:63–9.

30. Arnulf I, Konofal E, Merino-Andreu M, et al. Parkinson's disease and sleepiness. An integral part of PD. Neurology 2002;58:1019–24.

31. Sherif E, Valko PO, Overeem S, et al. Sleep benefit in Parkinson's disease is associated with short

sleep times. Parkinsonism Relat Disord 2014;20: 116–8.

32. Trenkwalder C, Kies B, Rudzinska M, et al. Rotigotine effects on early morning motor function and sleep in Parkinson's disease: a double-blind, randomized, placebo-controlled study (RECOVER). Mov Disord 2011;26:90–9.

33. Chaudhuri RK, Martinez-Martin P, Rolfe KA, et al. Improvements in nocturnal symptoms with ropinirole prolonged release in patients with advanced Parkinson's disease. Eur J Neurol 2012;19:105–13.

34. Zibetti M, Rizzone M, Merola A, et al. Sleep improvement with levodopa/carbidopa intestinal gel infusion in Parkinson disease. Acta Neurol Scand 2013;127:e28–32.

35. Iranzo A, Valldeoriola F, Santamaría J, et al. Sleep symptoms and polysomnographic architecture in advanced Parkinson's disease after chronic bilateral subthalamic stimulation. J Neurol Neurosurg Psychiatry 2002;72:661–4.

36. Breen DP, Vuono R, Nawarathna U, et al. Sleep and circadian rhythm regulation in early Parkinson disease. JAMA Neurol 2014;71:589–95.

37. Videnovic A, Noble C, Reid KJ, et al. Circadian melatonin rhythm and excessive daytime sleepiness in Parkinson disease. JAMA Neurol 2014;71: 463–9.

38. Tandberg E, Larsen JP, Karlsen K. Excessive daytime sleepiness and sleep benefit in Parkinson's disease: a community-based study. Mov Disord 1999;14:922–7.

39. Tan EK, Lum SY, Fook-Chong SM, et al. Evaluation of somnolence in Parkinson's disease: comparison with age and sex-matched controls. Neurology 2002;58:465–8.

40. Hobson DE, Lang AE, Martin WR, et al. Excessive daytime sleepiness and sudden-onset sleep in Parkinson Disease. A survey by the Canadian movement disorder group. JAMA 2002;287:455–63.

41. Fabbrini G, Barbanti P, Aurilia C, et al. Excessive daytime sleepiness in de novo and treated Parkinson's disease. Mov Disord 2002;17:1026–30.

42. Gjerstad MD, Aarsland D, Larsen JP. Development of daytime somnolence over time in Parkinson's disease. Neurology 2002;58:1544–6.

43. Stevens S, Comella CL, Stepanski EJ. Daytime sleepiness and alertness in patients with Parkinson disease. Sleep 2004;27:967–72.

44. Ghorayeb I, Loundou A, Auquier P, et al. A nationwide survey of excessive daytime sleepiness in Parkinson disease in France. Mov Disord 2007;22:1567–72.

45. Valko PO, Waldogavel D, Weller M, et al. Fatigue and excessive daytime sleepiness in idiopathic Parkinson's disease differently correlate with motor symptoms, depression and dopaminergic treatment. Eur J Neurol 2014;17:1428–36.

46. Yong MH, Fook-Chong S, Pavanni R, et al. Case control polysomnographic studies of sleep disorders in Parkinson's disease. PLoS One 2011;6(7): e22511.

47. Cochen De Cock V, Bayard S, Jaussent I, et al. Daytime sleepiness in Parkinson's disease: a reappraisal. PLoS One 2010;9(9):e107278.

48. Tholfsen LK, Larsen JP, Schulz J, et al. Development of excessive daytime sleepiness in early Parkinson disease. Neurology 2015;85:162–8.

49. Bliwise DL, Trotti LM, Wilson AG, et al. Daytime alertness in Parkinson's disease: potentially dose-dependent, divergent effects by drug class. Mov Disord 2012;27:1118–24.

50. Thannickal TC, Lai YY, Siegel JM. Hypocretin (orexin) cell loss in Parkinson's disease. Brain 2007;130:1586–95.

51. Fronczek R, Overeem S, Lee SY, et al. Hypocretin (orexin) loss in Parkinson's disease. Brain 2007; 130:1577–85.

52. Compta Y, Santamaria J, Ratti L, et al. Cerebrospinal hypocretin, daytime sleepiness and sleep architecture in Parkinson's disease dementia. Brain 2009;132:3308–17.

53. Frucht S, Rogers MD, Greene PE, et al. Falling asleep at the wheel: motor vehicle mishaps in persons taking pramipexole and ropinirole. Neurology 1999;52:1908–10.

54. Homann CN, Wenzel K, Suppan K, et al. Sleep attacks in patients taking dopamine agonists: review. BMJ 2002;324:1483–7.

55. Olanow CW, Schapira AH, Roth T. Waking up to sleep episodes in Parkinson's disease. Mov Disord 2000;15:212–5.

56. Möller JC, Stiasny K, Hargutt V, et al. Evaluation of sleep and driving performance in six patients with Parkinson's disease reporting sudden onset of sleep under dopaminergic medication: a pilot study. Mov Disord 2002;17:474–81.

57. Paus S, Brecht HM, Köster J, et al. Sleep attacks, daytime sleepiness, and dopamine agonists in Parkinson's disease. Mov Disord 2003;18:659–67.

58. Diederich NJ, Vaillant M, Leischen M, et al. Sleep apnea syndrome in Parkinson's disease. A case-control study in 49 patients. Mov Disord 2005;11: 1413–8.

59. Baumann C, Ferini-Strambi L, Waldvogel D, et al. Parkinsonism with excessive daytime sleepiness. J Neurol 2005;252:139–45.

60. Trotti LM, Bliwise DL. No increased risk of OSA in Parkinson's disease. Mov Disord 2010;25:2246–9.

61. Noradina AT, Karim NA, Hamidon BB, et al. Sleep-disordered breathing in patients with Parkinson's disease. Singapore Med J 2010;51:60–4.

62. Zeng J, Wei M, Li T, et al. Risk of OSA in Parkinson's disease: a meta-analysis. PLoS One 2013; 8(12):e82091.

63. Gagnon JF, Bédard MA, Fantini ML, et al. REM sleep behavior disorder and REM sleep without atonia in Parkinson's disease. Neurology 2002; 27(59):585–9.

64. Sixel-Döring F, Trautmann E, Mollenhauer B, et al. Associated factors for REM sleep behavior disorder in Parkinson disease. Neurology 2011;77:1048–54.

65. Gjestard MD, Boeve B, Wentzel-Larsen T, et al. Occurrence and clinical correlates of REM sleep behaviour disorder in patients with Parkinson's disease over time. J Neurol Neurosurg Psychiatry 2008;79:387–91.

66. Iranzo A, Santamaría J, Rye DB, et al. Characteristics of idiopathic REM sleep behavior disorder and that associated with MSA and PD. Neurology 2005; 65:247–52.

67. Postuma RN, Lang AE, Gagnon JF, et al. How does parkinsonism start? Prodromal parkinsonism motor changes in idiopathic REM sleep behaviour disorder. Brain 2012;27:617–26.

68. Romenets SR, Gagnon JF, Latreille V, et al. Rapid eye movement sleep behaviour disorder and subtypes of Parkinson disease. Mov Disord 2012;27: 996–1003.

69. Wetter TC, Trenkwalder C, Gershanik O, et al. Polysomnographic measures in Parkinson's disease: a comparison between patients with and without REM sleep disturbances. Wien Klin Wochenschr 2001;113:249–53.

70. De Cock VC, Vidailhet M, Leu S, et al. Restoration of normal muscle control in Parkinson's disease during REM sleep. Brain 2007;130:450–6.

71. Kumru H, Santamaria J, Tolosa E, et al. Relation between subtype of Parkinson's disease and REM sleep behavior disorder. Sleep Med 2007;8: 779–83.

72. Postuma RB, Gagnon JF, Vendette M, et al. REM sleep behavior disorder in Parkinson's disease is associated with specific motor features. J Neurol Neurosurg Psychiatry 2008;79:1117–21.

73. Fantini ML, Macedo L, Zibetti M, et al. Increased risk of impulse control symptoms in Parkinson's disease with REM sleep behaviour disorder. J Neurol Neurosurg Psychiatry 2015;86:174–9.

74. Postuma RB, Bertrand JA, Montplaisir J, et al. Rapid eye movement sleep behaviour disorder and risk of dementia in Parkinson disease. Mov Disord 2012;27:720–6.

75. Rijsman RM, Schoolderman LF, Rundervoort RS, et al. Restless legs syndrome in Parkinson's disease. Parkinsonism Relat Disord 2014;20(Suppl 1):S5–9.

76. Wong JC, Li Y, Schwarzschild MA, et al. Restless legs syndrome: an early clinical feature of Parkinson disease in men. Sleep 2014;37:369–72.

77. Walters AS, LeBrocq C, Passi V, et al. A preliminary look at the percentage of patients with restless legs syndrome who also have Parkinson's disease, essential tremor or Tourette syndrome in a single practice. J Sleep Res 2003;12:343–5.

78. Angelini M, Negrotti A, Marchesi E, et al. A study of the prevalence of restless legs syndrome in previously untreated Parkinson's disease patients: absence of co-morbid association. J Neurol Sci 2011;310:286–8.

79. Gjerstad MD, Tysnes OB, Larsen JP. Increased risk of leg motor restlessness but not RLS in early Parkinson disease. Neurology 2011;29(77):1941–6.

80. Lang AE, Johnson K. Akathisia in idiopathic Parkinson's disease. Neurology 1987;37:477–81.

81. Ondo WG, Dat Vuong K, Jankovic J. Exploring the relationship between Parkinson disease and restless legs syndrome. Arch Neurol 2002;59:421–4.

82. Khan SA, Sahota PK. A study look for the incidence of restless legs syndrome in patients with Parkinson's disease. Sleep 2002;25(Suppl):A378–9.

83. Tan EK, Lum SY, Wong MC. Restless legs syndrome in Parkinson's disease. J Neurol Sci 2002;196:33–6.

84. Krishnan PR, Bhatia M, Behari M. Restless legs syndrome in Parkinson's disease: a case-controlled study. Mov Disord 2004;18:181–5.

85. Braga-Neto P, Silva-Júnior FP, Monte FS, et al. Snoring and excessive daytime sleepiness in Parkinson's disease. J Neurol Sci 2004;217:41–5.

86. Nomura T, Inoue Y, Miyake M, et al. Prevalence and clinical characteristics of restless legs syndrome in Japanese patients with Parkinson's disease. Mov Disord 2006;21:380–4.

87. Loo HV, Tan EK. Case-control study of restless legs syndrome and quality of sleep in Parkinson's disease. J Neurol Sci 2008;266:145–9.

88. Lee JE, Shin HW, Kim KS, et al. Factors contributing to the development of restless legs syndrome in patients with Parkinson disease. Mov Disord 2009;24:579–82.

89. Calzetti S, Negrotti A, Bonavina G, et al. Absence of comorbidity of Parkinson disease and restless legs syndrome: a case-control study in patients attending a movement disorder clinic. Neurol Sci 2009;30:119–22.

90. Peralta CM, Frauscher B, Seppi K, et al. Restless legs syndrome in Parkinson's disease. Mov Disord 2009;24:2076–80.

91. Verbaan D, Rooden SM, van Hilten J, et al. Prevalence and clinical profile of restless legs syndrome in Parkinson's disease. Mov Disord 2010;25:2142–7.

92. Bhalsing K, Suresh K, Muthane UB, et al. Prevalence and profile of restless legs syndrome in Parkinson's disease and other neurodegenerative disorders: a case-control study. Parkinsonism Relat Disord 2013;19:426–30.

93. Ylikoski A, Martikainen K, Partinen M. Parkinson's disease and restless legs syndrome. Eur Neurol 2015;73:212–9.

94. Peeraully T, Yong MH, Chokroverty S, et al. Sleep and Parkinson's disease: a review of case-control polysomnography studies. Mov Disord 2012;27: 1729–37.

95. Kumru H, Santamaría J, Tolosa E, et al. Rapid eye movement sleep behavior disorder in parkinsonism with PARKIN mutations. Ann Neurol 2004; 56:599–603.

96. Adel S, Djarmati A, Kabakci K, et al. Co-occurrence of restless legs syndrome and Parkin mutations in two families. Mov Disord 2006;21:258–63.

97. Pont-Sunyer C, Iranzo A, Gaig C, et al. Sleep disorders in parkinsonian and nonparkinsonian LRRK2 mutation carriers. PLoS One 2015;10(7): e0132368.

98. Trotti LM, Bliwise DL. Treatment of the sleep disorders associated with Parkinson's disease. Neurotherapeutics 2014;11:68–77.

99. Neikrug AB, Liu L, Avanzino JA, et al. Continuous positive airway pressure improves sleep and daytime sleepiness in patients with Parkinson disease and sleep apnea. Sleep 2014;37:177–85.

100. Kumru H, Iranzo A, Carrasco E, et al. Lack of effects of pramipexole on REM sleep behavior disorder in Parkinson's disease. Sleep 2008;31:1418–21.

Sleep and Traumatic Brain Injury

Christian R. Baumann, MD

KEYWORDS

- Traumatic brain injury • Insomnia • Excessive daytime sleepiness • Pleiosomnia • Histamine

KEY POINTS

- Post-traumatic sleep–wake disturbances are frequent and often chronic complications after traumatic brain injury.
- The most prevalent sleep–wake disturbances are insomnia, excessive daytime sleepiness, and pleiosomnia (ie, increased sleep need).
- These disturbances are probably of multifactorial origin, but direct traumatic damage to key brain structures in sleep–wake regulation is likely to contribute.
- Diagnosis and treatment consist of standard approaches, but because of misperception of sleep–wake behavior in trauma patients, subjective testing alone may not always suffice.

Traumatic brain injury (TBI) occurs when an external force impacts the head and traumatically injures the brain. It is one of the most prevalent disorders affecting the brain. In the United States, about 1.7 million people sustain a TBI every year.[1] TBIs often produce long-term impairments that interfere with the return to normal life. In the previous 10 years, it has become evident that sleep–wake disturbances often complicate the course after TBI. In a meta-analysis comprising 21 studies, the authors found that about 50% of TBI patients suffer from sleep–wake disturbances.[2] This article provides a clinical guide on how to classify, diagnose, and treat post-traumatic sleep–wake disturbances.

CLASSIFICATION

There is no official classification of post-traumatic sleep–wake disturbances. Based on current literature and the International Classification of Sleep Disorders, third edition (ICSD-3), the proposed classification as given in **Table 1** can be used for clinical purposes.[3] Other sleep–wake disorders such as narcolepsy, sleep apnea, and sleep-related movement disorders have occasionally been reported after TBI, but because of the lack of stringent data, these were not included in **Table 1**.

POST-TRAUMATIC INSOMNIA
Definition

A chronic insomnia disorder is characterized by difficulty initiating and/or maintaining sleep and associated daytime symptoms including fatigue, sleepiness, cognitive deficits, mood disturbance, irritability, behavioral problems, impaired social performance, proneness for errors or accidents, and/or concerns about sleep.[3] These problems occur at least 3 times per week, have been present for at least 3 months, and cannot be attributed to inadequate sleep opportunities or circumstances.[3] For post-traumatic insomnia, these problems must be in temporal relation to the TBI and not related to other causes.

Epidemiology

Because of different assessments of insomnia after TBI, the reported prevalences differ markedly, with frequencies ranging from 5% to more

Disclosure Statement: The author has nothing to disclose.
Department of Neurology, University Hospital Zurich, University of Zurich, Frauenklinikstrasse 26, Zurich 8091, Switzerland
E-mail address: christian.baumann@usz.ch

Sleep Med Clin 11 (2016) 19–23
http://dx.doi.org/10.1016/j.jsmc.2015.10.004

Table 1
Best studied post-traumatic sleep–wake disturbances, their equivalent in the diagnostic international classification of sleep disorders, 3rd edition (ICSD-3), and a proposed definition for use in practice

Diagnosis	Equivalent in ICSD-3	Definition
Post-traumatic insomnia	Chronic insomnia disorder: Insomnia caused by a medical condition	Difficulty initiating sleep or maintaining sleep with related daytime symptoms such as fatigue, sleepiness, cognitive or mood disorders, behavioral or social problems, occurring after TBI and not related to other causes
Post-traumatic excessive daytime sleepiness	Hypersomnia caused by a medical disorder	Daily excessive daytime sleepiness or daytime lapses into sleep, occurring after TBI and not related to other causes
Post-traumatic pleiosomnia	(not existing in the ICSD-3)	Increased sleep need of at least 2 h per 24 h compared with pre-TBI conditions, with or without sleepiness, occurring after TBI and not related to other causes
Post-traumatic circadian sleep-wake disorders	Circadian sleep–wake disorders not otherwise specified	Circadian rhythm sleep–wake disorders, occurring after TBI and not related to other causes.

than 70% in TBI patient.[4] There is some evidence that insomnia may occur more likely in patients with mild TBI than in those with severe traumata.[5] In addition, in a military sample, Bryan[6] found that repeated TBI's enhance the risk of developing insomnia. To make things even more complicated, there is some evidence that TBI patients tend to overestimate insomnia problems; subjective measures reveal higher figures than objective testings.[7]

Etiology and Pathophysiology

In most patients, post-traumatic insomnia is most likely of multifactorial origin. **Box 1** summarizes potential contributors to post-traumatic insomnia.[8]

Diagnosis

Insomnia should be primarily assessed by structured interviews and with questionnaires such as the Pittsburgh Sleep Quality Index (PSQI) or the Insomnia Severity Index (ISI).[9] In most countries, sleep laboratory examinations including actigraphy or polysomnography are not reimbursed for the diagnosis of insomnia. Nevertheless, given the assumption that insomnia patients might overestimate their insomnia symptoms, the diagnosis of post-traumatic insomnia based on interviews or questionnaires alone must be interpreted with some caution.

Treatment

There is only sparse evidence on how to treat post-traumatic insomnia. Good sleep hygiene should be encouraged in all TBI patients, although this approach alone failed to produce significant improvements.[10] A more promising approach is probably cognitive–behavioral therapy, but solid scientific evidence from large-scale clinical trials is missing.[11,12] Regarding pharmacotherapy, benzodiazepine receptor agonists are effective to treat disrupted sleep, but these drugs should be used only during short periods (ie, up to 2 weeks).[13] In contrast to such recommendations, it has been observed that 1 out of 5 patients use hypnotics on average 9 years after TBI.[14]

Box 1
Potential contributors to post-traumatic insomnia

- Pain
- Analgesic pharmacotherapy
- Psychosocial factors
- Depression and anxiety
- Psycho-pharmacological treatment
- Neuroendocrine disturbances
- Medicolegal issues
- Post-traumatic epilepsy
- Anticonvulsive drugs
- Genetic predisposition
- Neuropsychological deficits
- Trauma-induced brain damage

POST-TRAUMATIC PLEIOSOMNIA
Definition

The term pleiosomnia has been introduced to prevent confusions with hypersomnia and excessive daytime sleepiness.[15] So far, there is no official definition of post-traumatic pleiosomnia. The author and colleagues used the working definition of a sleep need that is at least 2 hours per 24 hours longer compared with pre-TBI conditions.[16]

Epidemiology

So far, solid epidemiologic data on post-traumatic pleiosomnia are lacking. In a prospective study in 65 patients, 6 months after trauma, the author and colleagues found pleiosomnia in 22% of patients, irrespective of severity of trauma.[16] In another prospective and controlled study, they observed significantly longer sleeping times per 24 hours in TBI patients; compared with controls matched for age, sex, and sleep satiation, patients slept 1.2 hours longer.[17] This was associated with traumatic intracranial hemorrhage.

Etiology and Pathophysiology

There is some evidence that damage to wake-maintaining neuronal systems might contribute to post-traumatic pleiosomnia. In deceased TBI patients, there is a 41% loss of histamine-producing neurons in the tuberomammillary nucleus, when compared with matched controls.[18] The tuberomammillary nucleus is a major arousal-promoting and wake-maintaining system located in the posterior hypothalamus. Other wake-promoting neuronal populations such as the hypothalamic hypocretin (orexin) system or wake-promoting monoaminergic systems in the brainstem are less markedly damaged[18] (Valko et al, 2016, unpublished result). In a rodent model of TBI, increased sleep need was inversely correlated with the extent of histamine cell loss (Noain et al, 2016, unpublished result). This might indicate that deficient histaminergic signaling after TBI might be an important causative factor for pleiosomnia.

Diagnosis

Detailed history taking and actigraphy should be performed whenever possible. TBI patients markedly underestimate their sleep need, in contrast to controls.[17]

Treatment

There is no treatment option available for post-traumatic pleiosomnia.

POST-TRAUMATIC EXCESSIVE DAYTIME SLEEPINESS
Definition

In patients who suffer from daily episodes of irrepressible need to sleep or daytime lapses in to sleep that occur as a consequence of TBI (ie, in temporal relation to the trauma), post-traumatic excessive daytime sleepiness can be diagnosed.[3]

Epidemiology

As there is growing evidence that TBI patients underestimate sleep pressure during daytime, reliable epidemiologic data are not available. Studies in smaller series of patients suggest that excessive daytime sleepiness may occur in about 25% to 60% of TBI patients, irrespective of trauma severity.[16,17,19]

Etiology and Pathophysiology

Besides coexisting mood disorders, medication, and other comorbidities, trauma-associated damage to wake-promoting neuronal nuclei might contribute to excessive daytime sleepiness, as discussed previously. In addition, an earlier study revealed pain as an important factor in nocturnal sleep disruption and consecutive sleepiness.[20,21] Furthermore, sleep apnea and periodic limb movements might also contribute.[19–21]

Diagnosis

Several studies found evidence for underestimation of excessive daytime sleepiness in TBI cohorts. In a recent study, 19% of 42 TBI patients reported subjective sleepiness, as assessed with the Epworth sleepiness scale, but objective testing with multiple sleep latency tests revealed EDS in 57% of patients.[17] Therefore, the threshold toward objective examinations in a sleep laboratory should be low, given the considerable psychosocial and medicolegal consequences of post-traumatic sleepiness.[21]

TREATMENT

In a double-blind, randomized, placebo-controlled study over 6 weeks, 100 to 200 mg/d of modafinil significantly improved subjective excessive daytime sleepiness, as assessed with the Epworth sleepiness scale, and increased mean sleep latencies on the maintenance of wakefulness test.[22] Another study did not observe such an effect of modafinil in patients with TBI.[23] In a 12-week, randomized, double-blind study, armodafinil 250 mg significantly improved sleep latencies on the multiple sleep latency test in patients with excessive sleepiness associated with mild or moderate TBI.[24] Both efficacy and tolerability were sustained throughout a 12-month open-label extension. Finally, a randomized, placebo-controlled study revealed positive effects of blue light therapy on sleepiness after TBI.[25]

POST-TRAUMATIC CIRCADIAN SLEEP–WAKE DISORDERS
Definition

In the presence of delayed, advanced, or irregular sleep–wake rhythmicity that occurs after TBI, a post-traumatic circadian sleep–wake disorder may be diagnosed.

Epidemiology

There are no data available on the prevalence of post-traumatic circadian sleep–wake disorders. Delayed sleep phase syndrome and irregular sleep–wake pattern appear to be particularly common after TBI, and these disorders might be misdiagnosed as insomnia.[26]

Etiology and Pathophysiology

Apart from comorbid conditions such as depression or anxiety, reduced evening melatonin production may lead to disruption of circadian regulation of melatonin synthesis in TBI patients.[26,27]

Diagnosis

Apart from interviews and sleep logs, actigraphy, saliva melatonin measurements, and body temperature assessments are helpful to detect circadian sleep–wake disorders after TBI.

TREATMENT

There are no specific studies for the treatment of post-traumatic circadian sleep-wake disorders. Evening melatonin replacement and bright light exposure in the morning might be tried.

OTHER POST-TRAUMATIC SLEEP–WAKE DISORDERS

Sleep-related breathing disorders have been reported to be occurring more often in TBI compared with general populations, but literature is still inconsistent in this regard.[18] Recognition and treatment of sleep apnea in TBI patients are important, because it is significantly associated with excessive daytime sleepiness and fatigue.

Fatigue, a subjective experience comprising feelings such as tiredness, exhaustion, apathy, and a lack of energy, can be easily confused with excessive daytime sleepiness. It is also frequent after TBI, with reported frequencies from 16% up to 80%, and persists for many years after trauma.[28,29]

Post-traumatic narcolepsy is a controversial topic. Although it seems tempting to assume that hypocretin cell loss in the hypothalamus would lead to narcolepsy, there has not been any convincing report of post-traumatic narcolepsy with cataplexy in the literature.[30] Even in the presence of proven hypocretin deficiency in the cerebrospinal fluid and typical findings on multiple sleep latency tests, the symptoms in these patients are best described as a narcolepsy-like phenotype after TBI.[8]

Regarding parasomnias and related symptoms, literature is scant. In 2 retrospective studies on 184 and 60 TBI patients, interviews and questionnaires revealed parasomnias in up to 25% of patients, including somnambulism, hypnagogic hallucinations, sleep paralysis, and rapid eye movement sleep behavior disorder.[21,31]

REFERENCES

1. Faul M, Xu L, Wald MM, et al. Traumatic brain injury in the United States: emergency department visits, hospitalizations and deaths 2002–2006. Atlanta (GA): National Center for Injury Prevention and Control, Centers for Disease Control and Prevention; 2010.
2. Mathias JL, Alvaro PK. Prevalence of sleep disturbances, disorders, and problems following traumatic brain injury: a meta-analysis. Sleep Med 2012;13: 898–905.
3. American Academy of Sleep Medicine (AASM). The international classification of sleep disorders. 3rd edition. Darien (IL): American Academy of Sleep Medicine; 2014.
4. Zeitzer JM, Friedman L, O'Hara R. Insomnia in the context of traumatic brain injury. J Rehabil Res Dev 2009;46:827–36.
5. Ouellet MC, Beaulieu-Bonneau S, Morin CM. Insomnia in patients with traumatic brain injury: frequency, characteristics, and risk factors. J Head Trauma Rehabil 2006;21:199–212.
6. Bryan CJ. Repetitive traumatic brain injury (or concussion) increases severity of sleep disturbance among deployed military personnel. Sleep 2013;36:941–6.
7. Ouellet MC, Morin CM. Subjective and objective measures of insomnia in the context of traumatic brain injury: a preliminary study. Sleep Med 2006; 7:486–97.
8. Valko PO, Baumann CR. Sleep disorders after traumatic brain injury. In: Kryger MH, Roth T, Dement WC, editors. Principles and practice in sleep medicine. 6th edition. Elsevier, in press.

9. Mollayeva T, Kendzerska T, Colantonio A. Self-report instruments for assessing sleep dysfunction in an adult traumatic brain injury population: a systematic review. Sleep Med Rev 2013;17:411–23.

10. De La Rue-Evans L, Nesbitt K, Oka RK. Sleep hygiene program implementation in patients with traumatic brain injury. Rehabil Nurs 2013;38:2–10.

11. Ouellet MC, Morin CM. Cognitive behavioral therapy for insomnia associated with traumatic brain injury: a single-case study. Arch Phys Med Rehabil 2004;85: 1298–302.

12. Ouellet MC, Morin CM. Efficacy of cognitive–behavioral therapy for insomnia associated with traumatic brain injury: a single-case experimental design. Arch Phys Med Rehabil 2007;88:1581–92.

13. National Institutes of Health. National Institutes of Health state of the science conference statement on manifestations and management of chronic insomnia in adults, June 13–15, 2005. Sleep 2005; 28:1049–57.

14. Worthington AD, Melia Y. Rehabilitation is compromised by arousal and sleep disorders: results of a survey of rehabilitation centres. Brain Inj 2006;20: 327–32.

15. Sommerauer M, Valko PO, Werth E, et al. Excessive sleep need following traumatic brain injury. A case–control study of 36 patients. J Sleep Res 2013;22: 634–9.

16. Baumann CR, Werth E, Stocker R, et al. Sleep-wake disturbances 6 months after traumatic brain injury: a prospective study. Brain 2007;130:1873–83.

17. Imbach LL, Valko PO, Li T, et al. Increased sleep need and daytime sleepiness 6 months after traumatic brain injury: a prospective controlled clinical trial. Brain 2015;138:726–35.

18. Valko PO, Gavrilov YV, Yamamoto M, et al. Damage to histamine and other hypothalamic neurons with traumatic brain injury. Ann Neurol 2015;77:177–82.

19. Castriotta RJ, Wilde MC, Lai JM, et al. Prevalence and consequences of sleep disorders in traumatic brain injury. J Clin Sleep Med 2007;3:349–56.

20. Masel BE, Scheibel RS, Kimbark T, et al. Excessive daytime sleepiness in adults with brain injuries. Arch Phys Med Rehabil 2001;82:1526–32.

21. Guilleminault C, Yuen KM, Gulevich MG, et al. Hypersomnia after head–neck trauma: a medico-legal dilemma. Neurology 2000;54:653–9.

22. Kaiser PR, Valko PO, Werth E, et al. Modafinil ameliorates excessive daytime sleepiness after traumatic brain injury. Neurology 2010;75:1780–5.

23. Jha A, Weintraub A, Allshouse A, et al. A randomized trial of modafinil for the treatment of fatigue and excessive daytime sleepiness in individuals with chronic traumatic brain injury. J Head Trauma Rehabil 2008;23:52–63.

24. Menn SJ, Yang R, Lankford A. Armodafinil for the treatment of excessive sleepiness associated with mild or moderate closed traumatic brain injury: a 12-week, randomized, double-blind study followed by a 12-month open-label extension. J Clin Sleep Med 2014;10:1181–91.

25. Sinclair KL, Ponsford JL, Taffe J, et al. Randomized controlled trial of light therapy for fatigue following traumatic brain injury. Neurorehabil Neural Repair 2014;28:303–13.

26. Ayalon L, Borodkin K, Dishon L, et al. Circadian rhythm sleep disorders following mild traumatic brain injury. Neurology 2007;68:1136–40.

27. Shekleton JA, Parcell DL, Redman JR, et al. Sleep disturbance and melatonin levels following traumatic brain injury. Neurology 2010;74:1732–8.

28. Cantor JB, Gordon W, Gumber S. What is post TBI fatigue? Neurorehabilitation 2013;32:875–83.

29. Ponsford JL, Downing MG, Olver J, et al. Longitudinal follow-up of patients with traumatic brain injury: outcome at two, five, and ten years post-injury. J Neurotrauma 2014;31:64–77.

30. Poryazova R, Hug D, Baumann CR. Narcolepsy and traumatic brain injury: cause or consequence? Sleep Med 2011;12:811.

31. Verma A, Anand V, Verma NP. Sleep disorders in chronic traumatic brain injury. J Clin Sleep Med 2007;3:357–62.

Sleep and Epilepsy

Lynn Kataria, MD[a], Bradley V. Vaughn, MD[b],*

KEYWORDS

- Sleep • Epilepsy • Pharmacologic • Nonpharmacologic

KEY POINTS

- Epilepsy can fragment sleep and can change sleep architecture.
- Epilepsy therapies can influence sleep and produce sleep symptoms.
- Sleep can create a state that is conducive for some forms of epilepsy.
- Non-rapid eye movement sleep promotes interictal activity, whereas rapid eye movement sleep inhibits interictal activity.
- Sleep disorders such as obstructive sleep apnea make recurrent seizures more likely, and their treatment may help reduce recurrent seizures.

INTRODUCTION

Sleep and epilepsy have a complex relationship. This relationship has been recognized since early descriptions of Aristotle and Hippocrates. In the latter 1800s, Gower[1] studied the association between sleep and epilepsy and found that 21% of patients had seizures exclusively during sleep. The influence of sleep on epilepsy was later discovered to be sleep stage specific because interictal and ictal discharges were observed predominantly in non-rapid eye movement (NREM) sleep and suppressed during rapid eye movement (REM) sleep. This influence of sleep was also found to be a characteristic of some epilepsy syndromes such as benign childhood epilepsy with centrotemporal spikes or autosomal-dominant nocturnal frontal lobe epilepsy (ADNFLE). Furthermore, sleep disruption was also found to increase the likelihood of recurrent seizures.

Sleep deprivation can facilitate seizure occurrence, although it is unclear if this is due to the onset of sleep or activation from sleep loss.[2–4] Sleep architecture can also be disturbed in patients with epilepsy.[5–7] Increased seizure frequency can lead to sleep fragmentation, resulting in a constellation of symptoms impairing daytime function, and similarly, the therapies for epilepsy can produce sleep-related symptoms and substantially alter sleep architecture. Nonetheless, patients with epilepsy frequently have complaints regarding sleep primarily in the domains of excessive daytime sleepiness (EDS), insomnia, or other nocturnal events (**Box 1**).[8–10] Similar to the impact of voluntary sleep deprivation, questions arose as to the effect of primary sleep disorders on epilepsy. Studies of a common sleep disorder, obstructive sleep apnea (OSA), which causes sleep fragmentation and sleep deprivation, was found to increase recurrent seizures.[11] Further work showed that treatment with positive airway pressure (PAP) improved seizure frequency in patients with epilepsy and OSA.[12] Other sleep-related events such as parasomnias, or non-epileptic nocturnal events, can be difficult to distinguish from epileptic seizures and require clinicians' further investigation to distinguish. In this article, the dynamic interplay of sleep and epilepsy through the information gained from studies

[a] Sleep Medicine Section, Department of Neurology, Washington DC Veterans Affairs Medical Center, George Washington University School of Medicine, 50 Irving Street NW, Washington, DC 22042, USA; [b] Department of Neurology, University of North Carolina School of Medicine, Chapel Hill, NC, USA
* Corresponding author. 2122 Physician Office Building, CB # 7025 Department of Neurology, University of North Carolina School of Medicine, Chapel Hill, NC 27599-7025.
E-mail address: vaughnb@neurology.unc.edu

Sleep Med Clin 11 (2016) 25–38
http://dx.doi.org/10.1016/j.jsmc.2015.10.008
1556-407X/16/$ – see front matter © 2016 Elsevier Inc. All rights reserved.

Box 1
Sleep complaints in patients with epilepsy

- Insomnia
- Hypersomnia
- Nocturnal events

---

examining sleep stage, sleep deprivation, the effects of treatment regimen, and the impact of other sleep disorders are explored.

PATIENT EVALUATION OVERVIEW

The patient with epilepsy may have 3 major areas of concern for the clinician. For some patients, sleep may influence their epilepsy, and sleep-related complaints might indicate an underlying sleep disorder. For others, the epilepsy or the therapies may disturb sleep, and some may have nocturnal events. Each of these deserves clinical inspection, and the symptoms of such may not be readily offered.

Approximately one-third to one-half of patients with epilepsy will have a sleep-related complaint. A systematic approach should be taken when looking at sleep disturbances in patients with epilepsy (**Box 2**). A detailed clinical history should focus on both major aspects: the epilepsy and their sleep. In regards to their epilepsy, understanding the type of seizures, time of occurrence, seizure frequency and intensity, as well as the medication regimen is important. From the sleep perspective, the clinician will need to understand the patient's sleep complaint and what appears to influence the issues. The clinician will also want to gather the patient's sleep/wake schedule, including non-workday routines, the sleep environment, typical sleep habits, including other substance use (caffeine, alcohol, herbs, and so on), and a good description from bed partner history, including any unusual nocturnal events, snoring, and witnessed apneic events. Clinicians may garner circadian clues from knowing when patients prefer to sleep and when they feel their most awake. Patients also should describe their understanding of how sleep may influence their epilepsy. An occupational history may also give clues to sleep and circadian rhythm disorders, such as shift work disorder that may put one at risk for sleep deprivation. Lower melatonin levels have been found in patients with refractory epilepsy compared with healthy controls.[13] Seizures and medications used in the treatment of epilepsy can also attenuate or induce brief shifts in the circadian rhythm.[14]

Box 2
Approach to evaluating sleep complaints in patients with epilepsy

Sleep history
 Bedtimes and wake times
 Bedroom environment
 History of underlying sleep disorder such as OSA or RLS
 History of snoring or witnessed apneas
 Screening for maladaptive behaviors
 History from bed partner
 Presence of insomnia or hypersomnia (ESS)

Seizure history
 Frequency and duration
 AED dosage, timing, and adverse effects

Caffeine/alcohol/illicit drug history

Comorbid medical and psychiatric conditions

Review of active medications including over-the-counter medications

Occupational history

The presence of an underlying sleep disorder can affect seizure frequency. Patients with epilepsy should be questioned about the presence of other sleep disorders, such as OSA, restless legs syndrome (RLS), insomnia, and disorders of hypersomnia, such as narcolepsy. Although it has not been validated in epilepsy patients, the Epworth Sleepiness Scale (ESS) can be used in the evaluation of EDS in epilepsy patients for the presence of these sleep disorders. A score of 10 or greater represents clinically significant sleepiness. Malow and colleagues[9] showed that the elevated scores on the ESS were associated with symptoms of OSA and RLS as opposed to seizure frequency or number or type of antiepileptic medication.

Clinical manifestations of OSA include EDS, snoring, and witnessed apneic events by a bed partner. Polysomnography (PSG) is indicated for the confirmation of the diagnosis of OSA. OSA prevalence rates ranging from 4% to 33% have been reported in patients with epilepsy.[15,16] Given the high prevalence in patients with epilepsy, OSA should be strongly considered as part of the differential diagnosis in patients presenting with sleep disruption and EDS.

RLS involves patients having uncomfortable and unpleasant sensations in their legs primarily at night that are worse at rest and improved with movement. It is unclear what the prevalence of RLS is in patients with epilepsy. RLS can cause sleep disruption and can reduce overall total sleep time if not adequately treated and can thus cause significant comorbidity with epilepsy.

More than 15% of patients with epilepsy endorse having excessive sleepiness. Excessive sleepiness can commonly be related to underlying sleep deprivation, medication effect, a circadian rhythm issue, or something such as sleep apnea disrupting the nighttime sleep. Occasionally, when those causes have been eliminated, the clinician may be concerned with the possibility of a primary hypersomnia such as narcolepsy or idiopathic hypersomnia. Narcolepsy is associated with EDS; hypnagogic and/or hypnopompic hallucinations, sleep paralysis, and cataplexy may or may not be present. Overnight PSG displaying 6 hours of sleep followed by a multiple sleep latency test (MSLT) showing a mean sleep latency of less than 8 minutes with 2 sleep onset REM periods confirms the diagnosis. Cases of narcolepsy with cataplexy and epilepsy are rare.[17] Idiopathic hypersomnia is less common and similarly is diagnosed by the overnight polysomnogram followed by an MSLT showing a short, mean sleep latency without the presence of REM sleep during the naps; this too is uncommon in epilepsy.

Insomnia can also significantly affect patients with epilepsy. Many patients with epilepsy note difficulty with initiating and maintaining sleep. Arousals may be more likely due to the underlying epilepsy, medication effect, use of other substances such as caffeine, alcohol, or herbs, or fears associated with sleep. Some patients develop maladaptive behaviors that they think help their sleep but actually impair their ability to sleep. These behaviors include sleeping with the television or light on, sleeping in the living room, reading on a computer before bed, or having foods such as coffee in the evening. Frequent arousals

have been shown to be both a trigger and a manifestation of the seizure itself.[18–20] A detailed look at a patient's comorbidities may also prove fruitful because anxiety and depression have been shown to be prevalent in patients with epilepsy and frequently are associated with insomnia.[21,22]

Sleep stage also plays a crucial role in the propagation of seizures (**Table 1**). Most seizures occur during NREM sleep, thought in part because of the greater ability to recruit neurons than other states. Seizures that occur during NREM sleep may be due to the greater prevalence of neurons at resting state and thus more neurons available to join a synchronized firing pattern as opposed to REM sleep, which consists of a desynchronized electroencephalogram (EEG) and less neurons in the resting state. Within NREM sleep, most seizures occur during stage 2,[23] which may be in part due to greater facilitation of interictal discharges by thalamocortical relay neurons.[24] One study found that seizures arising out of slow-wave sleep were longer in duration than seizures coming from stage 2 sleep.[25] REM sleep, however, typically inhibits seizure transmission. A lower seizure threshold was found in electrically kindled cats in slow-wave sleep as opposed to REM sleep and wakefulness.[26] Kumar and Raju[27] conducted a study that increased the duration of REM sleep by injecting a cholinergic agonist, carbachol, into the pontine reticular formation in rats and found that there was a significant increase in the threshold current required to elicit an after-discharge in the amygdala. The same investigators demonstrated the antiseizure effects of REM, decreasing the likelihood of cortical seizure activity.

Epileptic seizures can affect the sleep state (**Box 3**). Many patients note postictal hypersomnolence, and this may extend into the day after a seizure.[25] Similarly, seizures can cause sleep disruption. Decreases in sleep efficiency, increases in sleep stage shifts, and periods of wakefulness have been reported in patients with primary generalized epilepsy or complex partial seizures compared with normal controls

Table 1		
Association between sleep state and seizure propagation		
Sleep State	**Effect on Interictal Discharges**	**Effects on Seizures**
NREM	More common and more locations	Increased seizure propagation with synchronized EEG
REM	Less frequent and more localized	Decreased seizure initiation and propagation with desynchronized EEG
Arousals	May have discharges just prior or during	Can provoke and also be a part of seizures itself

> **Box 3**
> **Reported possible effects of seizures on sleep state**
>
> - Postictal hypersomnolence
> - Decreased sleep efficiency
> - Increased wakefulness
> - Increased sleep stage shifts
> - Increased arousals
> - Increased sleep fragmentation
> - Reduction in REM (complex partial and generalized tonic clonic seizures)

particularly in patients with focal seizures.[28] These changes are seen on nights with seizures as well as seizure-free nights. Overall, these patients thus had increased sleep fragmentation and instability on seizure-free nights compared with nonepileptic controls.[28]

Many patients with epilepsy may present with nocturnal events that can be very similar to parasomnias, and NREM- and REM-related parasomnias can be difficult to differentiate from epilepsy for even a highly experienced clinician. Similar to the workup for epilepsy, a clear description of the events is paramount (**Table 2**). Historical features, such as time, duration and frequency of the events, the behavioral characteristics of the events, presence or absence of memory of the event, presence of dream mentation, and specific observed details (eyes being open or closed) are helpful in directing the evaluation. Other features, such as age of onset, family history, and settings with which the events occur, can also give clues

to the cause. For cases that involve the risk of injury or someone being harmed, symptoms of other sleep disorders, or concern that the history is atypical, patients should undergo video-PSG with extended EEG montage. NREM parasomnias consisting of the disorders of arousal, which include sleepwalking, sleep terrors, and confusional arousals, occur in the first half or third of the night, with variable behavior and are typically associated with minimal or partial memory of the event. Epileptic seizures are stereotypical and can be of variable in onset and duration throughout the night. REM sleep behavior disorder is an REM parasomnia that is associated with vivid dreams that patients may act out in their sleep that are often violent in nature and more common but not limited to the latter half of the night. Psychogenic events will display wakefulness on the EEG with eyes open.

Specific epilepsy syndromes are associated with sleep (**Table 3**). ADNFLE occurs almost entirely during sleep.[29] There can be 3 distinct subtypes observed, including paroxysmal arousals associated with brief and sudden recurrent motor behavior, nocturnal paroxysmal arousals associated with complex dystonic or dyskinetic postures, and episodic nocturnal wanderings associated with agitation and sterotyped behavior.[30] Understanding these variations can be helpful in distinguishing ADNFLE from parasomnias. Seizures in nocturnal frontal lobe epilepsy (NFLE) occur many times during the night, lasting approximately 30 seconds to 2 minutes in duration.[30–32] Typically, the daytime EEGs are normal in these individuals, but video-EEG or video-PSG with extended montage can help in the differentiation of NFLE from NREM

Table 2
Characteristics features of nocturnal events

Feature	Disorders of Arousal	REM Sleep Behavior Disorder	Nocturnal Seizures	Psychiatric Disorders
Time of night	First third to half of night	Latter half of sleep period during REM	Sporadic	Sporadic
Eye opening	Yes	No	No	Yes
Stereotypic movements	No	No	Yes	No
Memory	Partial or no memory	Vivid dream recall	Variable	Variable
Duration	Minutes	Seconds to minute	Minutes	Minutes to hours
Frequency	Typically 1 or less per night	Nightly events during REM	Sporadic to multiple per night	Sporadic
PSG findings	Arousal from slow-wave sleep	Excessive electromyography tone in REM	Epileptiform activity	Wake state before the event

Table 3
Effects of anticonvulsants on sleep architecture

Drug	Sleep Efficiency	Sleep Latency	Arousals	Stage 1	Stage 2	Stage 3	REM
Phenobarbital	↓	↓	↓	↑	↑	—	↓
Phenytoin	↓	↓	↓	↑	↓	↓/↑	↓
Carbamazepine	↑	↓	↓	—	—	↑	↓
Valproate	—	—	↑	↑	—	↑	—
Ethosuximide	↓	?	↑	↑	—	↓	↑
Felbamate	↓	?	↑	?	?	—	?
Gabapentin	↑	↓	↓	↓	?	↑	↑
Lamotrigine	—	—	—	—	↑	↓	↑
Topiramate	—	—	—	—	—	—	—
Vigabatrin	—	—	—	—	—	—	—
Tiagibine	↑	—	—	↓	—	↑	↓
Levetiracetam	↑	—	↓	—	↑	↑/↓	↓
Zonisamide	—	—	—	—	—	—	—
Pregabalin	↑	↓	↓	↓	—	↑	—
Oxcarbmazepine	?	?	?	?	?	?	?
Lacosamide	—	—	—	—	—	—	—
Clobazam	?	↓	?	↓	↑	↓	?

parasomnias, if an EEG discharge is seen, as well as demonstrating the stereotypic nature of the events. Derry and colleagues[20] developed an algorithm to examine characteristics that were specific for NREM parasomnias, which included interactive behavior, failure to wake after the event, and indistinct offset. This algorithm still contains significant overlap and should not be used in isolation to determine the diagnosis.

Benign childhood epilepsy with centrotemporal spikes (BECTS) is the most common focal epilepsy of childhood associated with clonic movements of the mouth with characteristic drooling, hemifacial and tonic body activity, and impairment of speech. Almost 70% to 80% of seizures with BECTS occur exclusively during sleep, having the characteristic high-amplitude centrotemporal spike pattern with a transverse dipole that is more common in sleep.[33] Similarly, benign nocturnal childhood occipital epilepsy, also known as Panayiotopoulos syndrome, presents with tonic eye deviation, vomiting, and nocturnal seizures with interictal occipital sharp waves present during NREM sleep.[34]

Juvenile myoclonic epilepsy and primary generalized seizures on awakening were initially described by Janz[35] as the "awakening epilepsies." Both present with myoclonic jerks or generalized tonic clonic seizures approximately 1 to 2 hours after awakening.[36] These patients have generalized spike and wave discharges most commonly in the 3.5- to 4.5-Hz range. Sleep deprivation can significantly exacerbate seizures and should be avoided. Differential diagnosis should include hypnic jerks, which occur at sleep onset, and periodic limb movements of sleep, which occur during NREM sleep.

Epilepsy with continuous spike and wave during slow-wave sleep presents predominantly with nocturnal focal motor seizures.[37] This devastating disorder is associated with significant cognitive decline, but some cases respond to treatment.[38] Landau Kleffner syndrome, potentially a milder form related to continuous spike and wave during sleep, is associated with significant neuropsychiatric sequelae including a decline in verbal fluency.[39–41] A study of 6 children who were found to have 1- to 2.5-Hz generalized spike and wave discharges during sleep also had cognitive and psychological deficits.[41]

Patients with epilepsy may underreport their sleep disruptions, viewing it as a normal part of their condition. It is critical that the clinician be knowledgeable about subtle signs that may indicate sleep disturbances in patients with epilepsy, including but not limited to an increased seizure frequency, behavioral changes, and changes in daily activities, such as increased naps. A thorough history is critical for successful management of these patients, which can help guide treatment options.

PHARMACOLOGIC TREATMENT OPTIONS

The overall goal for any patient with epilepsy is seizure freedom. Seizure freedom typically means the trial of anticonvulsants and subsequent dose adjustment until seizure freedom is attained or until untoward side effects are noted. Because many of the anticonvulsants have subjective and objective effects on sleep, one strategy could be to target the antiepileptic drug (AED) regimen for seizure control and treatment of the underlying sleep issues. Treatment of seizures with certain AEDs can cause significant sedation, whereas others may promote alertness. AEDs can also have direct effects on sleep architecture, and patients should be closely monitored and questioned about changes in sleep patterns. Medication selection can be tailored toward patient preferences based on their existing sleep complaints. Patients with difficulties sleeping at night may benefit from a higher dose of a sedating agent at night, and individuals with hypersomnia may benefit from alerting AEDs during the day.

AEDs can produce a variety of sleep architecture changes, and the changes may not be consistent across types of epilepsy nor are data gained in normal individuals necessarily applicable to patients with epilepsy (**Table 4**). Some AEDs can have more broad sleep-promoting effects. Gabapentin increases both REM and slow-wave sleep and reduces awakenings.[42,43] Pregabalin has also been shown to increase slow-wave sleep.[44,45] With other AEDs, the effects on sleep architecture can be mixed. Lamotrigine has been shown to increase REM sleep and decreases slow-wave

sleep in patients in which it was used as adjuvant therapy.[42,46,47] However, in newly diagnosed patients with epilepsy initiated on lamotrigine, no changes were found with respect to the sleep structure on PSG and MSLT.[48] Carbamazepine reduces REM sleep, sleep latency, and arousals and increases slow-wave sleep at doses ranging between 400 mg and 700 mg.[49–52] Similarly, phenytoin decreases REM sleep and causes decreased arousals, decreased sleep efficiency, and decreased latency.[53–55] Phenobarbital binds to the GABA receptor chloride channel complex and increases the duration of chloride channel opening. Phenobarbital has minimal effects on slow-wave sleep but can increase arousals and stage 2 sleep and decreases REM sleep and sleep latency.[53] Benzodiazepines also promote inhibition by binding to the GABA receptor and increasing the frequency of chloride channel opening. Benzodiazepines are known to increase stage 2 sleep and sleep spindle frequency and to decrease slow-wave sleep and sleep latency.[56,57] Valproate may increase arousals during sleep.[58,59] In a study of normal subjects, valproate was found to increase slow-wave sleep and decrease REM sleep.[60] Ethosuximide has been shown to reduce slow-wave sleep, although it increases REM sleep and stage 1 sleep.[61] In a randomized double-blind placebo-controlled trial, clobazam was found to decrease sleep latency, stage 1 sleep, slow-wave sleep, and wake after sleep onset and to increase stage 2 sleep.[62]

Some AEDs have minimal to no effects on the sleep architecture. Topiramate, vigabatrin, and

Table 4
Epilepsy syndromes and association with sleep

Epilepsy Syndrome	Association to Sleep/EEG Findings	Characteristic Features
ADNFLE	Occurs exclusively during sleep	• Paroxysmal arousals with recurrent motor behavior • Episodic stereotyped nocturnal wandering • Paroxysmal arousals with dystonic/dyskinetic postures
BECTS	70%–80% of seizures exclusively during sleep, centrotemporal spikes with transverse dipole	• Clonic movements of mouth with drooling • Hemifacial and tonic body activity • Speech impairment
Juvenile Myoclonic Epilepsy	3.5–4.5-Hz generalized spike and wave discharges	Myoclonic jerks 1–2 h after awakening
Epilepsy with Continuous Spike and Wave during Sleep	Continuous spike and wave discharges during sleep	• Nocturnal focal motor seizures • Cognitive decline

zonisamide have also been shown to have no significant changes on sleep architecture and daytime sleep on the MSLT.[63-65] In one study, levetiracetam was found to cause sleepiness and increase stage 2 sleep.[66] However, a later study found that levetiracetam has minimal to no effects on the structure of sleep.[67] Lacosamide was recently found to have no subjective or objective effects on sleep in healthy patients.[68] Given the varied effects of AEDs on sleep architecture, medication should be carefully chosen in patients with epilepsy and a concomitant sleep disorder.

NONPHARMACOLOGIC TREATMENT OPTIONS

Since the time of Aristotle, patients have been counseled on the importance of getting enough sleep because sleep deprivation is a known trigger for seizures.[69] Sleep deprivation and possibly oversleeping are associated with higher risk of seizures on the following day. In addition to total sleep time, the sleep schedule, sleep environment, daytime activities, and perceptions about sleep may also reveal clues that impact the control of epilepsy. Regular bedtimes and wake times are important to assuring adequate time dedicated to sleep to improve alertness and to help maintain a consistent circadian rhythm. Patients should limit consumption of caffeinated beverages especially close to bedtime because this can prolong sleep latency and contribute to sleep disruption. Correspondingly, technological devices, including television, video games, computers, tablets, and mobile phones, and light sources should be powered down before the onset of sleep because they may promote a delay in the circadian rhythm and cause more frequent arousals during the sleep period. Because light is the most powerful time cue for the circadian rhythm, patients should be exposed to bright light during the day to help reinforce the body clock. Opposite of light, melatonin is released in response to the initial onset of evening darkness. Individuals with epilepsy have lower melatonin levels, and thus, receive less signals to go to sleep.[13] Other time clues, such as activity, meals, and social activities, contribute to circadian entrainment and should be part of the routine to promote wakefulness during the day. Although the frequency of circadian rhythm disturbance in patients with epilepsy is unknown, it is the authors' experience that these patients respond to shifting the body by using these circadian clues as with other patients.

Nonpharmacologic therapies can also be applied to help patients with epilepsy who are suffering from insomnia. Maladaptive behaviors can perpetuate sleep complaints, and modifying these actions can very well be a difficult task. Stimulus control therapy can be applied to patients with epilepsy; however, sleep restriction is not routinely recommended given the potential risk of provoking seizures. One approach may be to consider addressing each issue or to set a few goals in a stepwise fashion so that patients can make changes in stages. A seizure-and-sleep diary can also prove very helpful in assessing how patients are progressing with prescribed changes and should be examined at each clinic visit. In addition, family members should be encouraged to attend clinic visits so as to reinforce the clinical importance of maintaining good sleep hygiene and can be helpful partners in facilitating and helping carrying out these lifestyle modifications.

Epilepsy patients presenting with EDS should be screened for the presence of an underlying sleep-related breathing disorder such as OSA because this is a common complaint. Although EDS is associated with OSA, many patients with epilepsy may not recognize or initially endorse the sign of sleepiness, and clinicians need to ask about other symptoms that may be associated with OSA, such as snoring, witnessed apneas, memory or concentration difficulties, uncontrolled headaches, treatment-resistant hypertension, and fatigue. The ESS score is a validated tool that is used in clinical settings to screen patients for the presence of OSA, with a score of 10 or greater being clinically significant. PSG can be used to confirm the diagnosis of OSA and continuous positive airway pressure (CPAP) is the most common treatment modality. There have been several studies that looked at the relationship between OSA and epilepsy. OSA has been found to be prevalent in patients with epilepsy.[70,71] One study reported OSA prevalence as high as 30% in patients with epilepsy, and increasing age and AED load were independent predictors of risk of OSA.[72] Malow and colleagues[15] also found 33% of patients with refractory partial epilepsy to have OSA. Simply the presence of OSA in one study of older adults with epilepsy was associated with worsening seizure control.[73]

Wyler and Weymuller[74] were the first to show improvement in generalized and partial seizures with treatment of OSA via tracheostomy. There have also been several studies that looked at the positive effects of CPAP use on seizure control.[11] Treatment of sleep-disordered breathing with CPAP has been associated with a reduction in interictal epileptogenic activity in 6 patients with partial epilepsy highlighting the benefits of sleep consolidation in reducing epileptogenicity.[75] This finding was further substantiated in a recent trial that examined 9 adults with medical refractory epilepsy whereby CPAP therapy was associated with a significant reduction in median spike rate overall, in wakefulness, and in NREM sleep but not REM sleep, in the absence of AED changes.[76] Patients with severe OSA in this trial were also found to have higher spike rates as well, again displaying the potential role of sleep fragmentation in epileptogenicity. Malow and colleagues[77] performed a randomized double-blind pilot trial comparing CPAP with sham treatment and found a greater seizure reduction in adults with refractory epilepsy using CPAP (n = 22) versus sham (n = 13) treatment, although the results were not significant because the study was not powered to measure the effect of PAP therapy on seizure control. Vendrame and colleagues[78] conducted a retrospective study that looked at the effects of CPAP compliance on seizure control and found that CPAP-compliant patients (n = 28) had a reduction in seizure frequency of 1.8 to 1 per month compared with no significant reduction in the noncompliant group (n = 13), with AED doses remaining constant after 6 months of CPAP use. A recent retrospective study looked at the effects of PAP on seizure control and found that the percentage of subjects with greater than 50% seizure reduction and the mean percentage of seizure reduction were greatest in the PAP-treated OSA group (≥4 h per night at least 5 nights per week) compared with patients with untreated OSA, although compliance was through self-report.[12]

All of these studies highlight the importance of treating OSA effectively. Although the mechanism is unclear, the association is mostly likely complex involving sleep deprivation and fragmentation models as well as the effects from oxygen desaturation. There is no doubt that stabilization and consolidation of sleep architecture with PAP and other effective therapies lead to beneficial aspects on sleep architecture and seizure frequency.

COMBINATION THERAPIES

A multimodal strategy should be used to treat patients with epilepsy and sleep disorders. Optimizing pharmacotherapy with AEDs to control seizures is of critical importance, along with control of the underlying sleep disorder. Depending on the type of sleep disorder they may have, therapy can be tailored toward the patient. One approach is to categorize epilepsy patients into whether they have insomnia or hypersomnia (**Figs. 1** and **2**). A thorough sleep history should then be conducted investigating the patient's bedtimes and wake times, number of awakenings at night, daytime caffeine and/or alcohol consumption, medication history, daytime effects from sleep disruption, and seizure history.

For the patient with epilepsy presenting with insomnia, the importance of good sleep hygiene and adherence to good circadian rhythm practices should be highly emphasized. A sleep diary can be a helpful tool in both determining and ultimately correcting a disrupted sleep schedule. Some patients may benefit from taking a hot shower in the evening to enhance the body temperature drop before sleep and taking exogenous melatonin in the early evening to accentuate the clues of the onset of darkness. Although cognitive behavioral therapy is considered the gold standard of therapy for patients with chronic insomnia, the sleep restriction component is contraindicated in patients with epilepsy because sleep deprivation may cause seizures to occur. Other techniques used in the treatment of chronic insomnia, including stimulus control therapy, progressive muscular relaxation techniques, and biofeedback, are viable options for patients with epilepsy. Epilepsy patients with insomnia on AEDs may benefit from higher somnogenic medications in the evening and more alerting medications, particularly felbamate, ethosuximide, lamotrigine, and zonisamide, in the morning; this may be of particular benefit in patients with frequent arousals at night because arousals may be a manifestation of epileptic events. Some patients with epilepsy may feel anxiety regarding sleep onset at night for fear of seizure occurrence during the sleep period. Some AED medications, such as gabapentin or pregabalin, can reduce and improve presleep anxiety. Similarly, gabapentin and pregabalin can be used in the treatment of RLS and can also be beneficial in treating neuropathic pain.[79,80] As affective disorders commonly coexist with epilepsy, patients with insomnia should be screened for the presence of an underlying psychiatric disorder that could cause and/or perpetuate of symptoms of insomnia. Treatment of the psychiatric disorder can be beneficial in patients with epilepsy.[81]

Epilepsy patients presenting with hypersomnia should have similar sleep history taken, as mentioned earlier, for patients with insomnia but also focusing on assuring adequate time for sleep and issues that may disturb sleep or inhibit wakefulness. In today's 24/7 society, many individuals opt to sleep less and thus are at risk for insufficient time dedicated to sleep. Similarly, both environmental and physiologic disturbances of sleep may also interfere with the person's ability to attain adequate rest. As noted above, several AEDs are known to have sedating effects and must be considered in the differential diagnosis of epilepsy

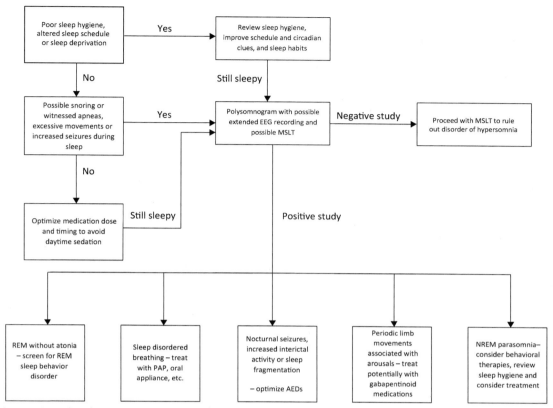

Fig. 1. Algorithm for the evaluation of epilepsy patients presenting with hypersomnia.

patients presenting with hypersomnia. For these patients, dosage adjustments can be considered or AEDs can be dosed before the sleep period. Alternatively, a less sedating AED can be considered for substitution to control seizures. Patients should also be screened for the presence of concomitant sleep disorders, particularly OSA. Although data are limited, patients being treated with stimulants for disorders of hypersomnia should be monitored closely for interactions with AEDs and effects on seizure frequency.

In patients with circadian rhythm disorders, a sleep diary or actigraphy may be helpful to identify the sleep-wake pattern. Patients may use appropriately timed bright light, exercise, or melatonin to shift the circadian phase; this may be beneficial in reducing seizure frequency.[82] To advance the circadian phase, exogenous melatonin can be given 2 to 6 hours before the desired bedtime.

A detailed seizure history should be taken from patients and bed partners because recurrent nocturnal seizures can contribute to sleep disruption and present as EDS.[83] Video-PSG with extended montage can be helpful for the detection and confirmation of events. Medication

adjustments can be made by dosing AEDs closer to sleep for recurrent nocturnal seizures.

SURGICAL TREATMENT OPTIONS

Surgery can also be considered for the treatment of OSA, and tonsillectomy and adenoidectomy are considered the first-line treatment for OSA in children. Surgery for sleep apnea in children was found to improve seizure frequency in a retrospective study, wherein 37% (n = 10) became seizure-free, 11% (n = 3) demonstrated seizure reduction, and 22% (n = 6) had an amelioration of seizure frequency.[84] A multivariate analysis in this study found a trend toward seizure freedom with elevated body mass index scores and apnea-hypopnea index (AHI) at the time of surgery.

In patients with medically refractory epilepsy, epilepsy surgery can potentially improve sleep outcomes through reductions in seizure frequency leading to less sleep fragmentation. Zanzmera and colleagues[85] conducted a prospective study that looked at 17 individuals with medically refractory epilepsy, and patients with good surgical outcomes were found to have a reduction in seizure

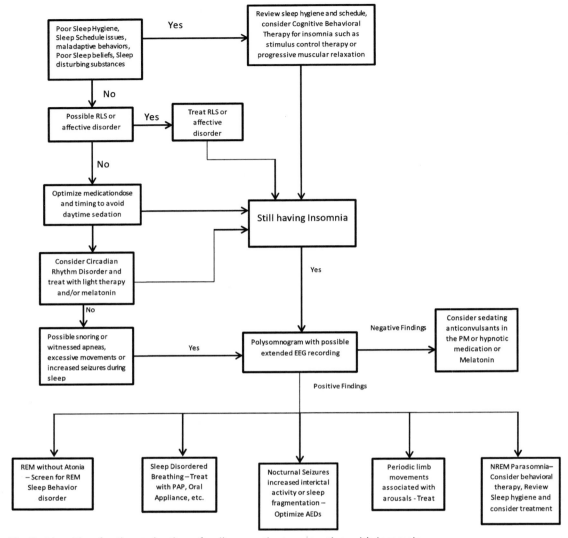

Fig. 2. Algorithm for the evaluation of epilepsy patients presenting with insomnia.

frequency, a reduction in arousal index, and an increase in total sleep time. This improvement may extend to sleep-related breathing control, as documented in a single case report demonstrating correction of OSA after left frontal lobe resection that also produced a marked reduction in spike rate.[86]

Vagus nerve stimulation (VNS) is another treatment modality in patients with epilepsy. Studies that looked at the effects on sleep from VNS have shown conflicting results. Malow and colleagues[87] found that VNS reduces daytime sleepiness in patients with epilepsy determined by increased sleep latency on the MSLT. Although another study found no change in the sleep latency overall, a subgroup analysis looked at

patients with treatment at low stimulus intensities of less than 1.5 mA and found a significant improvement in sleep latency that was observed on the MSLT.[88] One study reported that patients treated with VNS have increased slow-wave sleep and stage N1 sleep.[89] The variety of conflicting results may be attributed to the small sample sizes in these studies, leading to a lack of sufficient power to detect an effect size. In addition, maximal benefit for seizure reduction from VNS is not observed until 2 to 3 years later; thus, these short-term studies may not reflect longer-term influences.

Hypoglossal nerve stimulation (HNS) has been approved for the treatment of OSA in patients. A significant reduction in the AHI and the oxygen desaturation index was observed with HNS treatment in patients with moderate to severe OSA that were refractory to PAP therapy.[90] No studies have yet to formally look at the impact of HNS therapy on seizure control.

TREATMENT RESISTANCE/COMPLICATIONS

Many patients fail to respond to anticonvulsant medication. Although some nocturnal seizure types such as BECTS are easily responsive, others, such as NFLEs, are not as responsive to medical therapy. Patients who fail 2 or more medications should be considered for surgical evaluation. This evaluation may also include the determination of whether device therapy or other nonpharmacologic therapies should be considered. No matter how well controlled the seizures are, patients presenting with nocturnal seizures and their families should be counseled extensively on safety of the bedroom environment. Low-lying mattresses with bedrails should be used, and potentially hazardous objects should be located and removed from the bedroom to avoid injury. Families and patients should have a seizure emergency plan, whereby all individuals are counseled on dosing and administration of rescue medications, and when emergency medical services should be called.

For epilepsy patients with concomitant OSA on PAP, a good amount of time should be taken during the setup process on appropriate mask fitting and ease of removal so that patients do not get entrapped with equipment during seizures. Full face masks should be avoided in patients with a history of postictal vomiting. Oral appliances used for the treatment of OSA are contraindicated in patients with postictal vomiting as well. In addition, oral appliances should be tightly fitted in patients with epilepsy to avoid aspiration.

VNS has been associated with increased sleep disordered breathing in some cases.[91–93] A low level of stimulation intensity may be an alternative to counteract the apneas that occur at higher levels.

Amphetamines for the treatment of hypersomnia can increase in seizure frequency and should be carefully monitored in patients with epilepsy. Potential interactions with AEDs should also be considered when evaluating the initiation of stimulants in epilepsy patients.

EVALUATION OF OUTCOME AND LONG-TERM RECOMMENDATIONS

All patients with epilepsy should be screened in the clinical setting with respect to their sleep.

Patients should bring a family member to all visits to discuss the presence of any nocturnal symptoms including seizures that the patient may not be aware of. Patients with epilepsy should be instructed on the importance of maintaining a regular sleep schedule and avoiding sleep deprivation, which can provoke seizures. Circadian entrainment with zeitgebers such as bright light, regular meals, and social activities can facilitate this, and epilepsy patients should be encouraged to avoid a reclusive and sedentary lifestyle. Medications should be reviewed, and compliance should be emphasized. If an underlying sleep disorder is present, patients should be counseled on the importance of treating the disorder and the positive effects on seizure control.

SUMMARY

Sleep plays an intricate role in the disease process of epilepsy. Despite the complexity of this relationship, the prognosis is a favorable one for patients presenting with sleep disorders and epilepsy. Clinicians need to be vigilant about asking about and addressing sleep complaints in patients with epilepsy. Ultimately improving sleep and optimizing seizure control can have significant positive effects on the quality of life of these patients.

REFERENCES

1. Gowers W. Epilepsy and other chronic convulsive diseases. London: William Wood; 1885.
2. Foldvary-Schaefer N, Grigg Damberger M. Sleep and epilepsy. Semin Neurol 2009;29(4):419–28.
3. Matos G, Andersen M, do Valle AC, et al. The relationship between sleep and epilepsy: evidence from clinical trials and animal models. J Neurol Sci 2010;295:1–7.
4. Dinner DS. Effect of sleep on epilepsy. J Clin Neurophysiol 2002;19:504–13.
5. Kalevias J, Cruz M, Gorava J, et al. Spectrum of polysomnographic abnormalities in children with epilepsy. Pediatr Neurol 2008;39(3):170–6.
6. Crespel A, Coubes P, Baldy-Moulinier M. Sleep influence on seizures and epilepsy effects on sleep in partial frontal and temporal lobe epilepsies. Clin Neurophysiol 2000;111(Suppl 2):S54–9.
7. Zanzmera P, Shukla G, Gupta A, et al. Markedly disturbed sleep in medically refractory compared to controlled epilepsy—a clinical and polysomnographic study. Seizure 2012;21(7):487–90.
8. Khatami R, Zutter D, Siegel A, et al. Sleep-wake habits and disorders in a series of 100 adult-epilepsy patients—a prospective study. Seizure 2006;15:299–306.

9. Malow B, Bowes R, Lin X. Predictors of sleepiness in epilepsy patients. Sleep 1997;20(12):1105–10.

10. de Weerd A, de Haas S, Otte A, et al. Subjective sleep disturbance in inpatients with partial epilepsy: a questionnaire-based study on prevalence and impact on quality of life. Epilepsia 2004;45(11): 1397–404.

11. Vaughn BV, D'Cruz OF, Beach R, et al. Improvement of epileptic seizure control with treatment of obstructive sleep apnea. Seizure 1996;5:73–8.

12. Pornsriniyom D, Kim HW, Bena K, et al. Effect of positive airway pressure therapy on seizure control in patients with epilepsy and obstructive sleep apnea. Epilepsy Behav 2014;37:270–5.

13. Paprocka J, Dec R, Jamroz E, et al. Melatonin and childhood refractory epilepsy—a pilot study. Med Sci Monit 2010;16:CR389–96.

14. Quigg M. Seizures and circadian rhythms. Sleep and epilepsy: the clinical spectrum. 1st edition. Amsterdam: Elsevier Science; 2002. p. 127–42.

15. Malow BA, Levy K, Maturen K, et al. Obstructive sleep apnea is common in medically refractory epilepsy patients. Neurology 2000;55:1002–7.

16. Sonka K, Juklichova M, Preti M, et al. Seizures in sleep apnea patients: occurrence and time distribution. Sb Lek 2000;1(3):229–32.

17. Yang Z, Liu X, Dong X, et al. Epilepsy and narcolepsy-cataplexy in a child. J Child Neurol 2012;27(6):807–10.

18. Malow BA, Varma NK. Seizures and arousals from sleep—which comes first? Sleep 1995;18(9):783–6.

19. Nobili L, Sartori I, Terzhagi M, et al. Intracerebral recordings of minor motor events, paroxysmal arousals and major seizures in nocturnal frontal lobe epilepsy. Neurol Sci 2005;26(Suppl 3): s215–9.

20. Derry C, Harvey A, Walker M, et al. NREM arousal parasomnias and their distinction from nocturnal frontal lobe epilepsy: a video EEG analysis. Sleep 2009;32(12):1637–44.

21. Xu X, Brandenburg NA, McDermott AM, et al. Sleep disturbances reported by refractory partial-onset epilepsy patients receiving polytherapy. Epilepsia 2006;47(7):1176–83.

22. Stefanello S, Marin-Leon I, Fernandes PT, et al. Psychiatric comorbidity and suicidal behavior in epilepsy: a community-based control study. Epilepsia 2010;51(7):1120–5.

23. Minecan D, Natarajan A, Marzec M, et al. Relationship of epileptic seizures to sleep stage and sleep depth. Sleep 2002;25(8):899–904.

24. Steriade M, Amzica F. Sleep oscillations developing into seizures in corticothalamic systems. Epilepsia 2003;44(Suppl 12):9–20.

25. Bazil CW, Walczak TS. Effect of sleep and sleep stage on epileptic and nonepileptic seizures. Epilepsia 1997;38:56–62.

26. Sato M, Nakashima T. Kindling: secondary epileptogenesis, sleep and catecholamines. Can J Neurol Sci 1975;2(4):439–46.

27. Kumar P, Raju TR. Seizure susceptibility decreases with enhancement of rapid eye movement sleep. Brain Res 2001;922:299–304.

28. Touchon J, Baldy-Moulinier M, Billiard M, et al. Sleep organization and epilepsy. Epilepsy Res Suppl 1991;2:73–81.

29. Scheffer IE, Bhatia KP, Lopes-Cendes I, et al. Autosomal dominant nocturnal frontal lobe epilepsy. A distinctive clinical disorder. Brain 1995;118(Pt 1): 61–73.

30. Provini F, Piazzi G, Tinuper P, et al. Nocturnal frontal lobe epilepsy. A clinical and polygraphic overview of 100 consecutive cases. Brain 1999; 122(Pt 6):1017–31.

31. Derry CP, Davey M, Johns M. Distinguishing sleep disorders from seizures: diagnosing bumps in the night. Arch Neurol 2006;63(5):705–9.

32. Zucconi M, Ferini-Strambi L. NREM parasomnias: arousal disorders and differentiation from nocturnal frontal lobe epilepsy. Clin Neurophysiol 2000; 111(Suppl 2):S129–35.

33. Eeg-Olofsson O. Rolandic epilepsy. In: Bazil CA, Malow BA, Sammaritano MR, editors. Sleep and epilepsy: the clinical spectrum. Amsterdam: Elsevier Science; 2002. p. 257–63.

34. Loiseau P. Idiopathic and benign partial epilepsies. In: Wyllie E, editor. The treatment of epilepsy: principles and practice. Philadelphia: Lippincott, Williams and Wilkins; 2001. p. 475–84.

35. Janz D. The grand mal epilepsies and the sleep-waking cycle. Epilepsia 1962;3:69–109.

36. Reutens DC, Berkovic SF. Idiopathic generalized epilepsy of adolescence: are the syndromes clinically distinct? Neurology 1995;45(8):1469–76.

37. Tassinari CA, Rubboli G, Volpi L, et al. Encephalopathy with electrical status epilepticus during slow wave sleep or ESES syndrome including acquire aphasia. Clin Neurophysiol 2000;111(Suppl 2): S94–102.

38. Sinclair DB, Synder DJ. Corticosteroids for the treatment of Landua-Kleffner syndrome and continuous spike-wave discharge during sleep. Pediatr Neurol 2004;32(5):300–6.

39. Kothare SV, Kaleyias J. Sleep and epilepsy I children and adolescents. Sleep Med 2010;11(7): 674–85.

40. Baglietto MG, Battaglia FM, Nobili L, et al. Neuropsychological disorders related to interictal epileptic discharges during sleep in benign epilepsy of childhood with centrotemporal or Rolandic spikes. Dev Med Child Neurol 2001;43(6):407–12.

41. Patry G, Lyagoubi S, Tassinari A. A subclinical "electrical status epilepticus" induced by seep in children. Arch Neurol 1971;24:242–52.

42. Placidi F, Diomedi M, Scalise A, et al. Effect of anti-convulsants on nocturnal sleep in epilepsy. Neurology 2000;54:S25–32.

43. Foldvary-Schaefer N, De Leon Sanchez I, Karafa M, et al. Gabapentin increases slow-wave sleep in normal adults. Epilepsia 2002;43:1493–7.

44. Hindmarch I, Dawson J, Stanley N. A double-blind study in healthy volunteers to assess the effects on sleep of pregabalin compared with alprazolam and placebo. Sleep 2005;28:187–93.

45. Bazil CW, Dave J, Cole J, et al. Pregabalin increases slow wave sleep and may improve attention in patients with partial epilepsy and insomnia. Epilepsy Behav 2012;23:422–5.

46. Placidi F, Marciani MG, Diomedi M, et al. Effects of lamotrigine on nocturnal sleep, daytime somnolence and cognitive function in focal epilepsy. Acta Neurol Scand 2000;102:81–6.

47. Foldvary N, Perry M, Lee J, et al. The effects of lamotrigine on sleep in patients with epilepsy. Epilepsia 2001;42:1569–73.

48. Bonanni E, Massetani R, Gneri C, et al. Sleep pattern and daytime sleepiness in epileptic patients receiving pharmacological treatment. Epilepsia 1996;36(Suppl 3) [abstract:1.128].

49. Gann H, Riemann D, Hohagen F, et al. The influence of carbamazepine on sleep-EEG and the clonidine test in healthy subjects: results of a preliminary study. Biol Psychiatry 1994;35:893–6.

50. Gigli GL, Placidi F, Diomedi M, et al. Nocturnal sleep and daytime somnolence in untreated patients with temporal lobe epilepsy: changes after treatment with controlled release carbamazepine. Epilepsia 1997;38:696–701.

51. Riemann D, Gann H, Hohagen F, et al. The effect of carbamazepine on endocrine and sleep EEG variables in a patient with 48-hour rapid cycling, and healthy controls. Neuropsychobiology 1993;27:163–70.

52. Yang JD, Elphick M, Sharpley AL, et al. Effects of carbamazepine on sleep in healthy volunteers. Biol Psychiatry 1989;26:324–8.

53. Wolf P, Roder-Wanner UU, Brede M. Influence of therapeutic phenobarbital and phenytoin medication on the polygraphic sleep of patients with epilepsy. Epilepsia 1984;25:467–75.

54. Roder-Wanner UU, Noachtar S, Wolf P. Response of polygraphic sleep to phenytoin treatment for epilepsy. A longitudinal study of immediate, short- and long-term effects. Acta Neurol Scand 1987;76:157–67.

55. Legros B, Bazil CW. Effects of antiepileptic dugs on sleep architecture: a pilot study. Sleep Med 2003;4:51–5.

56. Sammaritano M, Sherwin A. Effect of anticonvulsants on sleep. Neurology 2000;54(5 Suppl 1):S16–24.

57. Copinschi G, Van Onderbergen A, L'Hermite-Baleriaux M, et al. Effects of the short-acting benzodiazepine triazolam, taken at bedtime, on circadian and sleep-related hormonal profiles in normal men. Sleep 1990;13:232–44.

58. Findji F, Catani P. The effects of valproic acid on sleep parameters in epileptic children. In: Sterman MB, Shouse MN, Passouant P, editors. Sleep and epilepsy. New York: Academic Press; 1982. p. 395–6.

59. Dadmehr N, Congbalay DR, Pakalnis A, et al. Sleep and waking disturbances in epilepsy. Clin Electroencephalogr 1987;18(3):136–41.

60. Harding GF, Alford CA, Powell TE. The effect of sodium valproate on sleep, reaction times, and visual evoked potential in normal subjects. Epilepsia 1985;26:597–601.

61. Wolf P, Inoue Y, Roder-Wanner UU, et al. Psychiatric complications of absence therapy and their relation to alteration of sleep. Epilepsia 1984;25(Suppl 1):S56–9.

62. Nicholson AN, Stone BM, Clarke CH. Effect of the 1,5-benzodiazepines, clobazam and triflubazam, on sleep in man. Br J Clin Pharmacol 1977;4:567–72.

63. Bonanni E, Galli R, Maestri M, et al. Daytime sleepiness in patients with epilepsy receiving topiramate monotherapy. Epilepsia 2004;45:333–7.

64. Bonanni E, Massetani R, Galli R, et al. A quantitative study of daytime sleepiness induced by carbamazepine and add-on vigabatrin in epileptic patients. Acta Neurol Scand 1997;95:193–6.

65. Romigi A, Izzi F, Placidi F, et al. Effects of zonisamide as add-on therapy on sleep-wake cycle in focal epilepsy: a polysomnographic study. Epilepsy Behav 2013;26:170–4.

66. Bell C, Vanderlinden H, Hiersemenzel R, et al. The effects of levetiracetam on objective and subjective sleep parameters in healthy volunteers and patients with partial epilepsy. J Sleep Res 2002;11:255–63.

67. Bazil CW, Battista J, Basner RC. Effects of levetiracetam on sleep in normal volunteers. Epilepsy Behav 2005;7:539–42.

68. Hudson JD, Guptil JT, Bynes W, et al. Assessment of the effects of lacosamide on sleep parameters in healthy subjects. Seizure 2015;25:155–9.

69. Degen R, Degen HE. Sleep and sleep deprivation in epileptology. Epilepsy Res Suppl 1991;2:235–60.

70. Devinsky O, Ehrenberg B, Barthlen GM, et al. Epilepsy and sleep apnea syndrome. Neurology 1994;44:2060–4.

71. Manni R, Terzaghi M, Arbasino C, et al. Obstructive sleep apnea in a clinical series of adult epilepsy patients: frequency and features of the comorbidity. Epilepsia 2003;44:836–40.

72. Foldvary-Schaefer N, Andrews ND, Pornsriniyom D, et al. Sleep apnea and epilepsy: who's at risk? Epilepsy Behav 2012;25:363–7.

73. Chihorek AM, Abou-Khalil B, Malow BA. Obstructive sleep apnea is associated with seizure occurrence in older adults with epilepsy. Neurology 2007;69: 1823–7.

74. Wyler AR, Weymuller EA. Epilepsy complicated by sleep apnea. Ann Neurol 1981;9:403–4.

75. Oliveira AJ, Zamagni M, Dolso P, et al. Respiratory disorders during sleep in patients with epilepsy: effect of ventilatory therapy on EEG interictal epileptiform discharges. Clin Neurophysiol 2000;111(Suppl 2):S141–5.

76. Pornsriniyom D, Shinlapawittayatorn K, Fong J, et al. Continuous positive airway pressure therapy for obstructive sleep apnea reduces interictal epileptiform discharges in adults with epilepsy. Epilepsy Behav 2014;37:171–4.

77. Malow BA, Foldvary Schaefer N, Vaughn BV, et al. Treating obstructive sleep apnea in adults with epilepsy: a randomized pilot trial. Neurology 2008;71: 572–7.

78. Vendrame M, Auerbach S, Loddenkemper T, et al. effect of continuous positive airway pressure treatment on seizure control in patients with obstructive sleep apnea and epilepsy. Epilepsia 2011;52: e168–71.

79. Lee DO, Zima RB, Perkins AT, et al. A randomized, double-blind, placebo-controlled study to assess the efficacy and tolerability of gabapentin encarbil in subjects with restless legs syndrome. J Clin Sleep Med 2011;7(3):282–92.

80. Misra UK, Kalita J, Kumar B, et al. Treatment of restless legs syndrome with pregabalin: a double-blind, placebo-controlled study. Neurology 2011;76(4):408.

81. Kanner AM, Palac S. Neuropsychiatric complications of epilepsy. Curr Neurol Neurosci Rep 2002; 2(4):365–72.

82. Goldberg-Stern H, Oren H, Peled N, et al. Effect of melatonin on seizure frequency in intractable epilepsy: a pilot study. J Child Neurol 2012;27(12): 1524–8.

83. Miller MT, Vaughn BV, Messenheimer JA, et al. Subjective sleep quality in patients with epilepsy. Epilepsia 1996;36(Suppl 4):43.

84. Segal E, Vendrame M, Gregas M, et al. Effect of treatment of obstructive sleep apnea on seizure outcomes in children with epilepsy. Pediatr Neurol 2012;46(6):359–62.

85. Zanzmera P, Shukla G, Gupta A, et al. Effect of successful epilepsy surgery on subjective and objective sleep parameters—a prospective study. Sleep Med 2013;14(4):333–8.

86. Foldvary-Schaefer N, Stephenson L, Bingaman W. Resolution of obstructive sleep apnea with epilepsy surgery? Expanding the relationship between sleep and epilepsy. Epilepsia 2008;49(8):1457–9.

87. Malow BA, Edwards J, Marzec M, et al. Vagus nerve stimulation reduces daytime sleepiness in epilepsy patients. Neurology 2001;57:879–84.

88. Galli R, Bonnani E, Pizzanelli C, et al. Daytime vigilance and quality of life in epileptic patients treated with vagus nerve stimulation. Epilepsy Behav 2003; 4:185–91.

89. Hallbook T, Lundgren J, Rosen I, et al. Beneficial effects on sleep of vagus nerve stimulation in children with therapy resistant epilepsy. Eur J Paediatr Neurol 2005;9:399–407.

90. Strollo PJ Jr, Soose RJ, Maurer JT. Upper airway stimulation for obstructive sleep apnea. N Engl J Med 2014;370(2):139–49.

91. Malow BA, Edwards J, Marzec M, et al. Effects of vagus nerve stimulation on respiration during sleep: a pilot study. Neurology 2000;55(10):1450–4.

92. Holmes MD, Chang M, Kapur V. Sleep apnea and excessive daytime sleepiness induced by vagal nerve stimulation. Neurology 2003;61(8):1126–9.

93. Marzec M, Edwards J, Sagher O, et al. Effects of vagus nerve stimulation on sleep-related breathing in epilepsy patients. Epilepsia 2003;44(7):930–5.

Sleep and Stroke

Kimberly Nicole Mims, MD[a], Douglas Kirsch, MD[b],*

KEYWORDS

- Stroke • Sleep • Obstructive sleep apnea • RLS/PLMS • Parasomnias • Cerebrovascular accident
- Central sleep apnea • Insomnia • Sleep duration

KEY POINTS

- Growing evidence suggests that sleep amount and sleep disorders may impact risk for stroke; conversely, the cerebrovascular events may change sleep drive and affect breathing patterns during sleep.
- Treatment of sleep disorders, whether causative of stroke or caused by stroke, will likely improve sleep-related symptoms and may improve further stroke risk and long-term outcomes.
- Sleep apnea, both obstructive and central, is strongly associated with increased cerebrovascular events.
- Other sleep disorders, including insomnia, RLS/PLMS, and parasomnias may also result in increased incidence of stroke.
- Short and long sleep duration increase cardiovascular events by increasing sympathetic tone and low-grade inflammation.
- Treatment of sleep disorders reduces sleep disruption and can improve functional stroke outcome as well as decrease stroke risk.

Strokes are one of the most common causes of death in the United States.[1] Growing evidence suggests that sleep amount and sleep disorders may impact risk for stroke; conversely, the cerebrovascular events may change sleep drive and affect breathing patterns during sleep. This article describes the most up-to-date information on the linkage between sleep and stroke and attempts to demonstrate how some physicians may use changes in sleep to limit the risk of stroke in some patients.

SLEEP APNEA AND STROKE

Sleep apnea is defined by decreased airflow occurring during sleep. Two main types of sleep apnea exist: obstructive and central. Obstructive sleep apnea (OSA) is the most common type of sleep apnea and consists of complete or partial occlusion of the airway, usually accompanied by an associated oxygen desaturation or arousal.

Central sleep apnea (CSA) occurs when respiratory effort is decreased or absent and is commonly associated with conditions such as heart failure. The most widely accepted epidemiologic data project that 4% of men and 2% of women suffer from OSA,[2] although more recent data suggest that the incidence of sleep apnea in highly developed countries could be as high as 20% in men and 10% in women.[3]

In patients with a history of stroke or transient ischemic attack, sleep apnea incidence is significantly higher than the general population, with estimates suggesting 72% for apnea-hypopnea index (AHI) >5/h and 38% for AHI >20/h.[4] In a small study evaluating sleep-disordered breathing (SDB) incidence in an inpatient stroke rehabilitation unit, 91% demonstrated AHI >10/h with a mean AHI of 32/h.[5] Furthermore, several prospective cohort studies indicate increased risk of cardiovascular events in patients with OSA; OSA serves as an independent risk factor for cardiovascular events.[6–9]

[a] Charlotte Medical Clinic, Carolinas HealthCare System, 1001 Blythe Boulevard, Suite 403, Charlotte, NC 28203, USA; [b] CHS Sleep Medicine, Carolinas HealthCare System, 1601 Abbey Place, Building 2, Suite 200, Charlotte, NC 28209, USA
* Corresponding author.
E-mail address: Douglas.Kirsch@carolinashealthcare.org

Sleep Med Clin 11 (2016) 39–51
http://dx.doi.org/10.1016/j.jsmc.2015.10.009

The American Heart Association recommends screening for OSA for stroke prevention and suggests treatment is reasonable, although its effectiveness for primary prevention of stroke remains unknown.[10]

The 2014 recommendations by the American Heart Association include stratification of antithrombotic therapy based on CHA_2DS_2-VASc score, which does not incorporate the presence of sleep apnea. A retrospective cohort study by Yaranov and colleagues[11] revealed that patients who had atrial fibrillation and OSA developed stroke more commonly than atrial fibrillation patients without OSA (odds ratio 3.84).

Pathology of Obstructive Sleep Apnea and Stroke

Although the specific causal mechanism linking sleep apnea to increased stroke risk has yet to be identified, several direct and indirect relationships contributing to atherosclerosis are known. Atherosclerosis, traditionally viewed as solely a disease of lipid storage, is now thought to be multifactorial, with several processes contributing to plaque development. Factors contributing to atherosclerotic development include hypertension, metabolic syndrome (diabetes, dyslipidemia), and smoking. Inflammatory mediators of atherosclerosis include markers of systemic inflammation (eg, interleukin [IL]-6, C-reactive protein [CRP], intracellular adhesion molecules [ICAMs]), fibrinogen, and lipoprotein (a).

OSA causes repetitive episodes of decreased oxygenation mimicking asphyxia and results in negative intrathoracic pressure. Increased arousals from sleep occur in response to decreased oxygen levels and increased circulating carbon dioxide levels. Arousals during sleep increase sympathetic activation, resulting in brief increases in blood pressure. Patients with OSA demonstrate increased incidence of refractory hypertension, perhaps as a result of the changed nocturnal blood pressure.[12] OSA may also cause insulin resistance resulting in diabetes mellitus type 2,[13] thought to be secondary to an increase in circulating cortisol. Leptin, a hormone released by adipocytes in response to food, is decreased in patients with OSA, lowering their metabolic rate, decreasing the sensation of fullness, and contributing to metabolic syndrome and increased weight gain.[14]

The predominant abnormality of OSA stems from intermittent hypoxia occurring during apnea and hypopnea events. In several mice models, intermittent hypoxia resulted in increased formation of fatty streaks in the aortic arch and acceleration in development of disease in those genetically prone to atherosclerosis.[15,16] Intermittent hypoxia has

been implicated in worsening dyslipidemia, oxidative stress, and endothelial dysfunction and inflammation. In addition, OSA is associated with a significant increase in carotid intima-media thickness and arterial stiffness evidenced as an early indication of atherosclerosis.

Intermittent hypoxia contributes to dyslipidemia by increasing levels of very low-density lipoprotein (VLDL) secretion. This increased secretion is mediated by upregulation of stearoyl coenzyme A desaturase 1, which increases in direct proportion to severity of nocturnal hypoxia.[17] Decreased lipoprotein clearance also contributes to an increase in circulating VLDL. Lipoprotein lipase contributes to clearing circulating lipoproteins, and intermittent hypoxia inhibits its activation. Patients with OSA who used positive pressure therapy as treatment had increased lipoprotein lipase activity.[18] However, several other studies contradict a relationship between OSA and dyslipidemia, and additional studies have been suggested to further investigate the relationship.[19]

Intermittent hypoxia resulting from OSA is highly associated with oxidative stress. Oxygen free radicals lead to lipid peroxidation, which are acquired more easily by macrophages; this causes macrophage foaming and provides a substrate for the progression of the atherosclerotic plaque.[17] Although most studies verify an increase in lipid peroxidation and oxidized low-density lipoprotein in patients with OSA, the lack of benefit seen with antioxidant therapy raises the question of whether oxidative stress is a result of vascular inflammation instead of atherosclerosis[20] (**Fig. 1**).

OSA is also correlated with an increase in inflammatory mediators and cytokines thought to contribute to endothelial dysfunction. A direct proportional relationship is observed with elevation of inflammatory markers in patients with increased AHI, resulting in increased serum levels of markers, including CRP and IL-6. Several studies indicated an increase in CRP was independently associated with OSA and nocturnal hypoxemia, although contradictory studies found increased CRP to be more independently associated with body mass index (BMI) than OSA severity. IL-6, responsible for CRP production by the liver, also increases in patients diagnosed with OSA compared with those without, although contradictory studies exist linking this mediator to BMI as well.[21] Intracellular adhesion molecules, which facilitate leukocyte adhesion to vascular endothelium, increase in OSA patients compared with controls, and they increase in direct proportion to nocturnal hypoxemia.[22] OSA and nocturnal hypoxemia severity also increase tumor necrosis factor-α with additional influence by age and BMI.[23] Although data are limited on IL-8,

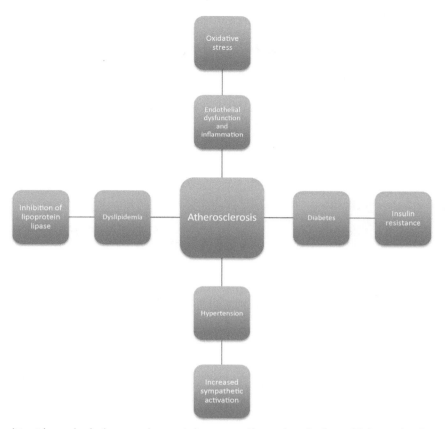

Fig. 1. Intermittent hypoxia during apneic events increases atherosclerosis via multiple mechanisms.

selectins, and vascular cell adhesion molecules, data suggest these markers are significantly elevated in patients with OSA, again associated with influence by age and BMI[21] (**Fig. 2**). In harvested endothelial cells in patients with OSA, the nuclear factor, NF-κB, increased, and nitric oxide synthase expression and activity decreased. These changes reversed after treatment of OSA with continuous positive airway pressure (CPAP) therapy.[24]

Stroke Subtypes

Several investigators questioned whether OSA predisposes to certain ischemic stroke types,

that is, large-vessel versus Small-vessel strokes. However, no studies have yet demonstrated a significant difference in type of ischemic stroke seen in patients diagnosed with sleep-disordered breathing (SDB) compared with those without. Although no significant relationship was seen between SDB and size of vessel occluded, a significant increase in cardioembolic strokes was observed in patients with SDB compared with those without.[25] Notably, most studies assessing this question rely on a diagnosis of SDB after stroke occurred.

Respiratory changes are commonly seen acutely after stroke and can be correlated to stroke location. Respiratory apraxia results from strokes in

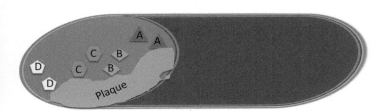

Fig. 2. OSA increases the risk of atherosclerosis and plaque formation by increasing inflammatory mediators, including (A) CRP, (B) IL-6, (C) ICAMs, and (D) tumor necrosis factor-α.

the frontal lobe, basal ganglia, or internal capsule. Neurogenic hyperventilation occurs after pontine strokes; apneustic respirations can result after strokes in the inferior medial posterior area of the pons; central alveolar hypoventilation syndrome (Ondine curse) can occur after medullary stroke, and medullary strokes at the level of C1 can impair voluntary respiration if stroke localizes posteriorly or automatic respiration if localized anteriorly. These respiratory patterns often lack significant prognostic implications, although low carbon dioxide can be associated with poorer prognosis. The mean prevalence of respiratory changes presenting in the acute poststroke period is 59%, with OSA being the most common respiratory disorder.[26]

Central sleep apnea

CSA is defined by a cessation or decrease of ventilatory effort during sleep and is usually associated with an oxygen desaturation. CSA is seen in up to 26% of patients following a stroke, but the CSA often improves as acuity of stroke decreases.[27] CSA is often a result of anterior circulation lesions.[28] In addition, the incidence of CSA increases in patients with larger strokes and strokes associated with significant mass effect.[29] The presence of CSA after stroke portends poorer prognosis despite higher minimum SaO_2 levels observed in patients with central respiratory events compared with those without central respiratory events.[28] Treatment of CSA after stroke includes CPAP therapy and adaptive servoventilation (ASV), although use of ASV is currently controversial in patients with predominant CSA, and moderate to severe congestive heart failure has recently been based on the mortality data from the SERV-HF study.[30]

Functional outcome after stroke

Several studies prove SDB increases incidence and recurrence of stroke as well as lowers mortality.[31] However, a dearth of studies exists detailing functional outcome after stroke in patients with sleep apnea. Recently, Aaronson and colleagues[32] investigated functional outcome of patients admitted to a neurorehabilitation unit. Within 4 weeks of admission, patients received several neuropsychiatric tests assessing vigilance, attention, memory, working memory, executive functioning, language, visuoperception, psychomotor ability, and intelligence. Within the first few weeks, an ambulatory overnight cardiorespiratory polygraphy was performed to generate an oxygen desaturation index (ODI, a surrogate index for sleep apnea severity). The investigators discovered patients with an elevated ODI demonstrate statistically worse impairment in attention, executive functioning, visuoperception, psychomotor ability,

and intelligence. These patients also had a significantly increased length of stay in the rehabilitation unit and were less functionally independent on discharge from the unit. There was no significant difference in levels of sleepiness, fatigue, depression, or anxiety between the patients with an elevated ODI and non-SDB patients.

Further sleep apnea and stroke studies

One of the most compelling and as of yet unanswered questions in terms of sleep apnea and stroke is whether treatment of sleep apnea improves neurologic outcome. Although there are several prospective cohort studies available demonstrating improved functional outcome with CPAP treatment of sleep apnea, the control population typically consists of nonadherent patients, thus introducing selection bias. No studies have been performed with sham CPAP treatments in this setting, arguably because of ethical consideration of nontreatment in diagnosed sleep apnea patients. A few studies are underway, most notably TOROS, to provide a reliable answer to whether treating sleep apnea significantly improves functional outcome after stroke.

Further studies are also necessary to assess the causal relationship between several correlative factors seen in stroke and sleep, including dyslipidemia, hypertension, and atrial fibrillation.

INSOMNIA AND STROKE

Insomnia is defined as persistent difficulty with sleep initiation, duration, consolidation, or quality that occurs despite adequate opportunity and circumstances for sleep and results in some form of daytime impairment.[33] It is the most common sleep disorder, affecting up to 22% of adults.[34] Insomnia varies in chronicity, but even in those with remission, 27% experiencing insomnia relapse within 3 years.[35]

Insomnia is associated with all-cause mortality and cardiovascular death, including stroke.[36] Insomnia incidence in patients who have had a stroke approaches 57%, with 38% reporting insomnia as a preceding symptom to the stroke.[37] In patients who have had a stroke, insomnia incidence is higher in women than in men.[38] Living alone and an older age also increase the risk of insomnia associated with stroke.[39]

Short sleep duration is also associated with increased atherosclerosis risk.[40] Postmenopausal women reporting short sleep demonstrated a distinct increased risk for stroke without an increase in clinically apparent cardiovascular disease.[41] A Japanese study demonstrated patients with short sleep time and higher nocturnal systolic blood pressures had a significant increase in cardiovascular events.[42] In a similar study on hypertensive patients, the presence of both diabetes and short sleep duration also correlated with increased cardiovascular disease than either independently[43] (**Figs. 3** and **4**).

Several studies indicate insomnia plays an important role in the development of cardiovascular disease, including stroke, and insomnia can affect poststroke outcome and quality of life, if left untreated. Insomnia increases the incidence rate of stroke as identified by a retrospective cohort study performed by Wu and colleagues.[44] Across all ages and both genders, patients with insomnia exhibited a higher incidence rate ratio of stroke compared with those without insomnia. The largest incidence rate ratio was identified in 18 to 34 year olds; the ratios then decreased with advancing age, although incidence of ischemic stroke increased with advancing age.[45] Overall, individuals with insomnia demonstrated a 54% increased likelihood of developing stroke compared with patients without insomnia. Wu and colleagues[44] also studied insomnia chronicity and discovered individuals with persistent insomnia had the highest risk of stroke, followed by individuals with relapsing insomnia. Subjects with insomnia in remission had the lowest increased rate of stroke compared with other subjects with insomnia but still demonstrated a hazards ratio exceeding that of those without insomnia.

Insomnia occurrence after stroke is also increased. Patients with right hemispheric strokes reported more insomnia symptoms than those with left hemispheric strokes in one study.[46] One brain area with insomnia as a prominent symptom includes the thalamus and brainstem, specifically the thalamomesencephalic region, pontomesencephalic region, and/or the pontine tegmentum, which can result in inversion of the sleep-wake cycle and nighttime agitation.[47] Insomnia commonly develops acutely after stroke, although usually with multifactorial cause, including complications of hospitalization, stroke, and/or medications.[26]

Poststroke insomnia also can also affect stroke recovery and quality of life. Insomnia increases the risk of subsequent stroke[48] and worsens psychological health with an associated increase in frequency of suicide.[49] Poststroke insomnia increases physical disability, dementia symptoms, and anxiety.[37] One study demonstrated patients with fewer days of insomnia positively correlated with improvement in overall health, energy, family roles, mobility, mood, personality, social roles, thinking, and work/productivity as reported by patients on a quality-of-life questionnaire.[38] The same study also demonstrated the converse: namely, that an increase in sleepless nights resulted in decreasing energy levels, concentration, and memory, similar to that reported in the general population.[50]

Pathology

Proposed mechanisms linking insomnia to stroke focus on the disruption of sleep seen in patients with insomnia. Increased arousals are implicated in increasing sympathetic activity at night compared with the typical lull in sympathetic activity seen during sleep, which results in nocturnal hypertension. In combination with increased activation of the hypothalamic-pituitary-adrenal axis, cortisol levels elevate, increasing the risk for vascular disease.[51]

In short sleep, nonrestorative sleep correlates with elevated levels of inflammatory cytokines, generating a low-grade inflammation state.[52] Gangwisch and colleagues[53] also demonstrated an association between elevation in sympathetic tone and short sleep.

Poststroke insomnia may localize to specific lesions based on certain symptoms. Supratentorial strokes decrease non-rapid eye movement (NREM) sleep, decrease total sleep time, and reduce sleep efficiency.[54] There is limited

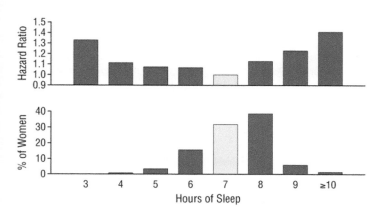

Fig. 3. U-shaped mortality curve for 636,095 women based on self-reported sleep duration. Hazard ratios represent all-cause mortality adjusted for covariates. (*From* Kripke DF, Garfinkel L, Wingard DL, et al. Mortality associated with sleep duration and insomnia. Arch Gen Psychiatry 2002; 59(2):131–6; with permission.)

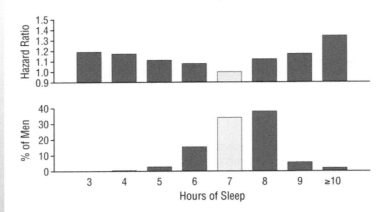

Fig. 4. U-shaped mortality curve for 480,841 men based on self-reported sleep duration. Hazard ratios represent all-cause mortality adjusted for covariates. (*From* Kripke DF, Garfinkel L, Wingard DL, et al. Mortality associated with sleep duration and insomnia. Arch Gen Psychiatry 2002;59(2):131–6; with permission.)

evidence that right hemispheric strokes reduce rapid eye movement (REM) and REM density, whereas left hemispheric strokes decrease NREM stages.[55] Strokes localized to the pontomesencephalic junction and the raphe nucleus may preferentially reduce NREM sleep without affecting REM sleep.[56] Paramedian thalamas strokes and strokes in the lower pons are associated with loss of slow wave sleep but preservation of REM sleep.[26] Conversely, several studies suggest strokes in the lower pons may also reduce REM sleep.[57,58] Finally, some studies suggest infratentorial strokes eliminate sleep spindles, K complexes, and/or vertex waves, thus changing the electroencephalography patterns of NREM sleep.[58] Finally, changes in sleep architecture associated with decreased functional recovery in stroke include decreased sleep efficiency, increased awakenings, decreased stage 2 sleep, decreased sleep spindles and K complexes, and increased stage 3 sleep.[59]

Diagnosis and Treatment of Insomnia

Diagnosis of insomnia is primarily clinical and often includes a detailed history, a 2-week sleep diary, identification of potential confounding medical and psychiatric illnesses, and occasionally, quality-of-life and daytime functioning questionnaires. Polysomnography is only indicated for patients with insomnia in instances of insomnia refractory to pharmacologic or cognitive treatment or if another sleep disorder is suspected. Actigraphy may be used to delineate sleep patterns, especially if the patient's sleep perception is difficult to discern.[60]

The simplest and perhaps most important treatment of insomnia after stroke involves encouraging appropriate sleep hygiene, including limiting exposure to nighttime stimulation and increasing exposure to daylight. Other important practices of appropriate sleep hygiene include

limiting exposure to "smart" devices (smartphone, tablet) and backlit screens in the bedroom, avoiding work or thinking about work in the bedroom, and maintaining a dark, quiet environment in the bedroom.

Psychological and behavioral modifications are indicated as first-line therapy for insomnia in all adults, either independently or coupled with other therapies including medications.[60] Cognitive behavioral therapy, including stimulus control therapy, sleep restriction therapy, and/or relaxation therapy, are recommended as standard of care for insomnia treatment.

Pharmacotherapy may supplement cognitive behavioral therapy but is recommended to be restricted to short-term use. The consensus statement of use of pharmacotherapy recommends choosing pharmacologic agents based on symptom pattern, treatment goals, past treatment responses, patient preference, cost, availability of other treatments, comorbid conditions, contraindications, concurrent medication interactions, and side effects.[60] In stroke patients, sedative hypnotics should generally be avoided if possible because of the risk of increased memory impairment, disorientation, and falls.

Other treatments specifically evaluated in stroke patients include acupuncture and problem-solving therapy. A double-blinded randomized control trial demonstrated utility of intradermal acupuncture in reducing insomnia in poststroke patients.[61] Problem-solving therapy with or without cognitive behavioral therapy also demonstrated efficacy in improving insomnia symptoms in stroke patients.[62] However, cognitive behavioral therapy remains the recognized standard of treatment for insomnia.

HYPERSOMNIA AND STROKE

Hypersomnia is defined as an "inability to stay awake and alert during the major waking episodes of the day, resulting in periods of irrepressible need for sleep or unintended lapses into drowsiness or sleep."[33] The prevalence of hypersomnia in the adult population is estimated at 20%.[63] In the stroke population, hypersomnia affects up to 27% of patients.[64] Studies investigating the association between short sleep duration and stroke abound, but studies addressing the relationship between long sleep duration and stroke are less prevalent. However, recent investigations reveal a U-shaped curve demonstrating increased mortality in both short and long sleepers, and a recent American Academy of Sleep Medicine consensus statement recommends at least 7 hours of sleep per night for adults, with a qualifier identifying unclear risk of increased mortality with sleep exceeding 9 hours.[65]

Several studies indicate that sleep exceeding 9 hours increases cardiovascular risk. The NOMAS study revealed an increased risk of cardiovascular outcomes but not myocardial infarction or nonvascular causes of death in patients with increased daytime sleepiness as measured by a modified Epworth sleepiness scale. This increased risk in cardiovascular events persisted after adjustment for covariates such as obesity, hypertension, and diabetes. The study further demonstrated a greater risk of mortality in excessively sleepy women compared with men but no significant difference when evaluating race or ethnicity.[66] Long sleepers demonstrated that increased mortality correlated strongly with socioeconomic status.[67] However, a study using data from the Nurses' Health Study failed to identify an independent relationship between daytime sleepiness and long sleep time and increased cardiovascular morbidity and mortality when controlling for confounding factors.[68]

The abnormality underlying the association between hypersomnia and stroke is not well understood, although several theories exist. The most prominent hypothesis focuses on demonstrable increased incidence in obesity and diabetes seen in patients with hypersomnia. A study investigating sleep in older women demonstrated decreased physical activity in patients with increased sleepiness and fatigue.[69] Long sleep is associated with increased development of diabetes also, although the underlying abnormality is unclear.[68] Metabolic syndrome, often seen in patients with obesity and diabetes, results in increased proinflammatory cytokines.[70] Proinflammatory cytokines induce sleep as an evolutionary response to promote rest and recovery from illness.[71] Another confounder often associated with hypersomnia is depression, which increases mortality and risk of heart disease.[72] A study investigating the relationship between hypersomnia and mortality discovered that depression attenuated the relationship between hypersomnia and increased mortality.[73]

Hypersomnia may present as a result of stroke as well. Lesions affecting the reticular activating system (RAS) often result in hypersomnia. These lesions include bilateral thalamic lesions, thalamo-mesencephalic lesions, upper and medial pontomedullary regions where RAS fibers are highly concentrated.[26] Lesions in the cerebral hemispheres tend to be less associated with hypersomnia because the RAS fibers are more diffuse, but large cerebral lesions, lesions affecting the left more than the right hemisphere, and lesions affecting the anterior more than the posterior regions result in increased hypersomnia.[74] Paramedian thalamic infarcts result in the most severe hypersomnia cases and typically present with sudden-onset stupor with preservation of responses to stimuli.[75]

Hypersomnia treatment is important especially during rehabilitation. A recent study demonstrated patients exhibiting hypersomnia symptoms in an acute rehabilitation unit were 10 times more likely to be discharged to a nursing facility and had significantly worse functional outcomes.[76] Treatment of hypersomnia in stroke patients differs little from standard treatment of hypersomnia. Mainstays of treatment involve use of amphetamines, modafinil, methylphenidate, and in some cases, levodopa therapy. One study demonstrated that levodopa and methylphenidate treatment improved arousal levels and poststroke outcome when administered in an acute rehabilitation center over a 3-week period.[77,78] Care should be taken when using amphetamines and their derivatives in patients with strokes given the potential for elevation of blood pressure and heart rate (**Table 1**).

OTHER SLEEP DISORDERS AND STROKE (RESTLESS LEG SYNDROME, PERIODIC LIMB MOVEMENTS IN SLEEP, PARASOMNIAS)

Among the sleep disorders, there are 2 types of leg movements that are regularly diagnosed. Restless leg syndrome (RLS) presents as a desire to move the legs that worsens at night and at rest, is partially relieved with movement, and worsens without movement.[33] Periodic limb movements in sleep (PLMS) are defined as leg movements seen during polysomnography that last 0.5 to 10 seconds and occur every 5 to 90 seconds, and at least 4 movements occur consecutively with at least an 8 uV increase in amplitude from baseline as seen in the limb movement leads.[79] Recent studies suggest a relationship between sleep-related leg movements and cardiovascular disease, including

Table 1
Stroke lesions and sleep disorders

	Stroke Lesions Associated with Sleep Disorder
Sleep apnea	Frontal lobe (respiratory apraxia), pontine stroke (neurogenic hypoventilation), inferomedial posterior pons (apneustic respirations), medullary stroke (Ondine curse)
Insomnia	Supratentorial stroke (decreased NREM, TST, SE), right hemisphere decreased REM, left hemisphere decreased NREM, paramedian thalamus strokes decreased NREM, infratentorial strokes eliminate sleep spindles, K complexes, and/or vertex waves
Hypersomnia	Reticular activating system, bilateral thalamic lesions, lesions affecting left more than right and anterior more than posterior, paramedian thalamic infarcts (present with sudden onset stupor)
RBD	Brainstem infarcts

Abbreviations: SE, sleep efficiency; TST, total sleep time.

stroke, although the association of the leg movements with possible vascular phenomena started with Ekbom in the 1940s.[80]

Several cohort studies, including the Wisconsin Sleep Cohort Study, demonstrated significantly increased incidence of hypertension and heart disease in those patients also reporting symptoms of RLS. The Sleep Heart Health Study also reported an increase in cardiovascular disease and coronary artery disease in patients with RLS, but only in RLS sufferers experiencing symptoms at least 16 times per month and with severe symptoms.[81] In a cohort study on older men, a PLMS arousal index exceeding 5 events per hour resulted in an increased risk for cardiovascular disease even after controlling for several comorbid conditions, including age and BMI.[82] According to a study performed by Siddiqui and colleagues,[83] elevated blood pressure following PLMS occurred in increasing and predictable ways based on type of PLMS. However, a few studies failed to find a correlation between hypertension and RLS, and the MEMO study demonstrated an inverse relationship between blood pressure and RLS.[84–86]

One theory suggests the relationship between sleep-related leg movements and cardiovascular disease including stroke relates to increased sympathetic activation seen with arousals associated with PLMS. Increased sympathetic activation is suggested by changes in pulse rate associated with PLMS. Interestingly, the pulse rate increase precedes the PLMS movement. A study by Winkelman[87] identified an increase in heart rate occurring 3 cardiac cycles before PLMS onset with peak at 4 cardiac cycles after PLMS onset. A study by Sforza and colleagues[88] found accelerations in heart rate were highest when PLMS induced a noticeable electroencephalogram (EEG) microarousal.

Published case studies describe increased PLMS and RLS incidence after stroke.[89,90] Lee and colleagues[91] identified an incidence of 12% of stroke patients presenting with RLS. Most patients develop bilateral symptoms of RLS, but a third complain of RLS affecting the contralateral side to the stroke. Conversely, a relationship has been identified suggesting PLMS can increase the risk for stroke. A study done in 26 subjects with RLS control-matched to 241 patients without RLS demonstrated a greater volume of subcortical lesions and cortical atrophy seen in the RLS group.[92] The above studies provide anecdotal evidence that RLS/PLMS may increase the risk of stroke, especially in the basal ganglia, internal capsule, or corona radiata.

Pathophysiology

The pathophysiology resulting in correlation between sleep-related leg movements and cardiovascular consequences such as stroke has yet to be identified definitively, but several theories exist. The most prominent theory linking leg movements to cardiovascular risks revolves around hypofunction of the A11 diencephalospinal pathway, which leads to increased sympathetic output to the periphery via somatic muscle fibers.[93] Typically, increased sympathetic activity results in heightened spinal sensory signaling via afferents from the muscle fibers back to the spinal cord, but this activity is dampened by A11 innervation at the dorsal horn. Theoretically, in RLS, the dopaminergic hypofunctioning of the A11 innervation results in a positive feedback loop, causing increased signaling of afferents back to the spinal cord, which also causes heightened sympathetic activation leading to increased RLS symptoms. This theory is supported by lesion creation in this pathway in rats that results in a restlessness that responds to pramipexole.[94] The A11 diencephalospinal pathway also links sympathetic activation to hypertension and increased risk of cardiovascular consequences like heart disease and stroke.

Comorbid conditions are also posited as a potential pathophysiology linking sleep-related leg movements to increased cardiovascular morbidity and mortality. Winkelman and colleagues[81] suggests that conditions such as anemia and renal failure may contribute to the association between cardiovascular risk and sleep-related leg movement. Many studies identified an association between sleep-related leg movements and OSA, a disorder that more clearly demonstrates increased cardiovascular risks, as described in an earlier section. Conversely, cardiovascular disease may increase the risk of sleep-related leg movements as seen in case studies.

Ferritin level and an iron panel should be a standard part of an RLS evaluation, and iron supplementation in patients with low ferritin with or without low total iron-binding capacity saturation can result in resolution of RLS symptoms. The standard pharmacologic treatment for sleep-related leg movements continues to be dopamine agonists, with the highest level of recommendation encouraging the use of pramipexole 0.5 to 1.5 mg and ropinirole 1 to 4 mg. Levodopa can be used for patients with intermittent and predictable instigating factors exacerbating RLS symptoms. However, levodopa is not recommended for use in patients needing chronic therapy due to the increased risk of augmentation. Gabapentin is increasingly used for RLS and PLMS with success, especially in those with painful RLS or RLS related to diabetic neuropathy. Opioids can also be used for painful RLS. Newer therapy like rotigotine delivered over a 24-hour period via a transdermal patch has been shown to be more effective than pramipexole and ropinirole but also increases the risk of side effects and had a higher discontinuation rate.[95] Gabapentin enacarbil, essentially a prodrug of gabapentin, is approved for use for RLS. Other off-label treatments for RLS and PLMS include pregabalin, carbamazepine, and clonidine, although the level of evidence is low.[96]

Parasomnias

Parasomnias are undesirable physical events or experiences that occur during entry into sleep, within sleep, or during arousal from sleep.[33] Parasomnias include dream enactment behaviors, sleepwalking, night terrors, and confusional arousals, among others. Most parasomnias present in children and adolescents and resolve by adulthood, but estimated incidence of parasomnias remains approximately 4% in the adult population.[97] Parasomnias may occur secondary to precipitating factors like medications (hypnotics like zolpidem), stress, underlying sleep disorders, or sleep deprivation. Sleepwalking exhibits a strong predilection in first-degree family members with a 10-fold increase in incidence compared with the general population.[98] Parasomnias may also be correlated with stroke.

Parasomnia pathophysiology consists of interruption in sleep stages. Sleep stage shifting occurs as a reorganization and transition of various neuronal centers until one exerts prominence and declares itself, and an arousal during this reorganization is hypothesized to increase complex motor and sensory behavior during sleep.[99]

In REM sleep behavior disorder (RBD) specifically, brainstem lesions are strongly correlated with the development of dream enactment behaviors. In the study by Schenk and Mahowald[100] described in later discussion, one patient developed RBD in response to an acute brainstem stroke and subsequently fractured her hip in the intensive care unit (ICU) during hospitalization. Bilateral pontine tegmental lesions create RBD in animal models. In a study performed in Hong Kong, 22% of patients with a brainstem stroke exhibited associated RBD and demonstrated lower brain volume involved in stroke compared with patients with stroke without RBD. Damage to pontine glutaminergic and medullary GABAergic neurons was implicated as the main abnormality resulting in RBD in this study.[101]

In one of the earliest published studies investigating the relationship of parasomnia behavior in ICU patients, parasomnias resulted from an acute neurologic disorder in 28.5% (4/14) patients. Only 3 of 20 patients identified in the study exhibited symptoms suggestive of NREM parasomnias; the remaining parasomnias consisted of RBD.[100] Of the 4 parasomnia patients in this study who previously had a stroke, all were diagnosed with RBD.

Although RBD is the most commonly associated parasomnia associated with stroke, other parasomnias have been described in association with strokes. Case studies described visual hallucinations especially at sleep onset associated with infarcts in the pontine tegmentum, midbrain, or paramedial thalamus.[47] Increased dreaming or nightmares and a syndrome resembling confusional arousal has been described following strokes in the thalamus, temporal, parietal, and occipital lobes.[102]

No clear evidence exists linking pre-existing parasomnias to the development of stroke; however, as mentioned previously in several sections, sleep disruption itself can result in increased sympathetic output during sleep, thereby increasing cardiovascular stress.

For definitive diagnosis of parasomnias, polysomnography may be required to distinguish between REM and NREM parasomnias and to evaluate for nocturnal seizures (which may require a full EEG montage).

Treatment of RBD typically consists of optimizing the bedroom environment to reduce risk of injury and treating underlying sleep disorders, such as OSA. Medication therapy for RBD includes clonazepam at 0.5 mg to 2 mg an hour before bedtime. If clonazepam is not well-tolerated or contraindicated, such as in patients with dementia or gait disorders, melatonin is indicated. Melatonin is a safe alternative to benzodiazepines that may also be effective for RBD treatment.[103]

Pramipexole may also be used in this population and has demonstrated effectiveness in some studies, although contradictory studies exist as well. Case studies demonstrated effective treatment with the following medications, although evidence is limited: zopiclone, benzodiazepines other than clonazepam, Yi-gan san, desipramine, clozapine, carbamazepine, and sodium oxybate.[104] Treatment of parasomnias other than RBD is similar, with clonazepam as the suggested initial treatment.

SUMMARY

Over the past decade, the importance of sleep disorders has grown within the medical community, increasingly recognized as being related to many medical conditions. This review has elucidated the bidirectional relationship of stroke with certain sleep disorders, with further research necessary to better understand these correlations. Treatment of sleep disorders, whether causative of stroke or caused by stroke, will likely improve sleep-related symptoms and may improve further stroke risk and long-term outcomes.

REFERENCES

1. Available at: http://www.cdc.gov/stroke/. Accessed July 14, 2015.
2. Young T, Palta M, Dempsey J, et al. The occurrence of sleep-disordered breathing among middle-aged adults. N Engl J Med 1993;32:1230–5.
3. Young T, Peppard PE, Gottlieb DJ, et al. The epidemiology of obstructive sleep apnea: a population health perspective. Am J Respir Crit Care Med 2002;165:1217–39.
4. Johnson KG, Johnson DC. Frequency of sleep apnea in stroke and TIA patients: a meta-analysis. J Clin Sleep Med 2010;6:131–7.
5. Brooks D, Davis L, Vujovic-Zotovic N, et al. Sleep disordered breathing in patients enrolled in an inpatient stroke rehabilitation program. Arch Phys Med Rehabil 2010;91(4):659–62.
6. Marin JM, Carrizo SJ, Vicente E, et al. Long-term cardiovascular outcomes in men with obstructive sleep apnea-hypopnea with or without treatment with continuous positive airway pressure: an observational study. Lancet 2005;365(9464):1046–53.
7. Young T, Finn L, Peppard PE, et al. Sleep disordered breathing and mortality: eighteen-year follow-up of the Wisconsin sleep cohort. Sleep 2008;31(8):1071–8.
8. Marshall NS, Wong KK, Cullen SR, et al. Sleep apnea and 20-year follow-up for all-cause mortality, stroke, and cancer incidence and mortality in the Busselton Health Study cohort. J Clin Sleep Med 2014;10(4):355–62.
9. Redline S, Yenokyan G, Gottlieb DJ, et al. Obstructive apnea-hypopnea and incident stroke: the Sleep Heart Health Study. Am J Respir Crit Care Med 2010;182(2):269–77.
10. Meschia JF, Bushnell C, Boden-Albala B, et al. Guidelines for the primary prevention of stroke: a statement for healthcare professionals from the American Heart Association/American Stroke Association. Stroke 2014;45:3754–832.
11. Yaranov DM, Smyrlis A, Usatii N, et al. Effect of obstructive sleep apnea on frequency of stroke in patients with atrial fibrillation. Am J Cardiol 2015;115:461–5.
12. Williams SK, Ravenell J, Jean-Louis G, et al. Resistant hypertension and sleep apnea: pathophysiologic insights and strategic management. Curr Diab Rep 2011;11:64–9.
13. Rasche K, Keller T, Tautz B, et al. Obstructive sleep apnea and type 2 diabetes. Eur J Med Res 2010;15(Suppl 2):152–6.
14. Tokuda F, Sando Y, Matsui H, et al. Serum levels of adipocytokines, adiponectin, and leptic, in patients with obstructive sleep apnea syndrome. Intern Med 2008;47:1843–9.
15. Jun J, Reinke C, Bedja D, et al. Effect of intermittent hypoxia on atherosclerosis in apolipoprotein E-deficient mice. Atherosclerosis 2010;209(2):381–6.
16. Savransky V, Nanayakkara A, Li J, et al. Chronic intermittent hypoxia induces atherosclerosis. Am J Respir Crit Care Med 2007;175(12):1290–7.
17. Savransky V, Jun J, Li J, et al. Dyslipidemia and atherosclerosis induced by chronic intermittent hypoxia are attenuated by deficiency of stearoyl coenzyme a desaturase. Circ Res 2008;103(10):1173–80.
18. Iesato K, Tatsumi K, Saibara T, et al. Decreased lipoprotein lipase in obstructive sleep apnea syndrome. Circ J 2007;71(8):1293–8.

19. Drager LF, Polotsky VY, Lorenzi-Filho G, et al. Obstructive sleep apnea: an emerging risk factor for atherosclerosis. Chest 2011;140(2):534–42.

20. Stocker R, Keaney JF Jr. Role of oxidative modifications in atherosclerosis. Physiol Rev 2004;84(4):1381–478.

21. Nadeem R, Molnar J, Madbouly EM, et al. Serum inflammatory markers in obstructive sleep apnea: a meta-analysis. J Clin Sleep Med 2013;9(10):1003–12.

22. Zamarron-Sanz C, Ricoy-Galbaldon J, Gude-Sampedro F, et al. Plasma levels of vascular endothelial markers in obstructive sleep apnea. Arch Med Res 2006;37:552–5.

23. Vgontzas AN, Papanicolaou DA, Bixler EO, et al. Elevation of plasma cytokines in disorders of excessive daytime sleepiness: role of sleep disturbance and obesity. J Clin Endocrinol Metab 1997;32:1313–6.

24. Jelic S, Lederer DJ, Adams T, et al. Vascular inflammation in obesity and sleep apnea. Circulation 2010;121(8):1014–21.

25. Brown DL, Mowla A, McDermott M, et al. Ischemic stroke subtype and presence of sleep-disordered breathing: the BASIC sleep apnea study. J Stroke Cerebrovasc Dis 2015;24(2):388–93.

26. Ferre A, Ribó M, Rodríguez-Luna D, et al. Strokes and their relationship with sleep and sleep disorders. Neurologia 2013;28(2):103–18.

27. Parra O, Arboix A, Bechich S, et al. Time course of sleep-related breathing disorders in first ever stroke or transient ischemic attack. Am J Respir Crit Care Med 2000;161:375–80.

28. Rowat AM, Dennis MS, Wardlaw JM, et al. Central periodic breathing observed during the acute assessment is associated with an adverse prognosis in conscious acute stroke patients. Cerebrovasc Dis 2006;21(5–6):340–7.

29. Rowat AM, Wardlaw JM, Dennis MS, et al. Abnormal breathing patterns in stroke: relationship with location of acute stroke lesion and prior cerebrovascular disease. J Neurol Neurosurg Psychiatry 2007;78(3):277–9.

30. Resmed. Available at: http://www.resmed.com/content/dam/resmed/global/documents/serve-hf/Patient_SERVE-HF_FAQs.pdf. Accessed July 17, 2015.

31. Elwood P, Hack M, Pickering J, et al. Sleep disturbance, stroke, and heart disease events: evidence from the Caerphilly cohort. J Epidemiol Community Health 2006;60:69–73.

32. Aaronson JA, van Bennekom CA, Hofman WF, et al. Obstructive sleep apnea is related to impaired cognitive and functional status after stroke. Sleep 2015;38(9):1431–7.

33. American Academy of Sleep Medicine. The International Classification of Sleep Disorders: diagnostic and coding manual. 2nd edition. Westchester (IL): American Academy of Sleep Medicine; 2005.

34. Phillips B, Mannino D. Correlates of sleep complaints in adults: the ARIC study. J Clin Sleep Med 2005;1:277–83.

35. Morin CM, Bélanger L, LeBlanc M, et al. The natural history of insomnia: a population-based 3-year longitudinal study. Arch Intern Med 2009;169(5):447–53.

36. Chien KL, Chen PC, Hsu HC, et al. Habitual sleep duration and insomnia and the risk of cardiovascular events and all-cause death: report from a community based cohort. Sleep 2010;33:177–84.

37. Leppavuori A, Pohjasvaara T, Vataja R, et al. Insomnia in ischemic stroke patients. Cerebrovasc Dis 2002;14:90–7.

38. Tang WK, Grace Lau C, Mok V, et al. Insomnia and health-related quality of life in stroke. Top Stroke Rehabil 2015;22(3):201–7.

39. Palomaki H, Berg A, Meririnne E, et al. Complaints of poststroke insomnia and its treatment with mianserin. Cerebrovasc Dis 2003;15:56–62.

40. Bassetti C, Aldrich MS. Sleep apnea in acute cerebrovascular diseases: final report on 128 patients. Sleep 1999;22:217–23.

41. Chen JC, Brunner RL, Ren H, et al. Sleep duration and risk of ischemic stroke in postmenopausal women. Stroke 2008;39:3185–92.

42. Eguchi K, Pickering TG, Schwartz JE, et al. Short sleep duration as an independent predictor of cardiovascular events in Japanese patients with hypertension. Arch Intern Med 2008;168(20):2225–31.

43. Eguchi K, Hoshide S, Ishikawa S, et al. Short sleep duration and type 2 diabetes enhance the risk of cardiovascular events in hypertensive patients. Diabetes Res Clin Pract 2012;98(3):518–23.

44. Wu MP, Lin HJ, Weng SF, et al. Insomnia subtypes and the subsequent risks of stroke: report from a nationally representative cohort. Stroke 2014;45:1349–54.

45. Huang WS, Tsai CH, Lin CL, et al. Nonapnea sleep disorders are associated with subsequent ischemic stroke risk: a nationwide, population-based, retrospective cohort study. Sleep Med 2013;14:1341–7.

46. Da Rocha PC, Barroso MT, Dantas AA, et al. Predictive factors of subjective sleep quality and insomnia complaint in patients with stroke: implications for clinical practice. An Acad Bras Cienc 2013;85(3):1197–206.

47. Basetti CL. Sleep and stroke. Semin Neurol 2005;25:19–32.

48. Hermann DM, Bassetti CL. Sleep-disordered breathing and stroke. Curr Opin Neurol 2003;16:87–90.

49. Paffenbarger RS Jr, Lee IM, Leung R. Physical activity and personal characteristics associated with depression and suicide in American college men. Acta Psychiatr Scand Suppl 1994;377:16–22.

50. Roth T, Ancoli-Israel S. Daytime consequences and correlates of insomnia in the United States: results of the 1991 national sleep foundation survey II. Sleep 1999;22:S354–8.

51. Vgontzas AN, Liao D, Bixler EO, et al. Insomnia with objective short sleep duration is associated with a high risk for hypertension. Sleep 2009;32:491–7.

52. Friedman EM. Sleep quality, social well-being, gender, and inflammation: an integrative analysis in a national sample. Ann N Y Acad Sci 2011; 1231:23–34.

53. Gangwisch JE, Heymsfield SB, Boden-Albala B, et al. Short sleep duration as a risk factor for diabetes incidence in a large US sample. Sleep 2007;30:1667–73.

54. Gasanov RL, Gitlevich TR, Lesnyak VN, et al. Structure of nocturnal sleep in patients with cerebral insult. Neurosci Behav Physiol 1998;28:325–9.

55. Korner E, Flooh E, Reinhart B, et al. Sleep alterations in ischemic stroke. Eur Neurol 1986; 25(Suppl 2):104–10.

56. Freemon FR, Salinas-Garcia RF, Ward JW, et al. Sleep patterns in a patient with a brain stem infarction involving the raphe nucleus. Electroencephalogr Clin Neurophysiol 1974;36:657–60.

57. Markand ON, Dyken ML. Sleep abnormalities in patients with brain stem lesions. Neurology 1976; 26:769–76.

58. Valldeoriola F, Santamaria J, Graus F, et al. Absence of REM sleep, altered NREM sleep, and supranuclear horizontal gaze palsy caused by a lesion of the pontine tegmentum. Sleep 1993;16: 184–8.

59. Vock J, Achermann P, Bischof M, et al. Evoluation of sleep and sleep EEG after hemispheric stroke. J Sleep Res 2002;11(4):331–8.

60. Schutte-Rodin S, Broch L, Buysse D, et al. Clinical guideline for the evaluation and management of chronic insomnia in adults. J Clin Sleep Med 2008;4(5):487–504.

61. Lee SY, Baek YH, Park SU, et al. Intradermal acupuncture on shen-men and nei-kuan acupoints improves insomnia in stroke patients by reducing the sympathetic nervous system activity: a randomized clinical trial. Am J Chin Med 2009;37: 1013–21.

62. Pech M, O'kearney R. A randomized controlled trial of problem-solving therapy compared to cognitive therapy for the treatment of insomnia in adults. Sleep 2013;36:739–49.

63. Young TB. Epidemiology of daytime sleepiness: definitions, symptomatology, and prevalence. J Clin Psychiatry 2004;65(Suppl 16):12–6.

64. Arzt M, Young T, Peppard PE, et al. Disassociation of obstructive sleep apnea from hypersomnolence and obesity in patients with stroke. Stroke 2010;41: e129–134.

65. Watson NF, Badr MS, Belenky G, et al. Recommended amount of sleep for a healthy adult: a joint consensus statement of the American Academy of Sleep Medicine and Sleep Research Society. J Clin Sleep Med 2015;11(6):591–2.

66. Boden-Albala B, Roberts ET, Bazil C, et al. Daytime sleepiness and risk of stroke and vascular disease. Circ Cardiovasc Qual Outcomes 2012;5: 500–7.

67. Patel SR. Social and demographic factors related to sleep duration. Sleep 2007;30(9):1077–8.

68. Gangwisch JE, Rexrode K, Forman JP, et al. Daytime sleepiness and risk of coronary heart disease and stroke: results from the Nurses' Health Study II. Sleep Med 2014;15:782–8.

69. Lambiase MJ, Gabriel KP, Kuller LH, et al. Temporal relationships between physical activity and sleep in older women. Med Sci Sports Exerc 2013;45:2362–8.

70. Wisse BE. The inflammatory syndrome: the role of adipose-tissue cytokines in metabolic disorders linked to obesity. J Am Soc Nephrol 2004;15: 2792–800.

71. Vgontzas AN, Chrousos GP. Sleep, the hypothalamic-pituitary-adrenal axis, and cytokines: multiple interactions and disturbances in sleep disorders. Endocrinol Metab Clin North Am 2002;31: 15–36.

72. Cuijpers P, Smit F. Excess mortality in depression: a meta-analysis of community studies. J Affect Disord 2002;72:227–36.

73. Patel SR, Malhotra A, Gottlieb DJ, et al. Correlates of long sleep duration. Sleep 2006;29:881–9.

74. Passouant P, Cadilhac J. Physiopathology of hypersomnias. Rev Neurol (Paris) 1967;116: 585–629.

75. Catsman-Berrevoets CE, von Harskamp F. Compulsive pre-sleep behavior and apathy due to bilateral thalamic stroke: response to bromocriptine. Neurology 1988;38:647–9.

76. Harris AL, Elder J, Schiff ND, et al. Post-stroke apathy and hypersomnia lead to worse outcomes from acute rehabilitation. Transl Stroke Res 2014; 5(2):292–300.

77. Scheidtmann K, Fries W, Müller F, et al. Effect of levodopa in combination with physiotherapy on functional motor recovery after stroke: a prospective, randomized, double-blind study. Lancet 2001;358:787–90.

78. Grade C, Redford B, Chrostowski J, et al. Methylphenidate in poststroke recovery: a double-blind, placebo-controlled study. Arch Phys Med Rehabil 1998;79:1047–50.

79. Iber C, Ancoli-Israel S, Chesson A, et al. The AASM manual for the scoring of sleep and associated events: rules, terminology and technical specifications. Westchester (IL): American Academy of Sleep Medicine; 2007.
80. Ekbom KA. Restless leg syndrome. Neurology 1960;10:868–73.
81. Winkelman JW, Shahar E, Sharief I, et al. Associations of restless leg syndrome and cardiovascular disease in the Sleep Heart Health Study. Neurology 2005;64:1920–4.
82. Koo BB, Blackwell T, Ancoli-Israel S, et al. Association of incident cardiovascular disease with periodic limb movements during sleep in older men; outcomes of sleep disorders in older men (MrOS) study. Circulation 2011;124(11):1223–31.
83. Siddiqui F, Strus J, Ming X, et al. Rise of blood pressure with periodic limb movements in sleep and wakefulness. Clin Neurophysiol 2007;118:1923–30.
84. Ulfberg J, Nyström B, Carter N, et al. Prevalence of restless leg syndrome among men aged 18 to 64 years: an association with somatic disease and neuropsychiatric symptoms. Mov Disord 2001;16:1159–63.
85. Hogl B, Kiechl S, Willeit J, et al. Restless leg syndrome: a community-based study of prevalence, severity, and risk factors. Neurology 2005;64:1920–4.
86. Rothdach AJ, Trenkwalder C, Haberstock J, et al. Prevalence and risk factors of RLS in an elderly population. Neurology 2000;54:1064–8.
87. Winkelman JW. The evoked heart rate response to periodic leg movements of sleep. Sleep 1999;22:575–80.
88. Sforza E, Nicolas A, Lavigne G, et al. EEG and cardiac activation during periodic leg movements in sleep: support for a hierarchy of arousal responses. Neurology 1999;52:786–91.
89. Kang SY, Sohn YH, Lee IK, et al. Unilateral periodic limb movement in sleep after supratentorial cerebral infarction. Parkinsonism Relat Disord 2004;10:429–31.
90. Lee JS, Lee PH, Huh K, et al. Periodic limb movements in sleep after a small subcortical infarct. Mov Disord 2005;20:260–1.
91. Lee SJ, Kim JS, Song IU, et al. Poststroke restless legs syndrome and lesion location: anatomical considerations. Mov Disord 2009;24:77–84.
92. Walters AS, Moussouttas M, Siddiqui F, et al. Prevalence of stroke in restless legs syndrome: initial results point to the need for more sophisticated studies. Open Neurol J 2010;4:73–7.
93. Walters A, Rye DB. Review of the relationship of restless leg syndrome and periodic limb movements in sleep to hypertension, heart disease, and stroke. Sleep 2009;32(5):589–97.
94. Ondo WG, He Y, Rajasekaran S, et al. Clinical correlates of 6-hydroxydopamine injections into A11 dopaminergic neurons in rats: a possible model for restless leg syndrome. Mov Disord 2000;15:154–8.
95. Sun Y, van Valkenhoef G, Morel T. A mixed treatment comparison of gabapentin enacarbil, pramipexole, ropinirole, and rotigotine in moderate-to-severe RLS. Curr Med Res Opin 2014;30(11):2267–78.
96. Aurora RN, Kristo DA, Bista SR, et al. The treatment of restless leg syndrome and periodic limb movement disorder in adults—an update for 2012: practice parameters with an evidence based systemic review and meta-analysis. Sleep 2012;35(8):1039–62.
97. Ohayon MM, Guilleminault C, Priest RG. Night terrors, sleep walking, and confusional arousals in the general population: their frequency and relationship to other sleep and mental disorders. J Clin Psychiatry 1999;60(4):268–76.
98. Kales A, Soldatos CR, Bixler EO, et al. Hereditary factors in sleepwalking and night terrors. Br J Psychiatry 1980;137:111–8.
99. Mahowald MW, Ettinger MG. Things that go bump in the night: the parasomnias revisited. J Clin Neurophysiol 1990;7(1):119–43.
100. Schenk CH, Mahowald W. Injurious sleep behavior disorders (parasomnias) affecting patients on intensive care units. Intensive Care Med 1991;17:219–24.
101. Tang WK, Hermann DM, Chen YK, et al. Brainstem infarcts predict REM sleep behavior disorder in acute ischemic stroke. BMC Neurol 2014;14:88.
102. Boller F, Wright DG, Cavalieri R, et al. Paroxysmal "nightmares". Sequel of stroke responsiveness to diphenylhydantoin. Neurology 1975;25:1026–8.
103. Boeve BF, Silber MH, Ferman TJ. Melatonin for treatment of REM sleep behavior disorder in neurologic disorders: results in 14 patients. Sleep Med 2003;4(4):281–4.
104. Aurora RN, Zak RS, Maganti RK, et al. Best practice guide for the treatment of REM sleep behavior disorder (RBD). J Clin Sleep Med 2010;6(1):85–95.

Sleep in Neuromuscular Diseases

Anna Monica Fermin, MD[a], Umair Afzal, MBBS[a], Antonio Culebras, MD[b],*

KEYWORDS

- Neuromuscular disease • Neuromuscular junction disorder • Motor neuron disease
- Amyotrophic lateral sclerosis • Myasthenia gravis • Spinal cord disorders • Phrenic nerve damage
- Myotonic dystrophy

KEY POINTS

- Patients with neuromuscular diseases should be routinely evaluated for symptoms of sleep dysfunction and sleep disordered breathing because these are treatable complications in an otherwise progressive disease process.
- Inspiratory vital capacity of less than 60% is a predictor of sleep disordered breathing in children and adolescents with neuromuscular disorders.
- The gold standard diagnostic test for patients with hypersomnia and nocturnal sleep disturbances is overnight polysomnogram, in some cases followed by a multiple sleep latency test.
- Sleep abnormalities of central origin are seen in myotonic dystrophy, which may not depend on the muscular deficit.
- Noninvasive ventilation has been shown to improve quality of life and mortality in patients with amyotrophic lateral sclerosis and other neuromuscular disorders.

INTRODUCTION

Sleep disorders are commonly seen in patients affected with neuromuscular diseases. However, the presence of sleep dysfunction is often overlooked because symptoms related to sleep disturbance are frequently attributed to the patient's underlying neurologic illness. It was not until the 1950s that clinicians became aware of sleep disorders and sleep-related respiratory compromise in patients with neuromuscular disease. Investigators crucial to highlighting sleep disorders in this patient population include Sarnoff and colleagues[1] who, in 1951 discussed hypoventilation in patients with poliomyelitis, and Benaim and Worster-Drought[2] who, in 1954, described alveolar hypoventilation in myotonic dystrophy.

Since the advent of clinical polysomnography, sleep disordered breathing and other sleep alterations, such as periodic limb movements of sleep (PLMS), have been uncovered in patients with neuromuscular and spinal cord disorders. In addition, widespread use of polysomnography has been able to quantify and show the beneficial effects of noninvasive positive breathing applications in this patient population.

In general, sleep disturbances in neuromuscular diseases are often caused by sleep-related ventilatory dysfunction; in some cases central hypersomnia, as in myotonic dystrophy, has also been observed. Damage to the anterior horn cell, motor root, peripheral nerve, neuromuscular junction, or the muscle fiber can result in thoracic, diaphragmatic, or oropharyngeal muscle weakness resulting in sleep dysfunction.

In addition to sleep-related respiratory compromise, patients with painful polyneuropathies and muscle pain in the setting of immobility often

[a] Upstate Medical University, 750 East Adams Street, Syracuse, NY 13210, USA; [b] Department of Neurology, Upstate Medical University, 750 East Adams Street, Syracuse, NY 13210, USA
* Corresponding author.
E-mail address: aculebras@aol.com

Sleep Med Clin 11 (2016) 53–64
http://dx.doi.org/10.1016/j.jsmc.2015.10.005
1556-407X/16/$ – see front matter © 2016 Elsevier Inc. All rights reserved.

sleep.theclinics.com

experience insomnia, sleep fragmentation, excessive daytime sleepiness, and symptoms of restless legs syndrome (RLS). Insufficient sleep can result in morning headaches, irritability, anxiety, depression, and impaired cognition.

It is important to identify symptoms of sleep dysfunction because treatment can be effective and improve quality of life. Early identification and treatment with noninvasive ventilation has been shown to improve not only quality of life but also survival in patients with amyotrophic lateral sclerosis (ALS).[3–5]

This article reviews the sleep disturbances found in spinal cord diseases (including poliomyelitis, ALS, and spinal cord injury), myopathies (including hereditary and inflammatory myopathies), neuropathies (including acute inflammatory demyelinating polyneuropathy), and neuromuscular junction disorders.

DIAGNOSTIC WORK-UP

A detailed sleep history is an essential component to the initial evaluation of patients with a suspected sleep disorder. It is advisable to perform the history in the presence of a family member such as a spouse or caregiver. These individuals can offer vital information because they often have a different insight into the patient's behavior during sleep or daytime functioning. For instance, many patients with PLMS are unaware of any nocturnal movements. However, their bed partners are typically affected by these symptoms and can provide details regarding nocturnal manifestations that may be unknown to the patient.

At times patients may not be aware that their daytime symptoms, such as morning headaches, fatigue, or cognitive impairment, may be related to a sleep disorder, and they often attribute these symptoms to their underlying neurologic illness. It is imperative that clinicians maintain a high index of suspicion for potential sleep disorders. Patients with neuromuscular diseases, particularly those with respiratory dysfunction, should specifically be screened for symptoms suggestive of sleep disordered breathing, such as snoring, witnessed apneas, or excessive daytime sleepiness. Episodes of nocturnal orthopnea should be investigated because this may be a sign of early respiratory muscle weakness and hypoventilation. Screening tools currently available include the Epworth Sleepiness Scale, STOP-BANG, and Pittsburgh Sleep Quality Index Scale. Concurrent medical issues, medication, and alcohol use should also be identified.

Nocturnal polysomnography is the test of choice to identify and quantify sleep disordered breathing.

In addition, the overnight study can uncover other sleep alterations commonly found in patients with neuromuscular disease, such as sleep onset insomnia, reduced sleep efficiency, and PLMS. All patients with positive screening for sleep disordered breathing, those with respiratory dysfunction, patients with bulbar weakness, and those with excessive daytime somnolence should undergo a diagnostic overnight polysomnogram.

A multiple sleep latency test (MSLT) should be performed in order to document the presence and severity of daytime sleepiness and to diagnose associated narcolepsy. In selected patients with respiratory weakness, electromyogram (EMG) and nerve conduction studies can be used to assess for phrenic and intercostal neuropathy.

Other tests, including pulmonary function tests to assess lung volume, gas exchange, and arterial blood gases, can be used to evaluate the integrity of the respiratory control system. Patients with symptoms of RLS should have iron studies performed and should be supplemented with iron if necessary.

SPECIFIC NEUROMUSCULAR CONDITIONS WITH SLEEP DISORDERS
Sleep Disorders in Motor Neuron Disease

ALS is the most common motor neuron disease. It is a neurodegenerative disorder characterized by progressive loss of motor neurons in the brain and spinal cord, resulting in the hallmark combination of upper and lower motor neuron signs and symptoms. Patients develop muscle weakness and paralysis, and eventually die of their disease. The median survival from the time of diagnosis is 3 to 5 years. Roughly 10% of patients survive 10 years or more. Presently the disease is incurable and management provides symptomatic treatment.

The most common cause of death in ALS is progressive neuromuscular respiratory failure. The loss of motor neurons in the brainstem and spinal cord results in pharyngeal, laryngeal, diaphragmatic, and intercostal muscle weakness that predisposes patients with ALS to respiratory dysfunction.[6] When respiratory compromise becomes severe, patients require tracheostomy and permanent ventilation. The deterioration of pulmonary function is highly predictive of mortality.[7,8]

Several studies have shown that breathing abnormalities during sleep often precede daytime respiratory dysfunction.[6,7,9] Patients with ALS develop sleep-related ventilatory abnormalities caused by the combination of central neurogenic dysfunction and peripheral muscle atrophy (**Box 1**).

Box 1
Frequently reported sleep-related symptoms in patients with ALS

Daytime symptoms

Excessive daytime sleepiness

Morning headaches

Fatigue

Poor concentration

Memory problems

Nighttime symptoms

Sleep fragmentation

Nocturia

Nocturnal cramps

Restless legs

Orthopnea

Snoring

Choking

Nightmares

Patients report nighttime symptoms, including insomnia, orthopnea, fragmented sleep, nightmares, snoring, choking, and restless legs. One study of 59 patients with ALS found that the most commonly reported nighttime complaints were nocturia (59%), sleep fragmentation (48%), and nocturnal cramps (45%).[10] Daytime symptoms included excessive daytime sleepiness, morning headaches, fatigue, poor concentration, and memory problems.[7] Daytime hypersomnolence can be attributed to nocturnal hypoventilation, hypoxemia, hypercapnia, repeated sleep-related apnea/hypopnea, and sleep fragmentation.

Sleep disordered breathing, including nocturnal hypoventilation, central apneas, and obstructive apneas, is found in 17% to 76% of patients with ALS.[7] The most commonly found abnormality is nocturnal hypoventilation, which is caused by weakness of the diaphragm and intercostal and accessory respiratory muscles, which are all affected in ALS.[11] As diaphragm weakness progresses, ventilation becomes dependent on intercostal and accessory respiratory muscles. Nocturnal hypoventilation becomes worse during rapid eye movement (REM) sleep as muscles become physiologically hypotonic. In addition, patients can also have apneic events, with central apneas predominating, a phenomenon caused by the combination of diaphragmatic and thoracic respiratory muscle weakness. Obstructive apneas occur because of upper airway hypotonia leading to a decrease in the airway lumen. The bulbar dysfunction seen in patients with ALS does not seem to increase the risk for obstructive sleep apnea.[12]

It is important to identify and treat patients with suspected sleep disorders because treatment can be effective and improve quality of life. Nocturnal pulse oximetry monitoring can be used as a screening tool to assess the degree of nocturnal hypoventilation and the need for noninvasive ventilation.[13] Overnight polysomnography remains the gold standard for diagnostic testing and should be done in all patients with ALS with respiratory dysfunction or reported sleep-related symptoms.

The most effective intervention to control sleep and respiratory dysfunction is noninvasive ventilation (ie, continuous positive airway pressure [CPAP], bilevel positive airway pressure), which has been shown to improve survival and quality of life.[3] In addition, sleep complaints in patients with ALS do not depend exclusively on respiratory dysfunction. One study involving 100 patients with ALS showed that sleep disturbance could be caused by other factors, such as poor mobility, muscle cramps, pain, and depression.[10] It is important to optimally treat these underlying conditions to improve the overall quality of sleep.

Postpolio Syndrome

Polio, also known as poliomyelitis, is a viral infection affecting the anterior horn cells of the spinal cord and cranial motor neurons, leading to muscle paralysis. During the first half of the twentieth century paralytic polio was a major cause of morbidity and mortality. In the United States alone, roughly 35,000 people each year were affected. One in 200 of those infected experienced irreversible muscle paralysis. Paralytic polio is classified into 3 types: spinal, bulbar, and bulbospinal. Spinal polio was the most common form, accounting for roughly 79% of cases. Patients developed asymmetric paralysis, most often involving the legs.[14] Bulbar polio, characterized by weakness of cranial nerve–innervated muscles, accounted for 2% of cases. Patients showing both bulbar and spinal symptoms were classified as having bulbospinal polio, which was roughly 19% of cases.[14] Patients with bulbar poliomyelitis are susceptible to respiratory and sleep dysfunction during the acute and convalescent stages.[15]

In the early 1950s, introduction of the polio vaccine was followed by a dramatic decline in new polio cases. According to the World Health Organization in 2014, only 3 countries (Afghanistan, Nigeria and Pakistan) remained polio endemic.

Although polio is not currently a major public health threat, patients previously affected by polio are at risk for new or progressive symptoms many years after the initial infection. Roughly 25% to 40% of polio survivors develop postpolio syndrome. The main clinical manifestations are new or progressive weakness, pain, fatigue, and sleep disturbances that develop decades after recovery from the initial attack.[16,17] The exact cause remains unclear but is thought to be progressive degeneration of reinnervated motor units, induction of autoimmunity with resulting destruction of neural structures, or a part of the normal aging process in patients who already have baseline poor neuromuscular reserve.[18]

Sleep disturbances are common, appearing in 13% to 48% of patients with postpolio, even in those with no prior bulbar involvement.[19–22] Symptoms reported include excessive daytime sleepiness, morning headaches, fatigue, and restless legs.[19,20] Some of the complaints typically attributed to postpolio, including increasing fatigue, may be the result of nocturnal respiratory dysfunction. Overnight polysomnography should be performed in patients with postpolio with respiratory manifestations and sleep disturbance.

Sleep apnea is commonly found in these patients. In one study, most of the respiratory events were obstructive apneas; however, central and mixed events were also seen.[23] Obstructive apneas are caused by pharyngeal and respiratory muscle weakness. Patients with bulbar polio most often had central apneic events, most likely caused by residual damage of the reticular formation.[24] There is favorable response to noninvasive positive airway ventilation, with improved sleep quality and improvement in daytime symptoms.[17,25]

Daytime fatigue can also be caused by difficulties in entering deeper stages of sleep. In a study involving 60 patients with postpolio, polysomnography revealed greater time spent in superficial sleep stages (73% of total sleep time [TST]) with much less time in slow wave sleep (7.8% of TST) and REM sleep (18.7% of TST).[23] These findings are thought to be caused by damage to the reticular formation caused by the polio virus. Difficulties in entering deeper stages of sleep were more pronounced in patients with bulbar involvement.[23]

Poor sleep quality can also be attributed to PLMS. Polysomnography performed on 99 patients with postpolio found PLMS index greater than 5 per hour in 16.6% of patients.[26] However, compared with patients without significantly increased PLMS index there was no difference in Apnea-Hypopnea Index, Awakening Index, TST, and sleep efficiency.[26] PLMS was unknown to patients during their clinical interview because their events did not cause full awakenings but instead resulted in microarousals. It is therefore important to obtain the clinical history in the presence of the patient's bed partner, because patients may not be aware of abnormal movements during sleep.[26]

In contrast with PLMS, in which the patients are often unaware of the symptoms, patients with RLS reported an uncontrollable urge to move their limbs. In a study of 10 patients with postpolio syndrome who reported symptoms of RLS, the investigators found a concomitant onset of symptoms for both RLS and postpolio syndrome, suggesting a possible underlying mechanism.[27] Patients with RLS responded well to dopaminergic agents.[28] As in PLMS, further studies with larger sample sizes are needed to better establish this relationship.

Myopathies

Primary muscle disorders or myopathies result in proximal muscle weakness with variable involvement of the respiratory musculature. Respiratory disturbances are generally noted in the advanced stage of the illness, but sometimes respiratory failure develops early in the disease. Sleep complaints and sleep-related respiratory dysfunctions are common in Duchenne muscular dystrophy, limb-girdle muscular dystrophy, and acid maltase deficiency; they may also occur in other congenital or acquired myopathies, mitochondrial encephalomyopathy, and polymyositis. Polysomnographic findings in Duchenne and other muscular dystrophies, as well as myotonic dystrophy, include increased number of awakenings, sleep fragmentation, and sleep disorganization, as well as reduced TST. Other findings include central, mixed, and upper airway obstructive sleep apneas or hypopneas associated with oxygen desaturation and nonapneic oxygen desaturation that become worse during REM sleep. In myopathies, multiple factors may play a role in causing nocturnal sleep disturbances and daytime hypersomnolence:

1. Impairment of chest bellows caused by weakness of the chest wall and respiratory muscles.
2. Increased work of breathing.
3. Functional impairment of medullary respiratory neurons caused by hyporesponsive or unresponsive chemoreceptors secondary to muscle diseases.
4. Excessive somnolence that is not corrected with ventilatory assistance, or is in excess, or occurs in the absence of a ventilatory impediment, suggesting a central form of hypersomnia.

Congenital and metabolic myopathies

Congenital and metabolic myopathies result in sleep disorders because of multiple factors, including respiratory muscle weakness, skeletal deformities, and alteration of respiratory chemosensitivity. In some forms of congenital myopathy, there is impairment of respiratory chemosensitivity with reduced sleep-related ventilatory drive independent of hypoxemia and hypercapnia, suggesting a central dysfunction.[29,30] The combination of ventilatory muscle dysfunction and reduced central ventilatory drive is a particularly dangerous situation.

Nocturnal hypoxia can present as poor sleep, nightmares, morning headache, and daytime sleepiness. Severe nocturnal respiratory failure has been described in 2 siblings with nemaline myopathy.[31] Nemaline myopathy involves all skeletal muscles, including the diaphragm. Both patients developed marked sleep inertia in the morning, with headaches, vomiting, and daytime lethargy. The nocturnal respiratory failure was primarily caused by disorder of central respiratory control with poor sensitivity to carbon dioxide. Symptoms resolved with nocturnal mechanical ventilation.

Duchenne muscular dystrophy

In a retrospective review[32] of 34 patients with Duchenne muscular dystrophy attending a tertiary pediatric sleep disorder clinic over a 5-year period, 22 (64%) patients reported sleep-related symptoms. Thirty-two patients had polysomnography, the results of which were diagnostic of obstructive sleep apnea in 10 patients (31%; median age, 8 years). A total of 11 patients (32%) showed hypoventilation (median age, 13 years) during the 5-year period. There was a significant improvement in the Apnea-Hypopnea Index (mean difference, 11.31; 95% confidence interval, 5.91–16.70; $P = .001$) following the institution of noninvasive ventilation.

The investigators concluded that the prevalence of sleep-related breathing disorders in Duchenne muscular dystrophy is high. There seems to be a bimodal presentation with obstructive sleep apnea found in the first decade and hypoventilation more commonly seen at the beginning of the second decade. In moderately advanced disease, there may be nocturnal hypoventilation with profound desaturation during REM sleep despite normal awake ventilation.[33] Restrictive lung disease develops with progression of muscle weakness and deformation of the rib cage. In advanced forms of the disease, there may be abundant fragmentation of nocturnal sleep, many sleep stage changes, and reduced REM sleep without evidence of nocturnal hypoxia.[34] Polysomnography is recommended in patients with Duchenne muscular dystrophy who have symptoms of obstructive sleep apnea, or who are at the stage of becoming wheelchair bound. Lung function is useful to predict nocturnal hypercapnia in patients with Duchenne muscular dystrophy. Polysomnography should be considered in Duchenne muscular dystrophy when the Pa_{CO_2} is greater than 45 mm Hg, particularly if the base excess is increased.[35] Daytime predictors of sleep hypoventilation in patients who have Duchenne muscular dystrophy are a forced expiratory volume of less than 40% and a base excess of greater than 4 mmol/L.[35] Moreover, a vital capacity less than 680 mL is sensitive to predict daytime hypercapnia.[36]

Myotonic dystrophy

Myotonic dystrophy is an autosomal dominant, multisystem disorder affecting the musculoskeletal, endocrine, and central nervous systems. There are 2 major forms: dystrophia myotonica I (DM1), also known as Steinert disease, and dystrophia myotonica II (DM2), recognized in 1994 as a milder version of DM1. Since the early description of alveolar hypoventilation in myotonic dystrophy,[2] many patients with myotonic dystrophy have been described with central, mixed, and upper airway obstructive sleep apneas; alveolar hypoventilation; daytime fatigue; and hypersomnolence.[37] Nocturnal oxygen desaturation accompanies alveolar hypoventilation and apneas, becoming worse during REM sleep. Excessive daytime sleepiness and dysregulation of REM sleep occur frequently in patients with DM1.[38] In a study of 29 patients with genetically proven DM2, only 6.9% had excessive daytime sleepiness, compared with 44.8% of patients with DM1 and 6.2% of population controls using the Epworth Sleepiness Scale, Pittsburgh Sleep Quality Index, and Checklist Individual Strength.[39] A study specifically targeting patients with DM2 revealed that RLS, excessive daytime sleepiness, and fatigue are frequent sleep disturbances, whereas obstructive sleep apnea and REM sleep behavior disorder are not.[40] Excessive daytime sleepiness was independently associated with DM2 diagnosis, suggesting a primary central nervous system hypersomnia mechanism, as noted by studies in DM1.

In myotonic dystrophy, weakness, and myotonia of the upper airway and other respiratory muscles, as well as an inherited membrane abnormality involving the respiratory and hypnogenic neurons in the brainstem, may be responsible for sleep and breathing disorders.[37] Nocturnal polysomnography in 11 patients with myotonic dystrophy uncovered alveolar hypoventilation in all patients, along with mild sleep disordered breathing of a central type in stage 1 and REM sleep.[41] Patients with myotonic dystrophy may also have intrinsic hypersomnia related to degeneration of nerve cells in dorsomedial nuclei of the thalamus and perhaps hypothalamus manifested by cytoplasmic eosinophilic inclusion bodies.[42] Laberge and colleagues,[43] in their series of patients with DM1, found characteristics similar to those encountered in patients with idiopathic hypersomnia. Excessive daytime somnolence was present in 33.1% of patients, with the intensity of somnolence correlating with the severity of muscular disease. Measurement of hypocretin levels in cerebrospinal fluid (CSF) in patients with myotonic dystrophy has shown a significantly lower content (<200 pg/mL) in 6 patients with myotonic dystrophy, suggesting a dysfunction of the hypothalamic hypocretin system.[44]

There is evidence that administration of up to 400 mg of modafinil daily to patients with myotonic dystrophy and hypersomnolence without sleep apnea disorder increases latencies in the MSLT and improves Epworth Sleepiness Scale scores[45] and sleepiness.[46,47] This favorable effect has been disputed by another small study using modafinil 300 mg/d conducted in an adult population with DM1 (n = 28) and a high prevalence of hypersomnia.[48] In this study, modafinil had no significant effect on daytime somnolence as measured with objective maintenance of wakefulness tests. In a placebo-controlled trial with a single dose of 20 mg of methylphenidate in 24 patients with myotonic dystrophy type 1 (12 men, 12 women), treatment with methylphenidate showed a favorable effect.[49] There was significant change in median scores on the Daytime Sleepiness Scale (−3.0 vs −0.5; $P = .003$) and the Epworth Sleepiness Scale (−3.0 vs −1.5; $P = .039$). There was no significant change in mean sleep latency test results. Three patients discontinued methylphenidate because of adverse events, including diarrhea, nervousness, and irritability. Loss of appetite, nausea, and palpitations were the most common adverse events reported by patients treated with methylphenidate. The investigators concluded that a single 20-mg dose of methylphenidate significantly reduced daytime sleepiness in this small, selected population of patients with myotonic dystrophy type 1.

Acid maltase deficiency

In glycogenosis type II, or acid maltase deficiency, a deficiency of acid alpha-glucosidase affects skeletal and cardiac muscles. The clinical spectrum ranges from very severe cases observed soon after birth to increasingly milder cases affecting infants, children, and adults.[50] Children and adults show a slowly progressing myopathy with decreased limb strength and respiratory impairment. Patients with glycogenosis type II may experience sleep disordered breathing and hypoventilation, particularly in REM sleep, as a result of diaphragmatic weakness.[51] Obstructive sleep apnea secondary to oropharyngeal muscle weakness has also been reported in glycogenosis type II.

Inflammatory myopathies

Inflammatory myopathies include polymyositis, dermatopolymyositis, and inclusion body myositis (IBM). In adult patients with inflammatory myopathies the frequency of obstructive sleep apnea is high.[52] These alterations may play a role in persistent fatigue in these patients. Diaphragmatic weakness can be seen in inflammatory myopathies, which is an independent risk factor for sleep disordered breathing. Teixeira and colleagues[53] studied diaphragmatic strength in 12 patients with polymyositis, 5 patients with dermatopolymyositis, and 6 patients with IBM. Eighteen patients (78%) had diaphragm weakness, with the most severe weakness found in dermatopolymyositis. Polysomnography in 15 patients with IBM revealed sleep disordered breathing (Apnea-Hypopnea Index, 23.4 ± 12.8 events/h) in all.[54] There was no consistency between the occurrence of sleep disordered breathing and the severity of peripheral muscle weakness. Asymptomatic impairment of respiratory function suggests that sleep studies should be performed routinely in inflammatory myopathies, irrespective of peripheral muscle function.

SPINAL CORD DISEASES AND PHRENIC NERVE DAMAGE

Sleep disturbances related to respiratory dysfunction can occur in patients with spinal cord diseases, particularly in those with upper cervical spinal cord lesions affecting the phrenic nerve nuclei. Conditions damaging the phrenic and intercostal motor neurons in the spinal cord are ALS, spinal cord tumors, spinal trauma, spinal surgery (eg, cervical cordotomy, or anterior spinal surgery), and nonspecific or demyelinating myelitis. Sleep disturbances in spinal cord diseases result from sleep-related respiratory alterations that cause sleep apnea-hypopnea or hypoventilation. The 2 respiratory controlling systems (the voluntary or behavioral system and the metabolic or automatic system) are integrated in the cervical spinal cord. The ventrolateral quadrant containing the automatic system and the dorsolateral quadrant containing the behavioral system control the final common respiratory motor neurons passing through the phrenic and intercostal nerves to the respiratory muscles. Direct dysfunction of these respiratory pathways in the spinal cord may result after cervical spinal surgery[55,56] and spinal trauma,[57] or may be caused by ALS, syringomyelia, cervical spinal cord tumor, or multiple sclerosis. Craniovertebral junction malformation and Chiari malformation in adults, with or without syringomyelia and basilar invagination, are associated with neuronal dysfunction of the brainstem, cerebellum, cranial nerves, and upper spinal cord. The incidence of sleep apnea-hypopnea syndrome is significantly higher in patients with craniovertebral junction malformation, especially if basilar invagination is present.[58] Hypercapnia in individuals with complete cervical cord injuries can induce arousals from sleep.[59]

Phrenic nerve damage may cause diaphragmatic paralysis. Unilateral paralysis is asymptomatic, but bilateral paralysis is invariably symptomatic and may be life threatening; paresis or weakness with partial diaphragmatic dysfunction may cause sleep-related ventilatory insufficiency. Bilateral paralysis underlies orthopnea with difficulty on inspiration out of proportion to the cardiopulmonary status. In the supine position, patients complain of profound difficulty breathing, which is the result of a reduction in lung volume and increased respiratory effort as the abdominal contents rise into the thorax. In severe or acute cases, patients present with nocturnal orthopnea, cyanosis, and fragmented sleep followed by morning headaches, vomiting, and daytime lethargy.[60]

EMG and nerve conduction studies may be necessary in patients with respiratory failure caused by dysfunction of the diaphragm, intercostal muscles, and other accessory muscles of respiration. In selected patients, EMG of the diaphragm and intercostal muscles may be necessary. Phrenic and intercostal nerve conduction studies can help diagnose phrenic and intercostal neuropathy in some patients.

An intriguing, but promising, finding has been the observation of a normal proportion of REM sleep in a series of patients with bilateral diaphragmatic paralysis.[61] This finding was attributed to inspiratory recruitment of extradiaphragmatic muscles in tonic and phasic REM sleep, suggesting brainstem reorganization of stimuli.

Treatment of sleep-related respiratory disturbances in spinal cord diseases should follow the same general principles as those suggested for neuromuscular disorders, and this includes noninvasive positive airway ventilation. A word of caution comes from a study[62] showing that patients with spinal cord injury who are on antispasticity medications and who are obese may have a higher risk of developing snoring and obstructive sleep apnea. The greatest risk was in patients taking diazepam or diazepam and baclofen in combination.

NEUROMUSCULAR JUNCTION DISORDERS

Disorders affecting the neuromuscular junction include myasthenia gravis, Lambert-Eaton myasthenic syndrome, botulism, and tick paralysis. Failure of transmission of the nerve impulses at the neuromuscular junction results in easy fatigability of muscles. When bulbar and respiratory muscles are involved this can result in respiratory failure, nocturnal hypoventilation, and sleep disordered breathing requiring assisted ventilation.

Myasthenia gravis is the most common of these disorders. Fatigue and weakness are the result of the action of antibodies against acetylcholine receptors in the postsynaptic membrane of the neuromuscular junction. There are 2 clinical forms: ocular and generalized. In ocular myasthenia gravis weakness is limited to the eyelids and extraocular muscles. In the generalized form ocular, bulbar, limb, and respiratory muscles are involved. These patients often have dysarthria, dysphagia, diplopia, and limb weakness worsened by repetitive muscle contraction. Roughly 30% of patients develop respiratory weakness. During wakefulness, symptoms can be mild but may deteriorate during the night, especially during REM sleep. Patients may have central, obstructive, and mixed apneas, and hypopneas associated with oxygen desaturation.[63] Most of the events are caused by hypoventilation related to diaphragmatic weakness.[63] However, one study showed an increased incidence of obstructive sleep apneas compared with controls.[64]

Risk factors for development of sleep disordered breathing in patients with myasthenia gravis are age, restrictive pulmonary disease, diaphragmatic weakness, daytime hypoventilation, and increased body mass index (BMI).[63] Disease severity may also be considered a risk factor but further studies are needed to determine the correlation. Studies also suggest that patients with well-controlled myasthenia gravis, without any daytime muscle dysfunction, may have abnormal breathing during sleep.[63]

Several studies show a high prevalence of sleep disturbances and decreased sleep quality among patients with myasthenia gravis.[63–65]

There are conflicting reports on the relationship between sleep disordered breathing and myasthenia gravis. The variability in findings is likely related to the fluctuating course and instability of myasthenia gravis. Nonetheless, it is important for clinicians to screen for sleep-related complaints (excessive daytime sleepiness, nocturnal awakenings) because adequate respiratory strength during sleep is often overlooked. Screening patients using the Pittsburgh Sleep Quality Index has been suggested.[65] Patients with sleep-related breathing disorders respond favorably to noninvasive ventilation. One case report showed that the use of CPAP therapy led to improvement of not only sleep disordered breathing but also of the ocular myasthenia symptoms.[66] Another treatment option is bilevel positive airway pressure ventilation, which is usually better tolerated by patients with neuromuscular disorders and at times can be more effective.[67]

In addition to sleep disordered breathing, patients with myasthenia gravis have an increased frequency of RLS. One study involving 73 patients with myasthenia gravis found RLS present in 43.2% of patients compared with 20% of controls; 9.4% of the patients reported RLS as their most disturbing health problem, whereas 46.9% reported that RLS was as problematic as other symptoms of the disease. This study also found a higher frequency of daytime sleepiness with higher mean Epworth Sleepiness Scale score in the myasthenia gravis group.

The study was unable to identify a relationship between the prevalence of RLS and the duration and type of myasthenia gravis therapy.[68] The management approach does not differ from the treatment options of RLS in patients who do not have myasthenia gravis.

There are limited reports on sleep disorders in the Lambert-Eaton myasthenic syndrome, botulism, and tick paralysis. The same principles and clinical approach used in myasthenia gravis can be applied to this patient population because respiratory muscle weakness predisposes all patients to sleep-related breathing disorders, particular during REM sleep.

Risks factors in developing sleep disordered breathing in patients with myasthenia gravis
Age
Increased BMI
Restrictive pulmonary disease
Diaphragmatic weakness
Daytime hypoventilation

NEUROPATHIES

Peripheral nerves are susceptible to damage from a variety of toxic, inflammatory, infectious, and hereditary factors. Clinical manifestations of peripheral nerve damage are typically symmetric and length dependent, including paresthesias, sensory loss, and muscle weakness. Most neuropathies are acquired and are the result of medical conditions such as diabetes, hypothyroidism, vitamin deficiencies, human immunodeficiency virus, amyloidosis, and Lyme disease.

Sleep disturbances are commonly reported in this patient population. Factors responsible for sleep dysfunction include, but are not limited to, pain and depression in diabetic neuropathy[69] and RLS in alcoholic neuropathy.[70]

Guillain-Barré Syndrome

Most neuropathies typically do not have a drastic effect on daytime or nocturnal respiratory function. One notable exception is Guillain-Barré syndrome (GBS), also known as acute inflammatory demyelinating polyneuropathy. It is an immune-mediated process resulting in a severe polyneuropathy with variable sensory and motor disability. Patients may have ocular, bulbar, and extremity weakness. Between 10% and 30% of patients develop severe respiratory muscle weakness requiring ventilatory support. Similar to other neuromuscular disorders with diaphragmatic weakness, patients with GBS have worsening hypoventilation during REM sleep.

In a questionnaire-based study involving hospitalized patients with GBS, more than half reported sleep disturbances, including increased sleep latencies, sleep fragmentation, and reduced sleep duration. Symptoms were most severe during the first week of hospitalization and improved thereafter.[71] Similar findings were reported in another group of patients with GBS admitted to the intensive care unit setting. Polysomnography revealed decreased sleep efficiency, increased sleep onset latency greater than 30 minutes, and increased arousals (>5 arousals per hour). Arousals were primarily caused by respiratory events and oxygen desaturation.[72]

Exact mechanisms of sleep disturbances in GBS remain unclear. The cause is thought to be multifactorial through a combination of sensory disturbances, motor weakness, and anxiety related to mental burden of disease. There is speculation that central mechanisms also play a role in sleep dysfunction because there have been reports of reduced CSF hypocretin-1 levels (a neuropeptide that is deficient in narcolepsy)[73,74] and narcolepsylike symptoms (hypnagogic and hypnopompic hallucinations).[75] GBS has also been associated with REM sleep behavior disorder, characterized as REM sleep without atonia, vivid dreams, and repeated episodes of sleep-related vocalizations and/or complex motor behaviors.[75]

Hereditary Motor Sensory Neuropathy or Charcot-Marie-Tooth Disease

Hereditary motor sensory neuropathy, also known as Charcot-Marie-Tooth (CMT) disease, is a spectrum of disorders caused by a mutation in myelin genes resulting in peripheral nerve dysfunction. CMT has been classified as CMT types 1 to 7. Classification is based on mode of inheritance, gene markers, metabolic defects, clinical characteristics, and electrophysiologic features. CMT type 1 and type 2 together are the most common hereditary peripheral neuropathies. Clinical manifestations include sensory impairments, foot deformities, distal motor weakness, muscle atrophy, and gait disturbances.

Sleep dysfunction, including sleep disordered breathing, RLS, and PLMS, has been reported in patients with CMT.[76,77] Sleep disordered breathing associated with CMT was first reported in severely affected patients with phrenic nerve dysfunction and diaphragmatic weakness.[78] Several studies since then have shown an increased prevalence of sleep apnea in CMT type 1A compared with matched controls.[73,76,79] Apneas were mainly obstructive because of a combination of diaphragm weakness and upper airway dysfunction in the form of pharyngeal neuropathy and vocal cord weakness. Severity correlated with neurologic disability caused by CMT.[76,79] Vocal cord dysfunction is thought to be the result of laryngeal nerve involvement, and is found in association with several CMT types. Symptoms can often mimic asthma.[67] Studies suggest that laryngeal symptoms are caused by slowly progressive neuropathy that seems to be length dependent.[80] Bilevel positive airway pressure therapy may be more appropriate than CPAP for the management of sleep apnea in patients with concomitant restrictive pulmonary impairment.[60]

RLS was initially reported mainly in patients with CMT type 2 but not with CMT type 1.[77] Recent studies reveal that RLS is highly prevalent not only in axonal subtypes of CMT (CMT type 2) but also in primarily demyelinating subforms (CMT type 1). RLS is highly associated with the presence of sensory symptoms in both subtypes. The presence and severity of RLS were associated with reduced sleep quality and impairment of health-related quality of life.[79]

RLS is often associated with PLMS, which are characterized by episodes of repetitive, highly stereotypical limb movements that occur during sleep.[81]

These movements often result in sleep disruptions (arousals) leading to daytime hypersomnolence. A recent study showed evidence that both the prevalence and number of PLMS are increased in patients with CMT type 1. However, the study failed to show any significant effect of the PLMS on polysomnography measures of sleep quality.[76] Further polysomnography-based studies on PLMS in patients with peripheral neuropathy are needed.

Treatment of RLS and PLMS in this patient population does not differ from traditional treatment options in patients without neuropathic dysfunction. Pharmacologic options include calcium channel alpha-2-delta ligands (ie, gabapentin), dopaminergic agents, benzodiazepines, and opioids.

SUMMARY

Sleep disturbances in neuromuscular disorders are secondary to weakness in respiratory and oropharyngeal muscles, phrenic and intercostal neuropathy, neuromuscular junction dysfunction, and abnormalities in the central respiratory drive. Central hypersomnias have been described in some cases (myotonic dystrophy, GBS).

Sleep disordered breathing is the most common sleep disorder. All patients with excessive daytime somnolence, respiratory dysfunction, or bulbar weakness should undergo overnight polysomnography. Polysomnography can identify and quantify sleep disordered breathing, nocturnal hypoventilation, and hypoxemia, and can uncover other sleep alterations. In some cases MSLT is indicated.

In addition to treating the underlying neurologic condition, treatment of sleep disorders can improve quality of life in this patient population. For instance, noninvasive ventilation has been noted to improve quality of life and mortality in patients with ALS.[3–5]

Patients with neuromuscular disease and sleep-related complications often attribute their symptoms to their underlying neurologic illness. Thus, it is imperative that clinicians maintain a high index of suspicion and screen all patients with neuromuscular disease for potential sleep disorders because these are treatable complications in an otherwise progressive disease process.

REFERENCES

1. Sarnoff SJ, Whittenberger JL, Affeldt JE. Hypoventilation syndrome in bulbar poliomyelitis. J Am Med Assoc 1951;147(1):30–4.

2. Benaim S, Worster-Drought C. Dystrophia myotonica with myotonia of the diaphragm causing pulmonary hypoventilation with anoxaemia and secondary polycythaemia. Med Illus 1954;8(4):221–6.

3. Barthlen GM, Lange DJ. Unexpectedly severe sleep and respiratory pathology in patients with amyotrophic lateral sclerosis. Eur J Neurol 2000;7(3):299–302.

4. Lyall RA, Donaldson N, Polkey MI, et al. Respiratory muscle strength and ventilatory failure in amyotrophic lateral sclerosis. Brain 2001;124(Pt 10): 2000–13.

5. Similowski T, Attali V, Bensimon G, et al. Diaphragmatic dysfunction and dyspnoea in amyotrophic lateral sclerosis. Eur Respir J 2000;15(2):332–7.

6. Labanowski M, Schmidt-Nowara W, Guilleminault C. Sleep and neuromuscular disease: frequency of sleep-disordered breathing in a neuromuscular disease clinic population. Neurology 1996;47(5):1173–80.

7. Gaig C, Iranzo A. Sleep-disordered breathing in neurodegenerative diseases. Curr Neurol Neurosci Rep 2012;12(2):205–17.

8. Chio A, Logroscino G, Hardiman O, et al. Prognostic factors in ALS: a critical review. Amyotroph Lateral Scler 2009;10(5–6):310–23.

9. Kimura K, Tachibana N, Kimura J, et al. Sleep-disordered breathing at an early stage of amyotrophic lateral sclerosis. J Neurol Sci 1999;164(1):37–43.

10. Lo Coco D, Mattaliano P, Spataro R, et al. Sleep-wake disturbances in patients with amyotrophic lateral sclerosis. J Neurol Neurosurg Psychiatry 2011;82(8):839–42.

11. Perrin C, Unterborn JN, Ambrosio CD, et al. Pulmonary complications of chronic neuromuscular diseases and their management. Muscle Nerve 2004; 29(1):5–27.

12. Arnulf I, Similowski T, Salachas F, et al. Sleep disorders and diaphragmatic function in patients with amyotrophic lateral sclerosis. Am J Respir Crit Care Med 2000;161(3 Pt 1):849–56.

13. Pinto A, de Carvalho M, Evangelista T, et al. Nocturnal pulse oximetry: a new approach to establish the appropriate time for non-invasive ventilation in ALS patients. Amyotroph Lateral Scler Other Motor Neuron Disord 2003;4(1):31–5.

14. Centers for Disease Control and Prevention. Postpolio syndrome. 2014. Available at: http://www.cdc.gov/polio/us/pps.html. Accessed July 5, 2015.

15. Chokroverty S. Sleep and breathing in neuromuscular disorders. Handb Clin Neurol 2011;99:1087–108.

16. Halstead LS, Rossi CD. Post-polio syndrome: clinical experience with 132 consecutive outpatients. Birth Defects Orig Artic Ser 1987;23(4):13–26.

17. Jubelt B, Drucker J. Poliomyelitis and the post-polio syndrome. Philadelphia: Lippincott Williams & Wilkins; 1999. p. 381–95.

18. Trojan DA, Cashman NR. Post-poliomyelitis syndrome. Muscle Nerve 2005;31(1):6–19.

19. McNalley TE, Yorkston KM, Jensen MP, et al. Review of secondary health conditions in postpolio syndrome: prevalence and effects of aging. Am J Phys Med Rehabil 2015;94(2):139–45.

20. van Kralingen KW, Ivanyi B, van Keimpema AR, et al. Sleep complaints in postpolio syndrome. Arch Phys Med Rehabil 1996;77(6):609–11.

21. Tersteeg IM, Koopman FS, Stolwijk-Swuste JM, et al. 5-year longitudinal study of fatigue in patients with late-onset sequelae of poliomyelitis. Arch Phys Med Rehabil 2011;92(6):899–904.

22. Cosgrove JL, Alexander MA, Kitts EL, et al. Late effects of poliomyelitis. Arch Phys Med Rehabil 1987; 68(1):4–7.

23. Silva TM, Moreira GA, Quadros AA, et al. Analysis of sleep characteristics in post-polio syndrome patients. Arq Neuropsiquiatr 2010;68(4):535–40.

24. Siegel H, McCutchen C, Dalakas MC, et al. Physiologic events initiating REM sleep in patients with the postpolio syndrome. Neurology 1999;52(3): 516–22.

25. Steljes DG, Kryger MH, Kirk BW, et al. Sleep in postpolio syndrome. Chest 1990;98(1):133–40.

26. Araujo MA, Silva TM, Moreira GA, et al. Sleep disorders frequency in post-polio syndrome patients caused by periodic limb movements. Arq Neuropsiquiatr 2010;68(1):35–8.

27. Marin LF, Carvalho LB, Prado LB, et al. Restless legs syndrome in post-polio syndrome: a series of 10 patients with demographic, clinical and laboratorial findings. Parkinsonism Relat Disord 2011;17(7):563–4.

28. Kumru H, Portell E, Barrio M, et al. Restless legs syndrome in patients with sequelae of poliomyelitis. Parkinsonism Relat Disord 2014;20(10):1056–8.

29. Carroll JE, Zwillich C, Weil JV, et al. Depressed ventilatory response in oculocraniosomatic neuromuscular disease. Neurology 1976;26(2):140–6.

30. Wilson DO, Sanders MH, Dauber JH. Abnormal ventilatory chemosensitivity and congenital myopathy. Arch Intern Med 1987;147(10):1773–7.

31. Maayan C, Springer C, Armon Y, et al. Nemaline myopathy as a cause of sleep hypoventilation. Pediatrics 1986;77(3):390–5.

32. Suresh S, Wales P, Dakin C, et al. Sleep-related breathing disorder in Duchenne muscular dystrophy: disease spectrum in the paediatric population. J Paediatr Child Health 2005;41(9–10):500–3.

33. Smith P, Edwards R, Calverley P. Ventilation and breathing pattern during sleep in Duchenne muscular dystrophy. Chest 1989;96(6):1346–51.

34. Redding GJ, Okamoto GA, Guthrie RD, et al. Sleep patterns in nonambulatory boys with Duchenne muscular dystrophy. Arch Phys Med Rehabil 1985; 66(12):818–21.

35. Hukins CA, Hillman DR. Daytime predictors of sleep hypoventilation in Duchenne muscular dystrophy. Am J Respir Crit Care Med 2000;161(1):166–70.

36. Toussaint M, Steens M, Soudon P. Lung function accurately predicts hypercapnia in patients with Duchenne muscular dystrophy. Chest 2007;131(2): 368–75.

37. Hansotia P, Frens D. Hypersomnia associated with alveolar hypoventilation in myotonic dystrophy. Neurology 1981;31(10):1336–7.

38. Yu H, Laberge L, Jaussent I, et al. Daytime sleepiness and REM sleep characteristics in myotonic dystrophy: a case-control study. Sleep 2011;34(2):165–70.

39. Tieleman AA, Knoop H, van de Logt AE, et al. Poor sleep quality and fatigue but no excessive daytime sleepiness in myotonic dystrophy type 2. J Neurol Neurosurg Psychiatry 2010;81(9):963–7.

40. Lam EM, Shepard PW, St Louis EK, et al. Restless legs syndrome and daytime sleepiness are prominent in myotonic dystrophy type 2. Neurology 2013;81(2):157–64.

41. Lopez-Esteban P, Peraita-Adrados R. Sleep and respiratory disorders in myotonic dystrophy of Steinert. Neurologia (Barcelona, Spain) 2000;15(3):102–8 [in Spanish].

42. Culebras A, Feldman RG, Merk FB. Cytoplasmic inclusion bodies within neurons of the thalamus in myotonic dystrophy. A light and electron microscope study. J Neurol Sci 1973;19(3):319–29.

43. Laberge L, Begin P, Montplaisir J, et al. Sleep complaints in patients with myotonic dystrophy. J Sleep Res 2004;13(1):95–100.

44. Martinez-Rodriguez JE, Lin L, Iranzo A, et al. Decreased hypocretin-1 (Orexin-A) levels in the cerebrospinal fluid of patients with myotonic dystrophy and excessive daytime sleepiness. Sleep 2003; 26(3):287–90.

45. Damian MS, Gerlach A, Schmidt F, et al. Modafinil for excessive daytime sleepiness in myotonic dystrophy. Neurology 2001;56(6):794–6.

46. Talbot K, Stradling J, Crosby J, et al. Reduction in excess daytime sleepiness by modafinil in patients with myotonic dystrophy. Neuromuscul Disord 2003;13(5):357–64.

47. MacDonald JR, Hill JD, Tarnopolsky MA. Modafinil reduces excessive somnolence and enhances mood in patients with myotonic dystrophy. Neurology 2002;59(12):1876–80.

48. Orlikowski D, Chevret S, Quera-Salva MA, et al. Modafinil for the treatment of hypersomnia associated with myotonic muscular dystrophy in adults: a multicenter, prospective, randomized, double-blind, placebo-controlled, 4-week trial. Clin Ther 2009;31(8):1765–73.

49. Puymirat J, Bouchard JP, Mathieu J. Efficacy and tolerability of a 20-mg dose of methylphenidate for the treatment of daytime sleepiness in adult patients with myotonic dystrophy type 1: a 2-center, randomized, double-blind, placebo-controlled, 3-week crossover trial. Clin Ther 2012;34(5):1103–11.

50. Bembi B, Cerini E, Danesino C, et al. Management and treatment of glycogenosis type II. Neurology 2008;71(23 Suppl 2):S12–36.

51. Mellies U, Ragette R, Schwake C, et al. Sleep-disordered breathing and respiratory failure in acid maltase deficiency. Neurology 2001;57(7):1290–5.

52. Selva-O'Callaghan A, Sampol G, Romero O, et al. Obstructive sleep apnea in patients with inflammatory myopathies. Muscle Nerve 2009;39(2): 144–9.

53. Teixeira A, Cherin P, Demoule A, et al. Diaphragmatic dysfunction in patients with idiopathic inflammatory myopathies. Neuromuscul Disord 2005; 15(1):32–9.

54. Rodriguez Cruz PM, Needham M, Hollingsworth P, et al. Sleep disordered breathing and subclinical impairment of respiratory function are common in sporadic inclusion body myositis. Neuromuscul Disord 2014;24(12):1036–41.

55. Krieger AJ, Rosomoff HL. Sleep-induced apnea. 1. A respiratory and autonomic dysfunction syndrome following bilateral percutaneous cervical cordotomy. J Neurosurg 1974;40(2):168–80.

56. Krieger AJ, Rosomoff HL. Sleep-induced apnea. 2. Respiratory failure after anterior spinal surgery. J Neurosurg 1974;40(2):181–5.

57. Short DJ, Stradling JR, Williams SJ. Prevalence of sleep apnoea in patients over 40 years of age with spinal cord lesions. J Neurol Neurosurg Psychiatry 1992;55(11):1032–6.

58. Botelho RV, Bittencourt LR, Rotta JM, et al. A prospective controlled study of sleep respiratory events in patients with craniovertebral junction malformation. J Neurosurg 2003;99(6):1004–9.

59. Ayas NT, Brown R, Shea SA. Hypercapnia can induce arousal from sleep in the absence of altered respiratory mechanoreception. Am J Respir Crit Care Med 2000;162(3 Pt 1):1004–8.

60. Culebras A. Sleep and neuromuscular disorders. Neurol Clin 2005;23(4):1209–23, ix.

61. Bennett JR, Dunroy HM, Corfield DR, et al. Respiratory muscle activity during REM sleep in patients with diaphragm paralysis. Neurology 2004;62(1): 134–7.

62. Ayas NT, Epstein LJ, Lieberman SL, et al. Predictors of loud snoring in persons with spinal cord injury. J Spinal Cord Med 2001;24(1):30–4.

63. Quera-Salva MA, Guilleminault C, Chevret S, et al. Breathing disorders during sleep in myasthenia gravis. Ann Neurol 1992;31(1):86–92.

64. Nicolle MW, Rask S, Koopman WJ, et al. Sleep apnea in patients with myasthenia gravis. Neurology 2006;67(1):140–2.

65. Martinez-Lapiscina EH, Erro ME, Ayuso T, et al. Myasthenia gravis: sleep quality, quality of life, and disease severity. Muscle Nerve 2012;46(2): 174–80.

66. Naseer S, Kolade VO, Idrees S, et al. Improvement in ocular myasthenia gravis during CPAP therapy for sleep apnea. Tenn Med 2012;105(9):33–4.

67. Culebras A. Sleep disorders associated with neuromuscular and spinal cord disorders. In: Greenamyre JT, editor. MedLink Neurology. San Diego: MedLink Corporation; 2006.

68. Sieminski M, Bilinska M, Nyka WM. Increased frequency of restless legs syndrome in myasthenia gravis. Eur Neurol 2012;68(3):166–70.

69. Zelman DC, Brandenburg NA, Gore M. Sleep impairment in patients with painful diabetic peripheral neuropathy. Clin J Pain 2006;22(8):681–5.

70. Pourfar M, Feigin A. The numb and the restless: peripheral neuropathy and RLS. Neurology 2009; 72(11):950–1.

71. Karkare K, Sinha S, Taly AB, et al. Prevalence and profile of sleep disturbances in Guillain-Barre syndrome: a prospective questionnaire-based study during 10 days of hospitalization. Acta Neurol Scand 2013;127(2):116–23.

72. Karkare K, Sinha S, Taly A, et al. Sleep abnormalities in Guillain Barre syndrome: a clinical and polysomnographic study. J Sleep Disord Ther 2013;2:109.

73. Nishino S, Kanbayashi T, Fujiki N, et al. CSF hypocretin levels in Guillain-Barre syndrome and other inflammatory neuropathies. Neurology 2003;61(6): 823–5.

74. Kanbayashi T, Ishiguro H, Aizawa R, et al. Hypocretin-1 (orexin-A) concentrations in cerebrospinal fluid are low in patients with Guillain-Barre syndrome. Psychiatry Clin Neurosci 2002;56(3):273–4.

75. Cochen V, Arnulf I, Demeret S, et al. Vivid dreams, hallucinations, psychosis and REM sleep in Guillain-Barre syndrome. Brain 2005;128(Pt 11): 2535–45.

76. Boentert M, Knop K, Schuhmacher C, et al. Sleep disorders in Charcot-Marie-Tooth disease type 1. J Neurol Neurosurg Psychiatry 2014;85(3):319–25.

77. Gemignani F, Marbini A, Di Giovanni G, et al. Charcot-Marie-Tooth disease type 2 with restless legs syndrome. Neurology 1999;52(5):1064–6.

78. Osanai S, Akiba Y, Nakano H, et al. Charcot-Marie-Tooth disease with diaphragmatic weakness. Intern Med (Tokyo, Japan) 1992;31(11):1267–70.

79. Dziewas R, Waldmann N, Bontert M, et al. Increased prevalence of obstructive sleep apnoea in patients with Charcot-Marie-Tooth disease: a case control study. J Neurol Neurosurg Psychiatry 2008;79(7): 829–31.

80. Benson B, Sulica L, Guss J, et al. Laryngeal neuropathy of Charcot-Marie-Tooth disease: further observations and novel mutations associated with vocal fold paresis. Laryngoscope 2010;120(2):291–6.

81. American Academy of Sleep Medicine. International classification of sleep disorders, 3rd edition. Darien (IL): American Academy of Sleep Medicine; 2014.

Occupational Sleep Medicine

Philip Cheng, PhD, Christopher Drake, PhD*

KEYWORDS

- Sleep • Sleepiness • Circadian rhythms • Work • Sleep disorders

KEY POINTS

- Occupational functioning can be affected by sleep loss, disordered sleep, and disruptions to circadian rhythms.
- Medical illnesses and medications can also affect sleep and sleepiness, resulting in added impairments to occupational functioning.
- The occupational consequences to disturbed sleep and sleepiness are numerous, although patients may lack insight into the ensuing consequences.

INTRODUCTION

The focus of occupational sleep medicine is predominantly organized around workplace productivity, safety, and health as influenced by sleep, circadian rhythms, and the assessment and treatment of sleep disorders. Sleepiness and sleep disturbance are common problems in the workplace and are associated with an array of adverse consequences, such as decreased productivity, increased risk for errors and accidents, and decrements in health and functioning. Depending on the occupational context, these consequences can be disastrous, as exemplified by historic accidents such as Chernobyl, Three Mile Island, and the Challenger explosion.

According to a national poll on adult sleep habits conducted by the National Sleep Foundation, sleep disturbance and sleepiness have become a significant problem in the working population.[1] Results from the poll found that more than one-third of the US workforce report daytime sleepiness, which amounts to approximately 5.7 million individuals, or roughly the entire population of Denmark. Similarly, 37% of working adults report symptoms that indicate risk for any sleep disorder.[2]

Although there are a multitude of causes for sleepiness and sleep disturbance, culprits can generally be organized into 5 overarching categories consisting of sleep deprivation, disordered sleep, disruptions in circadian rhythms, medical disorders, and medications. In addition to sleep duration, timing of sleep is also important to consider as sleep and alertness oscillate across 24 hours based on an internal biological clock. As such, sleepiness may also result when individuals are engaged in task performance at times when their biological clock is no longer actively promoting wakefulness, as occurs in the context of night shift work. Alternatively, sleepiness can also be a symptom of medical disorders involving dysregulations in the central nervous system, such as Parkinson's disease or narcolepsy, or may be a consequence of medications that influence central nervous system functioning, such as opiates or other sedating medications. We recommend that patients in occupational sleep medicine clinics are assessed on all 5 categories to achieve a comprehensive clinical landscape.

SLEEP AND WAKEFULNESS AS BIOLOGICAL PROCESSES

Sleep and wakefulness are governed by 2 biological processes that work in tandem.[3,4] The first process is often referred to as the *sleep-dependent process* (process S) and builds pressure for

Sleep Disorders and Research Center, Henry Ford Health System, Detroit, MI, USA
* Corresponding author.
E-mail address: cdrake1@hfhs.org

Sleep Med Clin 11 (2016) 65–79
http://dx.doi.org/10.1016/j.jsmc.2015.10.006
1556-407X/16/$ – see front matter © 2016 Elsevier Inc. All rights reserved.

sleep with each hour of extended wakefulness and dissipates during sleep (**Fig. 1**). As such, sleepiness may be consequential to the buildup of sleep pressure from prolonged wakefulness.

The second process is referred to as the *sleep-independent circadian process* (process C), which is reflected by a rhythmic variation of increased sleep propensity and enhanced alertness that is governed by a circadian oscillator.[4] This separate process explains why individuals undergoing total sleep deprivation often report a period of restored energy the following morning (because of the onset of a circadian alerting signal) despite a total lack of sleep. Importantly, this circadian process is calibrated/synchronized by a series of environmental cues, the most important of which is natural sunlight or bright artificial light.

SLEEP DEPRIVATION
Chronic Sleep Loss

The Sleep Research Society, American Academy of Sleep Medicine,[5] and the National Sleep Foundation[6] recently published recommendations for sleep duration for adults based on extensive review of sleep research and consensus among the leading experts in sleep medicine. The recommended amount of sleep for adults is between 7 and 9 hours of sleep. Based on this recommendation, a remarkably large number of individuals in the United States are chronically sleep deprived (regularly getting <7 hours of sleep a night). In fact, the 2002 Sleep in America poll found that 39% of adults in the United States report getting less than 7 hours of sleep during weeknights, and 22% continuing with less than 7 hours of sleep on weekends. Moreover, there is evidence that this number has been increasing since 1984.[7]

Assessment of sleepiness
Inadequate sleep satiation most commonly leads to sleepiness, which can be measured both subjectively and objectively. Increased subjective feelings of sleepiness can reflect an increased propensity for sleep (ie, sleep pressure). Measures of sleep propensity form the basis of assessments that index sleepiness using objective methods. Well-validated objective and subjective measures of sleepiness have been used successfully for decades, and are valuable tools for use in broad-based clinical practice settings (self-report, eg, Epworth Sleepiness Scale) and sleep medicine (electroencephalogram-based measures).

Importantly, individuals habituate to the feeling of sleepiness over time despite the buildup of performance deficits with accumulating sleep debt.[8] While subjective sleepiness is easily identified after acute sleep deprivation, habituation occurs following chronic sleep restriction, which can lead to inaccurate perception and self-report of sleepiness. For example, an early study indicated that sleep-deprived train operators were not able to accurately identify imminent dozing,[9] thereby reducing accurate self-assessment of accident risk (eg, falling asleep at the wheel).

Subjective measures of sleepiness Self-report measures of sleepiness can be completed via clinical interview, or using a range of validated sleepiness questionnaires. Because accidental dozing is a natural consequence of sleepiness, assessments can also capture reported likelihood of dozing across various situations, which can help reduce the subjectivity involved with clinical impression and provide normative data for comparison. The Epworth Sleepiness Scale[10] (ESS) is one such instrument that is standardized and validated. The ESS is commonly used to index sleepiness based on likelihood of dozing in situations such as "sitting and reading" or "in a car, while stopped for a few minutes in traffic." The ESS indexes sleepiness via estimated sleep propensity rather than perceived feelings of sleepiness, and is intended to capture a

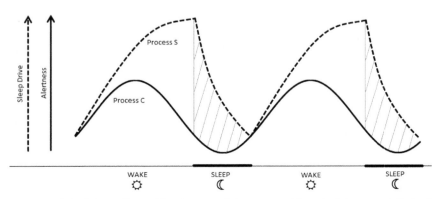

Fig. 1. Two-process model of sleep. Sleep drive (process S) increases with wakefulness and dissipates with sleep. The circadian signal (process C) oscillates rhythmically across day and night.

general level of sleepiness as opposed to reported sleepiness at a particular point in time. The ESS has also been used extensively in the context of sleep disorders, such as obstructive sleep apnea. A score of 0 to 9 on the ESS corresponds to normal levels of sleepiness,[11] and a score of 10 or greater suggests excessive daytime sleepiness of potential clinical significance.

Objective measures of sleepiness Objective measures of sleepiness are also available, and the 2 most widely used measures use the rapidity of sleep onset to determine the degree of sleepiness. Such tests are administered during the daytime and include the Multiple Sleep Latency Test (MSLT) and the Maintenance of Wakefulness Test (MWT). The MSLT measures the mean latency to sleep on at least 4 separate trials, where participants are asked to try to sleep during the day. Individuals who show an average sleep-onset latency of 8 minutes or less are considered excessively sleepy, which is consistent with a disorder of hypersomnolence. Note that the presence of excessive sleepiness is not a diagnostic procedure but rather an important assessment tool that is used to guide clinical diagnoses within the context of a thorough clinical sleep evaluation, including overnight polysomnography (PSG) and patients' descriptions of nocturnal sleep (see Vaughn and Giallanza[12] for a review of PSG assessment procedures).

Although the MSLT is commonly used as the gold standard objective measure of sleepiness, its ecological validity is sometimes challenged, particularly for the purposes of occupational medicine. Specifically, it is argued that although the MSLT measures propensity to fall asleep, it lacks the face validity of assessing one's ability to remain awake. The latter may have more ecological validity with respect to maintaining alertness while performing occupational tasks. Thus, the MWT is often presented as a preferred alternative to the MSLT because it assesses the ability to remain awake.[13] Both the MWT[14] and the MSLT[15] have been shown to predict driving performance and documented vehicular accidents. Normative data are also available for both measures.[15,16]

The American Academy of Sleep Medicine recommends that MWT be used when the primary outcome is ability to remain awake, and that each MWT should last for 40 minutes.[13] The MSLT should be used when disorders of excessive somnolence (narcolepsy, idiopathic hypersomnolence) are critically important to rule out in the context of an assessment. However, data obtained during the overnight PSG (ie, nocturnal REM onset) can often be used to confirm the presence of such disorders.[17]

DISORDERED SLEEP

Although some individuals may choose to curtail sleep duration for various reasons, others suffer sleep disturbances consequent to disordered sleep. Among the various sleep disorders as outlined in the International Classification of Sleep Disorders,[18] insomnia and obstructive sleep apnea are most common.

Insomnia

Insomnia is the most prevalent of all sleep disorders, and insomnia in adults is characterized by persistent difficulties initiating and maintaining sleep, or waking up earlier than desired. The disturbance(s) to sleep results in consequences during wakefulness, such as fatigue, attentional difficulties, impaired social or occupational performance, mood disturbance, sleepiness, behavioral problems, reduced motivation, and concerns or dissatisfactions about sleep. Symptoms are frequent and persistent, defined by the International Classification of Sleep Disorders as occurring at least 3 times per week and lasting for at least 3 months.

The burden of insomnia on occupational functioning is widely documented. In a large sample of 948 individuals randomly recruited from a national census,[19] participants reporting clinically significant insomnia were at increased likelihood to also report more frequent and varied health care utilization compared with good sleepers, including general practitioners, psychiatrists, social workers, psychologists, pharmacists, acupuncturists, homeopaths, and massage therapists. Additionally, those with clinically significant insomnia were also more likely to use medications for mood disturbance, anxiety, disorders of bone/muscle/conjunctive tissues, and infectious/parasitic diseases. Not surprisingly, those with clinically significant insomnia also missed an average of 9 more hours of paid work in the previous 3 months and reported less productivity. The collective monetary value of absenteeism and lost productivity was estimated at $41.1 billion,[20] which is approximately twice the amount of the annual federal revenue derived from business taxes.

Assessment of insomnia can include clinical interview in conjunction with validated instruments. The Insomnia Severity Index[21] is a commonly used 7-item instrument to assess risk and severity of insomnia and can also be used to track improvements throughout treatment. The Insomnia Severity Index assesses for difficulties with sleep initiation, sleep maintenance, and waking too early, and scores at or greater than 15 are considered clinically significant. Assessment also commonly includes 1 to 2 weeks of sleep diaries.[22] Chesson and colleagues[23] detail recommendations of assessment for insomnia as put forth by the American Academy for Sleep Medicine (AASM).

Although patients with insomnia report sleepiness/fatigue, objective measures of sleepiness are more likely to indicate hyperarousal of the central nervous system (for review, see Riemann and colleagues[24]). As such, sleepiness is often distinguished from fatigue, which is better characterized by a state of low energy. Patients with insomnia commonly report fatigue but are unable to achieve efficient and consolidated sleep because of hyperarousal and have reduced levels of sleepiness as assessed using objective measures.[25]

Treatment for insomnia can include use of hypnotic medications (eg, zolpidem), psychosocial interventions (eg, cognitive-behavioral therapy for insomnia), or a combination of both. Morgenthaler and colleagues[26] review the psychological and behavioral treatment of insomnia as recommended by the AASM.

Currently, nonbenzodiazepine hypnotics such as zolpidem, eszopiclone, and zaleplon are commonly prescribed for insomnia. Benzodiazepines such as alprazolam, lorazepam, and clonazepam are also used at times as a sleep aid (for review, see Rosini and Dogra[27] and Rouch and colleagues[28]). Both nonbenzodiazepine GABA receptor agonists and benzodiazepines, while generally considered safe, have been associated with concerns including psychomotor control and increased arousal thresholds. Other adverse events may include nausea, dizziness, malaise, agitation, and headaches.[29,30]

A wide range of other medications are also used to treat insomnia, many of which include off-label use. Since the mid 1980s, there has been a rise in the off-label use of low-dose antidepressants in treating insomnia, particularly with trazodone. Doxepin in low doses (1, 3, and 6 mg) has also been shown to increase sleep maintenance in insomnia,[31] and has recently received approval to treat insomnia by the US Food and Drug Administration (FDA). Doxepin has been purported to have less impairing effects on arousal (which impacts awakening arousal threshold, balance, memory, etc) compared to other sleep aids,[32] though further comparative research is needed. Over the counter (OTC) sleep aids are also used. These are often anti-histaminergic agents, which are usually longer acting and therefore increase next-morning hang-over effects.[33] Notably, tolerance may develop quickly for many sleep aids, such as trazodone and diphenhydramine. Newer

pharmacological approaches include use of ramelteon and suvorexant. Ramelteon is FDA approved to treat insomnia characterized by difficulty with sleep onset, and is a chronobiotic that acts as a selective melatonin receptor agonist to regulate sleep-wake timing.[34] Finally, suvorexant is the first orexin (hypocretin) receptor antagonist and has received FDA approval to treat insomnia.[35] Suvorexant acts as an oxrein receptor antagonist in order to dampen wakefulness and promote sleep.

Obstructive Sleep Apnea

Another common culprit of sleep disturbance and excessive sleepiness is obstructive sleep apnea (OSA), which results from disordered breathing during sleep, often in the form of total or partial occlusions in the upper airway. When apneic events occur repeatedly throughout the night, sleep continuity is disrupted, and the restorative properties of sleep are reduced, resulting in excessive daytime sleepiness and impairments in occupational functioning.[36] Of note, OSA patients are particularly vulnerable to vehicular accidents (see later discussion).

Common assessments for OSA include the ESS, the Stop Bang questionnaire,[37] and additional medical assessment for micrognathia, retrognathia, or narrowed posterior oropharynx, often using the Mallampati classification.[38] However, a diagnosis of OSA can only be confirmed using either in-laboratory PSG or home testing with portable monitors. Positive airway pressure therapies are widely used for improving sleep and alertness in OSA, with evidence indicating that use of continuous positive airway pressure (CPAP) results in decreased risk for automobile accidents.[39,40] For further guidelines on the assessment and management of OSA, see recommendations published by the AASM.[41]

CIRCADIAN RHYTHMS

Timing of sleep and wakefulness is also influential to health and functioning. Although human beings generally exhibit nocturnal sleep and diurnal wakefulness, evidence also indicates that a range of individual differences exist for preferential timing of sleep and peak times for alertness and performance. When individuals are engaged in task performance at times that are at odds with their circadian phase, there can be adverse consequences to both performance and health.

Chronotype

Although individuals commonly have a preference for sleep between midnight and 8 AM,[42] some deviate significantly from this range. Some individuals exhibit tendencies toward later sleep and wake times (ie, night owls), whereas others have a preference for earlier sleep and wake times (ie, morning larks). Chronotype can be assessed using validated questionnaires, including the Morningness-Eveningness Questionnaire,[43] the Munich Chronotype Questionnaire,[44] or the Composite Scale of Morningness.[45]

A large epidemiologic study of chronotype found that 8.2% of the population show a preference of initiating sleep at or after 3 AM on free days, suggesting that these individuals are likely phase delayed in timing of both sleep and alertness in reference to most workers.[42] For these individuals, performance during the regular work day (9 AM to 5 PM) may be less productive either because of sleep curtailment (due to their late bed time) or a delayed circadian signal for alertness during the work day.

Interestingly, research on school start times may shed light on the mismatch between chronotype and work schedule. Despite the fact that adolescents commonly exhibit a delayed sleep phase that is part of normal development, school start times are often quite early (approximately 7:30 AM). When school start times are delayed, improvements in performance are observed, including increased attendance, decreased lateness from oversleeping, decreased reports of sleepiness, reduced sleeping during morning classes, reduced depression, and reduced sick days (for review, see Au and colleagues[46]).

Delayed Sleep-Wake Phase Disorder

At the extreme, variations in individuals' chronotype become too discrepant with societal norms, leading to reduced occupational functioning. Deviations toward a later circadian phase is more common, and, when clinically significant, is referred to as delayed sleep-wake phase disorder (DSWPD). DSWPD is characterized by a significant delay in preferred sleep-wake rhythms as evidenced by a chronic or recurrent complaint of inability to fall asleep and difficulty awakening at a desired or required clock time. Furthermore, when allowed to sleep ad libitum, patients should show a delayed sleep phase that is of better sleep quality.

Assessment of DSWPD may include clinical interview in conjunction with two weeks of 24-hour sleep diaries. Various treatments are available for DSWPD, some which address the symptoms of sleepiness, and others that target the endogenous circadian timing. Prescribed sleep-wake scheduling is often used to make incremental adjustments until the desired sleep-wake schedule is reached. This is sometimes supplemented with the use of a hypnotic.[47] Treatments that directly target circadian timing may include use of melatonin and/or bright light to advance the intrinsic circadian rhythm. Administration of melatonin (dose ranges from 0.3 to 5 mg) prior to bed time (30 minutes to 6 hours depending on dose) can engender advances in circadian timing.[48,49] Alternatively, exposure to bright light (2000–10,000 lux) following awakening can also result in advances in circadian timing.

Notably, the American Academy of Sleep Medicine recently published an updated clinical practice guideline for the treatment of intrinsic circadian rhythm sleep-wake disorders,[50] in which strategically timed melatonin administration was the only treatment recommended due to a paucity of existing high grade evidence. As such, further research is needed in order to clearly assess the effectiveness of the available treatments.

Individuals with DSWPD typically experience difficulties waking in time for work and school, leading to frequent lateness and subsequent penalties. This lateness often causes interruptions that lead to prolonged periods of schooling, or difficulty maintaining steady employment. Even when punctuality is addressed, performance is often compromised because of sleep deprivation or reduced circadian alertness. As such, it may also follow that workers with a delayed sleep phase may benefit from flexibility in delaying their work schedule.

Shift Work Disorder

Approximately 20% of the population in the United States (about 30 million people) is engaged in shift work, which is defined as any work schedule that occurs outside of the traditional 9 AM to 5 PM work day. In approximately 10% of the US workforce (about 3 million workers), the severity of sleep disturbance and sleepiness meets criteria for shift work disorder (SWD).[51] As determined by the International Classification of Sleep Disorders (3rd edition),[18] SWD is characterized by insomnia or excessive sleepiness during wakefulness accompanied by a reduction of total sleep time not due to voluntary sleep restriction. Symptoms should be related temporally to a shift work schedule that overlaps with usual sleep time before starting shift work and has been present for at least 3 months. Assessment of shift work disorder can be conducted via clinical interview or the 4-item SWD screening questionnaire[52] in conjunction with actigraphy and sleep diaries for at least 14 days to demonstrate a disturbed sleep-wake pattern.

Circadian misalignment

Symptoms of disturbed sleep and excessive sleepiness can be attributed in part to the misalignment of biological rhythms and work schedule. This misalignment occurs because workers are attempting sleep during the day when their circadian signal for wakefulness is increasing, and working during the night when their circadian signal is promoting sleep. As a result, shift workers are often sleep deprived because of fragmented and curtailed daytime sleep, which is compounded by reduced circadian alertness during the night shift.

Although workers with SWD experience similar difficulties in health and productivity as those with insomnia, individuals may also experience additional impairments caused by excessive sleepiness (as opposed to hyperarousal) during work (for review, see Cheng and Drake[53]). Because shift work frequently includes safety-sensitive operations such as transportation, medicine, and emergency response, accidents caused by sleepiness can be especially catastrophic and symptoms should be addressed immediately at the time of identification using both acute (ie, alertness-enhancing medications) or long-term treatments (ie, behavioral circadian interventions).

Treatment of circadian misalignment

Symptoms of sleep and sleepiness are often addressed via hypnotic medications and wake-promoting agents (see later discussion). Caffeine has also been indicated to enhance alertness during the night shift, although care must be taken in the timing of use to avoid impairing daytime sleep. Research using simulated shift work has indicated that caffeine (dose of 4 mg/kg of body weight) administered at approximately 22:30 improved alertness and performance.[54] Alternatively, naps before or during the night shift also effectively improve alertness and performance during the shift.[55] Other studies have found that naps in combination with caffeine use can also reduce workplace sleepiness and improve work performance.[56]

Although addressing symptoms of insomnia and sleepiness in shift work or other circadian rhythm disorders can improve functioning, it does not directly address circadian misalignment as a causal mechanism. This finding is important because internal desynchrony of body clocks may also be associated with medical morbidities.[57–59] As such, it may also be important to consider interventions that reduce circadian misalignment.

Exposure to bright light is the primary mechanism for circadian entrainment, and interventions that target circadian misalignment typically use specifically timed exposure to light and darkness. Interventions using specifically timed exposure to bright light (2000–10,000 lux at the cornea) have gained empirical support. Light exposure shows effectiveness at various doses,[55] which may be determined based on the intended effect of improving momentary alertness or shifting circadian rhythms. The use of light-blocking goggles in the morning (approximately 6–11 AM) is critical when shifting circadian rhythms, especially because shift workers may be exposed to natural sunlight before their scheduled sleep time. Similarly, light-blocking shades should be installed in the sleeping environment to prevent exposure to sunlight during daytime sleep and supplemented with earplugs to reduce the impact of environmental noise.

Currently, there are no US Food and Drug Administration–approved medications that have been found to adjust circadian rhythms in night shift workers. However, use of melatonin as a chronobiotic intervention has shown promise in controlled studies of simulated shift work.[60,61] Investigations indicate that the impact of melatonin on shifting circadian rhythms is phase dependent, with administration in the morning resulting in phase delays, and administration in the evening resulting in phase advances.

COMMON MEDICAL ILLNESSES THAT AFFECT SLEEP AND SLEEPINESS

Although sleep disorders are prevalent, they are not the only disorders that impact occupational functioning. In fact, sleep disorders are likely a small fraction of more prevalent occupational illnesses, such as musculoskeletal disease, mental illness, or traumatic injuries. However, sleep disruption and sleepiness also commonly manifest as symptoms of medical illness. Assessment of sleep disturbance and sleepiness is particularly important in these circumstances because these symptoms occur in addition to the primary medical problem, resulting in significant adverse consequences to occupational functioning, or serve as complications to interventions.

Brain-related injuries and disorders are highly prevalent, and often result in disturbed sleep and excessive sleepiness. As a result, traumatic workplace injuries have been identified as a key priority by the National Institute for Occupational Safety and Health.[62] Traumatic brain injuries and stroke often lead to insomnia, hypersomnia, sleep-disordered breathing, and excessive daytime sleepiness (for review, see Vermaelen and colleagues[63]), which add to the impact of the cognitive impairments from the injury.

Brain injuries also increase the risk of neurodegenerative illnesses.[64,65] Excessive sleepiness is often observed in neurodegenerative illnesses[66] such as Parkinson's disease,[67] Alzheimer's disease, and dementia with Lewy bodies.[68] Common sleep-related problems associated with these diseases include sleep fragmentation and nighttime wakefulness, increased light sleep, and reduced deep sleep.

Patients with chronic pain (eg, fibromyalgia) also commonly report impaired sleep, which further increases pain sensitivity.[69] Sleepiness is often a common symptom of infectious diseases, which can affect sleep and sleepiness through the increased production of inflammatory cytokines or activation of the hypothalamic–pituitary–adrenal axis (for review, see Pollmächer and colleagues[70]). Other medical conditions associated with sleepiness include metabolic syndrome/obesity,[71] asthma,[72] nocturnal gastroesophageal reflux,[73] and psychiatric disorders.[74]

MEDICATIONS THAT AFFECT SLEEP AND SLEEPINESS

Medications that act on the central nervous system are also likely to influence sleep and alertness, which in turn impact occupational functioning. Some medications are prescribed to assuage symptoms of sleep disturbance and sleepiness, and should be used in a way that minimizes impact on work performance and safety. For example, individuals experience hangover effects from some hypnotics that can increase risk for vehicular accidents, particularly in the elderly.[75,76] As such, timing of hypnotic use may be important to consider.

Sleepiness can also result from medications that have sedating side effects (**Box 1**), and a comprehensive assessment of medication use is often helpful in identifying contributors to excessive sleepiness. Often, the timing of sedating medications may be altered to reduce its interference with functioning during wakefulness. For example, antidepressant medications such as mirtazapine can often have sedating side effects and, therefore, can be used prior to bed time.

Stimulants and wake-promoting agents are commonly used to increase wakefulness in occupational settings. Wake-promoting agents such as modafinil and armodafinil are a newer class of alerting medications that have recently become first-line agents for excessive sleepiness because of the lower potential for abuse.[77] The timing for use of alerting medications is important, as they can interfere with sleep. For example, methylphenidate (ie, Concerta) can have an effect for up to

12 hours, which can result in disrupted sleep if intake occurs later in the day.

Other medications may also have side effects that disrupt sleep. These medications may disrupt sleep through their impact on the central nervous system (eg, alterations to sleep architecture from certain antidepressant medications) or through the peripheral nervous system (eg, nighttime coughing from angiotensin-converting enzyme inhibitors). Some medications such as analgesics or appetite suppressants may also contain caffeine, which may disrupt sleep if taken within proximity to bedtime (5 PM or later). Diuretic medications can also fragment sleep by increasing nighttime urination. **Box 2** contains a list of common medications that disrupt sleep and can have alerting side effects.

There may be circumstances in which timing of medications may not be easily altered to accommodate sleep or wakefulness. For example, benzodiazepines may be used for its anxiolytic effect to support job performance, but the resulting drowsiness may also detract from its intended purpose. In such cases, alternative medications may be considered, or an alerting medication may also be used when appropriate. The interactional effects of multiple medications may be unknown, and is an important consideration.

CONSEQUENCES OF DISTURBED SLEEP AND SLEEPINESS

Because sleep is so essential for survival and healthy functioning, the consequences of inadequate sleep are numerous and pervasive.

Box 1
List of some common medications that have sedating side effects

First-generation antihistamines (eg, Benadryl)

Sedating antidepressants (eg, mirtazapine, trazodone, amitriptyline)

Anxiolytics (eg, diazepam, lorazem)

Pain medications (eg, opiates, narcotics)

Sedating anticonvulsants (eg, gabapentin, carbamazepine)

Antipsychotics (eg, quetiapine, risperidone, olanzapine)

Hypnotics (eg, benzodiazepines, nonbenzodiazepine hypnotics, melatonin agonists)

Dopamine agonists for Parkinson's disease (eg, pramipexole, ropinirole, pergolide)

Some muscle relaxants (eg, cyclobenzoprine)

Box 2
List of some common medications that have alerting side effects and can disrupt sleep

---

Alerting antidepressants (eg, selective serotonin reuptake inhibitors, tricyclic)

Corticosteroids   (eg,   prednisone, methylprednisolone)

Smoking cessation medications (eg, nicotine patches)

Angiotensin-converting enzyme inhibitors

Diuretics

Ephedrine and pseudoephedrine

Some immunosuppressants (eg, tacrolimus, ciclosporin)

Antineoplastic agents

Attention-deficit   hyperactive   disorder medications

Thyroid medications (eg, aminophylline)

However, sleep-deprived individuals may not necessarily have insight into the ensuing consequences, and may therefore underestimate their risk for errors and accidents. In a study in which performance on a critical thinking task was examined, sleep-deprived individuals reported higher confidence in their performance than sleep-satiated individuals, despite having objectively lower scores.[78] These results suggest that workers who are sleep deprived may not readily recognize their sleep debt and may also have limited insight into any consequential deficits in performance. As such, patients may benefit from education regarding the commonly observed consequences, which often affect cognitive functioning, affective functioning, safety, and health.

Excessive Sleepiness

For individuals working at night, excessive sleepiness may be a major challenge to occupational performance and safety. Although the prevalence of excessive sleepiness varies based on the operational definition, most studies find that at least 75% of shift workers report excessive sleepiness during work,[79] which is notably higher than the 7.7% reported in day workers.[80] Naturally, excessive sleepiness during shift work also leads to increased accidental sleeping during work. A study comparing nurses working various shifts reported that as many as 35.3% of nurses working nights reported accidentally falling asleep compared with only 2.7% of accidental sleeping reported in nurses working days.[81]

Cognitive Performance

Vigilance

Perhaps the most reliable experimentally demonstrated impairment caused by sleep loss is decreased vigilance.[82,83] Vigilance is of particular interest and importance because it is critical for error detection and prevention in safety-sensitive operations. One study of threat detection performance on a simulated luggage screening task (similar to that conducted by the Transportation Security Administration agents at airports) compared performance in individuals who were sleep deprived versus those who were sleep satiated.[84] Results showed that those who were deprived of sleep were less able to maintain vigilance throughout the task, and exhibited faster decreases in accuracy and less total time spent on the task.

Errors

One of the most critical indicators of reduced cognitive performance is the occurrence of errors. Research examining errors in the medical setting found that shift work in interns is related to increased serious diagnostic and medication errors (errors in ordering or administration of pharmaceutical agents, intravenous fluids, or blood products) as well as increased rates of patient death.[85,86] Similarly, another study comparing nurses on rotating shifts and day or evening shifts found that rotators were twice as likely to commit work-related accidents or errors and 2.5 times more likely to have near-miss accidents.[81] Moreover, there is also evidence suggesting that shift workers may exhibit impairments not only for error detection, but also reduced capacity for error correction.[87]

Processing speed

Sleepy individuals also show reduced speed in information processing, evidenced by slower response times on myriad tasks (for review see Durmer and Dinges[88]). Reduced reaction time in tasks for which speed is critical, such as emergency response (police officers, emergency medical technicians) can have fatal consequences, particularly when combined with the effects of sleep inertia.[89]

Logical reasoning

Logical reasoning is also found to vary across the circadian period, and is thus affected in shift work. In reasoning tasks where individuals are asked to evaluate the accuracy of statements at varying semantic complexities, response accuracies declined starting at approximately 1 AM and reached a low point at 5 AM.[90] Response times also followed a similar trend, with time for trial completion increasing at approximately 1 AM, and the longest response times occurring in the morning hours between 6 and 8 AM. This suggests that night shift workers may take longer to make decisions involving reasoning and may also be more prone to reasoning errors during their shift.

Learning and memory

The ability to learn and retain information is critical for effective performance across a range of occupations. Research indicates that sleep also plays an important role in the strengthening and consolidation of previously encoded memories, as indicated by sleep-dependent improvements on memory tasks for both declarative (ie, knowledge based on declarable fact) and implicit memory tasks (eg, performance of a skills).[91,92]

Unsurprisingly, sleep-deprived individuals also show deficits related to memory formation and consolidation. Not only do individuals lose the benefit of offline memory consolidation, loss of sleep further impacts encoding of new information. As demonstrated in a neuroimaging study in sleep-deprived individuals, deficits in hippocampal activity during episodic memory encoding was detected and associated with decreased recall.[93] This finding suggests that workers who are sleep deprived may not only be less able to encode new information or procedures, they may also be less able to retain the information that was initially encoded. Finally, sleep-deprived individuals also appear to have decreased ability to modify existing memories,[94] which is necessary when occupational procedures are changed or updated.

Insight

In a widely cited study in which performance on a novel task was tested, volunteers were randomly assigned into 3 conditions: 8 hours of nocturnal sleep, nocturnal wakefulness, or daytime wakefulness.[95] Improvement on this task occurs gradually with practice, although significant gains in performance may also be achieved if a hidden abstract rule was discovered. Volunteers were not informed of the existence of this short cut. Results showed that twice as many individuals in the nocturnal sleep condition demonstrated spontaneous insight into the short cut compared with both conditions of extended wakefulness. This study suggests sleepy workers may be at a disadvantage in gaining insight for solution to work-related challenges.

Creativity

Creativity is also often important in successful work performance and requires cognitive flexibility. In a study of shift workers with shift work disorder, use of armodafinil significantly improved performance on the Remote Associates Test, which is a task measuring creativity via word association.[96] Results showed that creativity improved after use of armodafinil, indicating that sleepy workers may show deficits in creative thinking.

Psychomotor Functioning

Research also shows circadian variation in psychomotor control, which can impact performance in tasks requiring manual labor or complex psychomotor tasks, such as surgery and driving. Manual dexterity was previously found to decrease after 11 PM and reached a nadir at approximately 5 AM,[90] which also coincides with circadian nadir of alertness. This finding suggests that shift workers may be at increased risk for manual errors or even injuries related to equipment operation. Not surprisingly, this finding was confirmed in a study showing that night shift medical interns were at higher risk of self-injury from used needles compared with day shift interns.[97] Furthermore, of all percutaneous injuries with at least one contributing factor cited, fatigue was implicated in 56% of incidents, and lapses in attention were implicated in 62%.

Emotion Regulation

It has long been established that sleep and emotional health are intimately related, as is evident by the heightened risk of psychopathology after the development of insomnia. Emotional functioning is an important construct in workplace psychology because it often guides decision making and impacts workplace morale and relationships (for review on the impact of sleepiness in the workplace, see Mullins and colleagues[98]).

Research has found that sleep loss results in compromised brain functioning in areas responsible for emotion and emotion regulation. In particular, sleep loss is related to increased negative affect, such as hostility, and decreased positive affect, such as cheerfulness or joviality.[99] As a result, individuals experiencing chronic sleep loss may appear cantankerous, and in turn experience a reduction in positive relations with others. This can significantly decrease workplace morale, which can subsequently impact efficiency and productivity.

Additionally, neuroimaging research found that sleep loss reduces brain function in areas responsible for emotion and emotion regulation, indicating that sleep-deprived individuals may experience emotions more intensely, particularly with negatively valenced emotions.[100] This suggests that sleep-deprived workers may not only be more affected by stress but also less able to engage in stress management and regulation.

Drowsy Driving

One major area of risk resulting from sleep deprivation is drowsy driving. Traffic accidents are an increasing cause of death and injury in the world, and epidemiologic studies estimate that up to 25% of fatal vehicular accidents are sleep related.[101–103] Sleep deprivation is found to be common among professional drivers. An earlier study on professional truck drivers found that the mean duration of sleep was 4.78 hours a day,[104] which is significantly lower than the 7 hour minimum recommended for adults.

Box 3
Summary of updated recommendations regarding the clinical management of driving risk in patients with suspected or confirmed OSA

Recommendation 1

Assess for daytime sleepiness, accidental dozing during inappropriate times, and recent vehicular accidents or near misses attributable to sleepiness, fatigues, or inattention. Patients displaying these characteristics are regarded as high-risk drivers and should be educated and warned about the potential risks of driving until effective intervention has been instituted.

Recommendation 2

Inquire about additional potential causes of sleepiness (eg, inadequate sleep time, use of alcohol, or sedating medications), comorbid neurocognitive impairments (eg, neurologic disorders, depression), and diminished physical skills.

Recommendation 3

Initial visits for patients with suspected OSA include symptom severity, driving risk, and previous treatments received. Subsequent visits should routinely elicit information on adherence and response to treatments, with repeated driving risk assessment for high-risk drivers.

Recommendation 4

Education regarding risks of drowsy driving and behavioral methods of reducing such risks should also extend to patients' families when possible.

Recommendation 5 (weak)

For patients with high risk for OSA and deemed high-risk drivers, assessment (PSG or home portable monitoring, based on patient characteristics) and treatment (when indicated) should be initiated as soon as possible, preferably within 1 month of initial visit.

Recommendation 6 (weak)

Empiric CPAP should not be used in patients with suspected OSA and deemed as high-risk driver for the sole purpose of reducing driving risk.

Recommendation 7 (strong)

For patients with confirmed OSA, CPAP therapy to reduce driving risk is strongly recommended over no treatment.

Recommendation 8 (weak)

For patients with suspected or confirmed OSA and deemed high-risked drivers, wake promoting or stimulant medications should not be prescribed for the sole purpose of reducing driving risk.

Recommendation 9

Health providers should be familiar with the presentation and complications of excessive sleepiness and local and state statutes or regulations regarding the compulsory reporting of high-risk drivers with OSA. In states with permissive reporting mechanisms, the Department of Motor Vehicles should be notified if the highest-risk patients (eg, severe daytime sleepiness and previous vehicular accident or near miss) insist on driving before the condition has been successfully treated, or fail to comply with treatment requirements.

See official publication[112] for additional clarification and underlying rationale.

Data from Strohl KP, Brown DB, Collop N, et al. An official American thoracic society clinical practice guideline: sleep apnea, sleepiness, and driving risk in noncommercial drivers. An update of a 1994 Statement. Am J Respir Crit Care Med 2013;187(11):1259–66.

Sleepiness while driving has also been documented. A 2012 National Sleep Foundation poll of transportation professionals found that 15% of truck drivers, 26% of train operators, and 10% of bus/taxi/limo drivers reported that their job performance was affected by sleepiness at least once a week. Furthermore, a study monitoring encephalography of truck drivers on the job found that more than half of the drivers showed signs of physiologically verified drowsiness while driving, and 2 drivers demonstrated one occasion of entering stage 1 sleep while driving.[104] In another study on commercial truck drivers, more than 20% reported dozing at least twice in the past 3 months while driving.[105]

Apart from the apparent dangers of falling asleep at the wheel, drowsy drivers also experience other impairments that increase risk for accidents, including delayed reaction time, lapses in attention, and impaired decision making.[106] In fact, driving performance on a simulator after 21 hours of wakefulness was comparable to performance when intoxicated (as defined by the legal limit of 0.08% blood alcohol concentration).[107] The impairments include increased variation in speed, decreased ability to drive in the center of the lane, and increased variation in lane position (eg, weaving).

Not surprisingly, drowsy driving leads to a higher rate of vehicular accidents or near misses. In a large sample of approximately 4000 randomly selected drivers, habitually sleepy drivers reported more than 13 times the risk for vehicular accidents compared with nonsleepy drivers.[108] Another study found that near misses caused by accidental dozing had occurred in 17% of drivers.[105] Similarly, medical professionals are also at increased risk for accidents, especially after extended work shifts, which confer more than twice the risk for a vehicular accident and almost 6 times the risk for near misses.[109]

Obstructive sleep apnea and drowsy driving

OSA (see previous discussion) has been identified as an important risk factor for drowsy driving. Prior research show that patients with an apnea-hypopnea index (average apnea events per hour) of 10 or higher have a 2- to 6-fold higher risk for vehicular accidents compared with those without OSA.[110,111] This has resulted in discussions regarding the importance of screening and management of driving risk in OSA.

To date, there is still limited empirical evidence that speaks clearly and comprehensively to the clinical management of drowsy driving in OSA. Nevertheless, the American Thoracic Society has published updated recommendations based on available research and expert opinions (**Box 3**).[112]

Health and Productivity

In addition to performance outcomes, chronic sleep deprivation also leads to adverse health outcomes, which results in increased absenteeism and increased utilization of health services and workers' compensation. Sleep deprivation is also found to increase the perception of pain,[113] impair glucose tolerance,[114] and compromise immune functioning,[115] ultimately leading to increased risk for morbidities such as obesity, diabetes, hypertension, and overall reduced longevity.

Disorders involving inadequate sleep duration or sleep quality also tend to be highly comorbid with other illnesses. For example, insomnia is highly comorbid with psychiatric and medical disorders such as depression, anxiety, and hypertension.[116–118] Similarly, individuals with OSA are also at risk for medical morbidities, including cardiovascular illness,[119,120] obesity,[121] and diabetes,[122] which may contribute to the 6-fold increase in all-cause mortality associated with OSA.[123]

REFERENCES

1. National Sleep Foundation. 2002 Sleep in America poll: adult sleep habits. Washington, DC: The Foundation; 2002.

2. Swanson LM, Arnedt J, Rosekind MR, et al. Sleep disorders and work performance: findings from the 2008 National Sleep Foundation Sleep in America poll. J Sleep Res 2011;20(3):487–94.

3. Achermann P. The two-process model of sleep regulation revisited. Aviat Space Environ Med 2004;75(Supplement 1):A37–43.

4. Borbély A. A two process model of sleep regulation. Hum Neurobiol 1982;1(3):195–204.

5. Watson NF, Badr MS, Belenky G, et al. Recommended amount of sleep for a healthy adult: a joint consensus statement of the American academy of sleep medicine and sleep research society. J Clin Sleep Med 2015;11(6):591–2. Available at: http://www-ncbi-nlm-nih-gov.proxy.lib.umich.edu/pubmed/25979105.

6. Hirshkowitz M, Whiton K, Albert SM, et al. National Sleep Foundation's sleep time duration recommendations: methodology and results summary. Sleep Health 2015;1(1):40–3.

7. National Center for Health Statistics. Quick-Stats: percentage of adults who reported an average of≤ 6 hours of sleep per 24-hour period, by sex and age group—United States, 1985 and 2004. MMWR Morb Mortal Wkly Rep 2005;54:933.

8. Van Dongen H, Maislin G, Mullington JM, et al. The cumulative cost of additional wakefulness: dose-response effects on neurobehavioral functions and sleep physiology from chronic sleep restriction and total sleep deprivation. Sleep 2003;26(2):117–29.

9. Åkerstedt T, Torsvall L, Fröberg JE. A questionnaire study of sleep/wake disturbances and irregular work hours. Sleep Res 1983;12:358.

10. Johns MW. A new method for measuring daytime sleepiness: the Epworth sleepiness scale. Sleep 1991;14(6):540–5.

11. Johns MW. Sleepiness in different situations measured by the Epworth Sleepiness Scale. Sleep 1994;17(8):703–10.

12. Vaughn BV, Giallanza P. Technical review of polysomnography. Chest 2008;134(6):1310–9.

13. Littner M, Kushida C, Wise M, et al. Practice parameters for clinical use of the multiple sleep latency test and the maintenance of wakefulness test. Sleep 2005;28(1):113–21.

14. Sagaspe P, Taillard J, Chaumet G, et al. Maintenance of wakefulness test as a predictor of driving performance in patients with untreated obstructive sleep apnea. Sleep 2007;30(3):327.

15. Drake C, Roehrs T, Breslau N, et al. The 10-year risk of verified motor vehicle crashes in relation to physiologic sleepiness. Sleep 2010;33(6):745.

16. Doghramji K, Mitler MM, Sangal RB, et al. A normative study of the maintenance of wakefulness test (MWT). Electroencephalogr Clin Neurophysiol 1997;103(5):554–62.

17. Andlauer O, Moore H, Jouhier L, et al. Nocturnal rapid eye movement sleep latency for identifying patients with narcolepsy/hypocretin deficiency. JAMA Neurol 2013;70(7):891–902.

18. American Academy of Sleep Medicine. The international classification of sleep disorders: diagnostic and coding manual. Darien (IL): American Academic of Sleep Medicine; 2014.

19. Daley M, Morin CM, LeBlanc M, et al. Insomnia and its relationship to health-care utilization, work absenteeism, productivity and accidents. Sleep Med 2009;10(4):427–38.

20. Daley M, Morin CM, LeBlanc M, et al. The economic burden of insomnia: direct and indirect costs for individuals with insomnia syndrome, insomnia symptoms, and good sleepers. Sleep 2009;32(1):55.

21. Bastien CH, Vallières A, Morin CM. Validation of the insomnia severity Index as an outcome measure for insomnia research. Sleep Med 2001;2(4):297–307.

22. Carney CE, Buysse DJ, Ancoli-Israel S, et al. The consensus sleep diary: standardizing prospective sleep self-monitoring. Sleep 2012;35(2):287–302.

23. Chesson A, Hartse K, McDowell WA, et al. Practice parameters for the evaluation of chronic insomnia. Sleep 2000;23(2):237–42.

24. Riemann D, Spiegelhalder K, Feige B, et al. The hyperarousal model of insomnia: a review of the concept and its evidence. Sleep Med Rev 2010;14(1):19–31.

25. Roehrs T, Randall S, Harris E, et al. MSLT in primary insomnia: stability and relation to nocturnal sleep. Sleep 2011;34(12):1647.

26. Morgenthaler T, Kramer M, Alessi C, et al. Practice parameters for the psychological and behavioral treatment of insomnia: an update. An American Academy of sleep medicine report. Sleep 2006;29(11):1415.

27. Rosini JM, Dogra P. Pharmacology for insomnia: consider the options. Nursing 2015;45(3):38–45 [quiz: 45–6].

28. Rouch I, Wild P, Ansiau D, et al. Shiftwork experience, age and cognitive performance. Ergonomics 2005;48(10):1282–93.

29. Glass J, Lanctôt KL, Herrmann N, et al. Sedative hypnotics in older people with insomnia: meta-analysis of risks and benefits. BMJ 2005;331(7526):1169.

30. Hajak G, Bandelow B. Safety and tolerance of zolpidem in the treatment of disturbed sleep: a post-marketing surveillance of 16944 cases. Int Clin Psychopharmacol 1998;13(4):157–67.

31. Roth T, Rogowski R, Hull S, et al. Efficacy and safety of doxepin 1 mg, 3 mg, and 6 mg in adults with primary insomnia. Sleep 2007;30(11):1555.

32. Roth T, Durrence H, Tran M, et al. Arousability of insomnia patients and healthy volunteers is not impacted by the sleep-specific doses of Doxepin (3 mg and 6 mg), but is impacted in healthy volunteers using Zolpidem 10 mg. Presented at the annual meeting of the Association of Professional Sleep Societies. Denver, CO, 2016.

33. Zhang D, Tashiro M, Shibuya K, et al. Next-day residual sedative effect after nighttime administration of an over-the-counter antihistamine sleep aid, diphenhydramine, measured by positron emission tomography. J Clin Psychopharmacol 2010;30(6):694–701.

34. Roth T, Stubbs C, Walsh JK. Ramelteon (TAK-375), a selective MT1/MT2-receptor agonist, reduces latency to persistent sleep in a model of transient insomnia related to a novel sleep environment. Sleep 2005;28(3):303–7.

35. Herring WJ, Snyder E, Budd K, et al. Orexin receptor antagonism for treatment of insomnia A randomized clinical trial of suvorexant. Neurology 2012;79(23):2265–74.

36. Jurado-Gámez B, Guglielmi O, Gude F, et al. Workplace accidents, absenteeism and productivity in patients with sleep apnea. Arch Bronconeumol 2015;51(5):213–8.

37. Chung F, Yegneswaran B, Liao P, et al. Validation of the Berlin questionnaire and American Society of

Anesthesiologists checklist as screening tools for obstructive sleep apnea in surgical patients. Anesthesiology 2008;108(5):822–30.

38. Nuckton TJ, Glidden DV, Browner WS, et al. Physical examination: mallampati score as an independent predictor of obstructive sleep apnea. Sleep 2006;29(7):903.

39. Findley L, Smith C, Hooper J, et al. Treatment with nasal CPAP decreases automobile accidents in patients with sleep apnea. Am J Respir Crit Care Med 2000;161(3):857–9.

40. George CFP. Reduction in motor vehicle collisions following treatment of sleep apnoea with nasal CPAP. Thorax 2001;56(7):508–12.

41. American Academy of Sleep Medicine. Clinical guideline for the evaluation, management and long-term care of obstructive sleep apnea in adults. J Clin Sleep Med 2009;5(3):263.

42. Roenneberg T, Kuehnle T, Juda M, et al. Epidemiology of the human circadian clock. Sleep Med Rev 2007;11(6):429–38.

43. Horne JA, Ostberg O. A self-assessment questionnaire to determine morningness-eveningness in human circadian rhythms. Int J Chronobiol 1975; 4(2):97–110.

44. Roenneberg T, Wirz-Justice A, Merrow M. Life between clocks: daily temporal patterns of human chronotypes. J Biol Rhythms 2003;18(1):80–90.

45. Smith CS, Reilly C, Midkiff K. Evaluation of three circadian rhythm questionnaires with suggestions for an improved measure of morningness. J Appl Psychol 1989;74(5):728.

46. Au R, Carskadon M, Millman R, et al. School start times for adolescents. Pediatrics 2014;134(3): 642–9.

47. Ito A, Ando K, Hayakawa T, et al. Long-term course of adult patients with delayed sleep phase syndrome. Jpn J Psychiatry Neurol 1993;46:563–7.

48. Mundey K, Benloucif S, Harsanyi K, et al. Phase-dependent treatment of delayed sleep phase syndrome with melatonin. Sleep 2005;28(10):1271.

49. Kayumov L, Brown G, Jindal R, et al. A randomized, double-blind, placebo-controlled crossover study of the effect of exogenous melatonin on delayed sleep phase syndrome. Psychosom Med 2001;63(1):40–8.

50. Auger RR, Burgess HJ, Emens JS, et al. Clinical practice guideline for the treatment of intrinsic circadian rhythm sleep-wake disorders. J Clin Sleep Med 2015;11(10):1199–236.

51. Drake C, Roehrs T, Richardson G, et al. Shift work sleep disorder: prevalence and consequences beyond that of symptomatic day workers. Sleep 2004;27(8):1453–62.

52. Barger LK, Ogeil RP, Drake CL, et al. Validation of a questionnaire to screen for shift work disorder. Sleep 2012;35(12):1693–703.

53. Cheng P, Drake C. Shiftwork and work performance. In: Wagner D, editor. Work and sleep. Oxford (United Kingdom): Oxford University Press; 2015, in press.

54. Walsh JK, Muehlbach MJ, Schweitzer PK. Hypnotics and caffeine as countermeasures for shift-work-related sleepiness and sleep disturbance. J Sleep Res 1995;4(S2):80–3.

55. Morgenthaler T, Lee-Chiong T, Alessi C, et al. Practice parameters for the clinical evaluation and treatment of circadian rhythm sleep disorders: an American Academy of Sleep Medicine report. Sleep 2007;30(11):1445.

56. Schweitzer PK, Randazzo AC, Stone K, et al. Laboratory and field studies of naps and caffeine as practical countermeasures for sleep-wake problems associated with night work. Sleep 2006; 29(1):39–50.

57. Morris CJ, Yang JN, Scheer FAJL. The impact of the circadian timing system on cardiovascular and metabolic function. Prog Brain Res 2012;199: 337–58.

58. McHill AW, Melanson EL, Higgins J, et al. Impact of circadian misalignment on energy metabolism during simulated nightshift work. Proc Natl Acad Sci 2014;111(48):17302–7.

59. Garaulet M, Gómez-Abellán P. Timing of food intake and obesity: A novel association. Physiol Behav 2014;134:44–50.

60. Sharkey KM, Eastman CI. Melatonin phase shifts human circadian rhythms in a placebo-controlled simulated night-work study. Am J Phys 2002; 282(2):R454–63.

61. Sharkey KM, Fogg LF, Eastman CI. Effects of melatonin administration on daytime sleep after simulated night shift work. J Sleep Res 2001;10(3):181–92.

62. Stout N, et al. Traumatic Occupational Injury Research Needs and Priorities A Report by the NORA Traumatic Injury Team. In ASSE Professional Development Conference and Exhibition. American Society of Safety Engineers. 1999. Available at: https://www-onepetro-org.proxy.lib.umich.edu/conference-paper/ASSE-99-063. Accessed June 16, 2015.

63. Vermaelen J, Greiffenstein P, deBoisblanc B. Sleep in traumatic brain injury. Crit Care Clin 2015;31(3): 551–61. Available at: http://www.sciencedirect.com.proxy.lib.umich.edu/science/article/pii/S0749070415000287.

64. Gavett BE, Stern RA, Cantu RC, et al. Mild traumatic brain injury: a risk factor for neurodegeneration. Alzheimers Res Ther 2010;2(3):18.

65. Sivanandam TM, Thakur MK. Traumatic brain injury: a risk factor for Alzheimer's disease. Neurosci Biobehav Rev 2012;36(5):1376–81.

66. Stroe AF, Roth T, Jefferson C, et al. Comparative levels of excessive daytime sleepiness in common medical disorders. Sleep Med 2010;11(9):890–6.

67. Rye DB, Bliwise DL, Dihenia B, et al. Daytime sleepiness in Parkinson's disease. J Sleep Res 2000;9(1):63–9.

68. Grace JB, Walker MP, McKeith IG. A comparison of sleep profiles in patients with dementia with lewy bodies and Alzheimer's disease. Int J Geriatr Psychiatry 2000;15(11):1028–33.

69. Roehrs T, Roth T. Sleep and Pain: interaction of two vital functions. Semin Neurol 2005;25(01): 106–16.

70. Pollmächer T, Schuld A, Kraus T, et al. Experimental immunomodulation, sleep, and sleepiness in humans. Ann N Y Acad Sci 2000;917(1):488–99.

71. Vgontzas AN, Bixler EO, Chrousos GP. Obesity-related sleepiness and fatigue. Ann N Y Acad Sci 2006;1083(1):329–44.

72. Koinis Mitchell D, Kopel SJ, Williams B, et al. The association between asthma and sleep in urban adolescents with undiagnosed asthma. J Sch Health 2015;85(8):519–26.

73. Chen C-L, Robert JJ, Orr WC. Sleep symptoms and gastroesophageal reflux. J Clin Gastroenterol 2008;42(1):13–7.

74. Benca RM, Obermeyer W, Thisted R. Sleep and psychiatric disorders: a meta-analysis. Arch Gen Psychiatry 1992;49(8):651–68.

75. Betts TA, Birtle J. Effect of two hypnotic drugs on actual driving performance next morning. Br Med J 1982;285(6345):852.

76. Dassanayake T, Michie P, Carter G, et al. Effects of benzodiazepines, antidepressants and opioids on driving. Drug Saf 2011;34(2):125–56.

77. Gowda CR, Lundt LP. Mechanism of action of narcolepsy medications. CNS Spectr 2014;19(Suppl 1):25–33 [quiz: 25–7, 34].

78. Pilcher JJ, Walters AS. How sleep deprivation affects psychological variables related to college students' cognitive performance. J Am Coll Health 1997;46(3):121–6.

79. Åkerstedt T, Wright KP. Sleep loss and fatigue in shift work and shift work disorder. Sleep Med Clin 2009;4(2):257–71.

80. Roehrs T, Carskadon MA, Dement WC, et al. Daytime sleepiness and alertness. In: Kryger M, Roth T, Dement WC, editors. Principles and practice of sleep medicine. 5th edition. Philadelphia: Saunders; 2011. p. 784–98.

81. Gold DR, Rogacz S, Bock N, et al. Rotating shift work, sleep, and accidents related to sleepiness in hospital nurses. Am J Public Health 1992;82(7): 1011–4.

82. Dinges DF, Pack F, Williams K, et al. Cumulative sleepiness, mood disturbance and psychomotor vigilance performance decrements during a week of sleep restricted to 4-5 hours per night. Sleep 1997;20(4): 267–77. Available at: http://psycnet.apa.org.proxy. lib.umich.edu/psycinfo/1997-06077-003.

83. Van Dongen H, Dinges DF. Sleep, circadian rhythms, and psychomotor vigilance. Clin Sports Med 2005;24(2):237–49.

84. Basner M, Rubinstein J, Fomberstein KM, et al. Effects of night work, sleep loss and time on task on simulated threat detection performance. Sleep 2008;31(9):1251–9.

85. Barger LK, Ayas NT, Cade BE, et al. Impact of extended-duration shifts on medical errors, adverse events, and attentional Failures. PLoS Med 2006;3(12):e487.

86. Landrigan CP, Rothschild JM, Cronin JW, et al. Effect of reducing interns' work hours on serious medical errors in intensive care units. N Engl J Med 2004;351(18):1838–48.

87. Hsieh S, Tsai C-Y, Tsai L-L. Error correction maintains post-error adjustments after one night of total sleep deprivation. J Sleep Res 2009;18(2):159–66.

88. Durmer JS, Dinges DF. Neurocognitive consequences of sleep deprivation. Semin Neurol 2005; 25:117–29. Available at: http://faculty.vet.upenn. edu/uep/user_documents/dfd3.pdf.

89. Wertz AT, Ronda JM, Czeisler CA, et al. Effects of sleep inertia on cognition. JAMA 2006;295(2): 159–64.

90. Monk T, Buysse D, Reynolds Iii C, et al. Circadian rhythms in human performance and mood under constant conditions. J Sleep Res 1997;6(1):9–18.

91. Diekelmann S, Wilhelm I, Born J. The whats and whens of sleep-dependent memory consolidation. Sleep Med Rev 2009;13(5):309–21.

92. Stickgold R. Sleep-dependent memory consolidation. Nature 2005;437(7063):1272–8.

93. Yoo S-S, Hu PT, Gujar N, et al. A deficit in the ability to form new human memories without sleep. Nat Neurosci 2007;10(3):385–92.

94. Hagewoud R, Havekes R, Tiba PA, et al. Coping with sleep deprivation: shifts in regional brain activity and learning strategy. Sleep 2010;33(11):1465.

95. Wagner U, Gais S, Haider H, et al. Sleep inspires insight. Nature 2004;427(6972):352–5.

96. Drake C, Gumenyuk V, Roth T, et al. Effects of armodafinil on simulated driving and alertness in shift work disorder. Sleep 2014;37(12):1987–94.

97. Ayas N, Barger B, Cade B, et al. Extended work duration and the risk of self-reported percutaneous injuries in interns. JAMA 2006;296(9):1055–62.

98. Mullins HM, Cortina JM, Drake CL, et al. Sleepiness at work: a review and framework of how the physiology of sleepiness impacts the workplace. J Appl Psychol 2014;99(6):1096.

99. Scott BA, Judge TA. Insomnia, emotions, and job satisfaction: a multilevel study. J Manag 2006; 32(5):622–45.

100. Yoo S-S, Gujar N, Hu P, et al. The human emotional brain without sleep — a prefrontal amygdala disconnect. Curr Biol 2007;17(20):R877–8.

101. Centers for Disease Control and Prevention. Drowsy driving and risk behaviors — 10 states and Puerto Rico, 2011–2012. MMWR Morb Mortal Wkly Rep 2011;60(8):239–42.

102. Connor J, Norton R, Ameratunga S, et al. Driver sleepiness and risk of serious injury to car occupants: population based case control study. BMJ 2002;324(7346):1125.

103. Horne JA, Reyner LA. Sleep related vehicle accidents. BMJ 1995;310(6979):565–7.

104. Mitler MM, Miller JC, Lipsitz JJ, et al. The sleep of long-haul truck drivers. N Engl J Med 1997; 337(11):755–62.

105. Häkkänen H, Summala H. Sleepiness at work among commercial truck drivers. Sleep 2000; 23(1):49–57.

106. Jackson ML, Croft RJ, Kennedy GA, et al. Cognitive components of simulated driving performance: sleep loss effects and predictors. Accid Anal Prev 2013;50:438–44.

107. Arnedt JT, Wilde GJS, Munt PW, et al. How do prolonged wakefulness and alcohol compare in the decrements they produce on a simulated driving task? Accid Anal Prev 2001;33(3):337–44.

108. Masa JF, Rubio M, Findley LJ. Habitually sleepy drivers have a high frequency of automobile crashes associated with respiratory disorders during sleep. Am J Respir Crit Care Med 2000; 162(4):1407–12.

109. Barger LK, Cade BE, Ayas NT, et al. Extended work shifts and the risk of motor vehicle crashes among interns. N Engl J Med 2005;352(2):125–34.

110. Amra B, Dorali R, Mortazavi S, et al. Sleep apnea symptoms and accident risk factors in Persian commercial vehicle drivers. Sleep Breath 2012; 16(1):187–91.

111. Teran-Santos J, Jimenez-Gomez A, Cordero-Guevara J. The association between sleep apnea and the risk of traffic accidents. N Engl J Med 1999;340(11):847–51.

112. Strohl KP, Brown DB, Collop N, et al. An official American Thoracic Society Clinical Practice Guideline: sleep apnea, sleepiness, and driving risk in noncommercial drivers. An update of a 1994 statement. Am J Respir Crit Care Med 2013; 187(11):1259–66.

113. Roehrs T, Hyde M, Blaisdell B, et al. Sleep loss and REM sleep loss are hyperalgesic. Sleep 2006; 29(2):145.

114. Spiegel K, Leproult R, Van Cauter E. Impact of sleep debt on metabolic and endocrine function. Lancet 1999;354(9188):1435–9.

115. Besedovsky L, Lange T, Born J. Sleep and immune function. Pflugers Arch 2011;463(1):121–37.

116. Dolsen MR, Asarnow LD, Harvey AG. Insomnia as a transdiagnostic process in psychiatric disorders. Curr Psychiatry Rep 2014;16(9):471.

117. Taylor DJ, Mallory LJ, Lichstein KL, et al. Comorbidity of chronic insomnia with medical problems. Sleep 2007;30(2):213.

118. Vgontzas AN, Fernandez-Mendoza J, Liao D, et al. Insomnia with objective short sleep duration: the most biologically severe phenotype of the disorder. Sleep Med Rev 2013;17(4):241–54.

119. Nieto FJ, Young TB, Lind BK, et al. Association of sleep-disordered breathing, sleep apnea, and hypertension in a large community-based study. JAMA 2000;283(14):1829–36.

120. Peppard PE, Young T, Palta M, et al. Prospective study of the association between sleep-disordered breathing and hypertension. N Engl J Med 2000; 342(19):1378–84.

121. Anstead M, Phillips B. The spectrum of sleep-disordered breathing. Respir Care Clin N Am 1999;5(3):363–77.

122. Reichmuth KJ, Austin D, Skatrud JB, et al. Association of sleep apnea and type II diabetes: a population-based study. Am J Respir Crit Care Med 2005;172(12):1590–5.

123. Marshall NS, Wong KKH, Liu PY, et al. Sleep apnea as an independent risk factor for all-cause mortality: the Busselton health study. Sleep 2008;31(8):1079.

Sleep Duration and Cardiovascular Disease Risk
Epidemiologic and Experimental Evidence

Naima Covassin, PhD*, Prachi Singh, PhD

KEYWORDS

- Sleep duration • Cardiovascular disease • Sleep deprivation • Hypertension
- Coronary heart disease • Stroke

KEY POINTS

- Inadequate sleep has become increasingly pervasive, and its impact on health and quality of life remains to be fully understood.
- Both extremes of sleep duration have been associated with increased prevalence and incidence of cardiovascular diseases, including hypertension, coronary heart disease, and stroke.
- Aberrations in physiologic functions induced by abnormal sleep may explain this association, along with enhanced prevalence of established cardiovascular risk factors.

INTRODUCTION

According to outcome-based recommendations issued recently by the National Sleep Foundation, the appropriate sleep duration for adults lies between 7 and 9 hours per night.[1] Notably, only 48% of the US adult population reports a habitual sleep time falling within that range,[2] whereas 26% average 6 to 7 hours of sleep per night, and 20% sleep less than 6 hours per night.

The time allotted to sleep has gradually declined over the past decades, with similar trends observed in multiple Western countries.[3] A growing proportion of individuals are curtailing their sleep in response to increasing demands and lifestyle changes, such as prolonged working hours, increased environmental lighting, and introduction of new communication technologies, which enable living "around the clock."

Nevertheless, changes in sleep habits are not without consequences. Deviations from optimal sleep duration may pose a substantial threat to health, with the detrimental effects of abnormal sleep on physical and psychological well-being only beginning to be unraveled. In this review, available data on the relationship between abnormal sleep duration and risk of prevalent and incident cardiovascular disease, the leading cause of morbidity and mortality, are presented. The putative physiologic mechanisms underlying the observed associations and potential confounders are also discussed.

EPIDEMIOLOGIC EVIDENCE
Hypertension

Hypertension is widespread, affecting approximately one-third of the adult population in the

Disclosure Statement: The authors have nothing to disclose.
The authors were supported by the American Heart Association (AHA 13POST16420009 and AHA 11SDG7260046) and by the National Institutes of Health (RO1 HL114676).
Division of Cardiovascular Diseases, Mayo Clinic, 200 First Street, Rochester, MN 55905, USA
* Corresponding author.
E-mail address: covassin.naima@mayo.edu

Sleep Med Clin 11 (2016) 81–89
http://dx.doi.org/10.1016/j.jsmc.2015.10.007

United States, and is a prominent risk factor for other cardiovascular and cerebrovascular diseases.[4] Epidemiologic evidence indicates that the relationship between customary sleep duration and risk of hypertension is better described as a curvilinear phenomenon, with both extremes of the sleep length distribution independently associated with enhanced likelihood of prevalent hypertension in the general population.[5–7]

A U-shaped relationship between self-reported sleep length and hypertension has been documented in a large (N = 71,455) national representative sample (National Health Interview Survey, NHIS),[6] with both ends of the tail exhibiting larger age-standardized prevalences of hypertension (<6 hours/night: 32.4%; ≥10 hours/night: 32.5%) compared with the referent category (8 hours/night, 23.2%). Similarly, the lowest risk of hypertension in the Sleep Heart Health Study[7] was observed in those subjects sleeping 7 to 7.9 hours per night, whereas a progressive increase was seen when moving away from this reference. The greater hazard conferred by both short and long sleep withstood multivariable adjustments for lifestyle, clinical, and sleep-related covariates (adjusted odds ratio [OR] = 1.66, 95% confidence interval [CI] = 1.35–2.04 for <6 hours/night; OR = 1.30, 1.04–1.62 for ≥9 hours/night). Large population studies have replicated this pattern.[5,8]

Although both ends of sleep duration have been cross-sectionally related to hypertension, the prospective contribution of long sleep is less compelling. As concluded by a recent meta-analysis,[9] current longitudinal data mainly support a role of short sleep as an independent marker of incident hypertension.

Indeed, it has been estimated that individuals sleeping less than 6 hours per night are 20% to 32% more likely to develop hypertension compared with those sleeping 7 to 8 hours.[8,10] Gangwisch and colleagues[10] studied the incidence of hypertension over an 8- to 10-year time span using the first National Health and Nutrition Examination Survey (NHANES I) dataset. In the pooled cohort comprising 4810 participants, fully adjusted probability of high blood pressure (BP) was more elevated in those sleeping 5 hours per night or less (adjusted hazard ratio [HR] = 1.32, 1.02–1.71) than in normal sleepers (7–8 hours/ night). Nevertheless, age-stratified analysis revealed that those who were 32 to 59 years old and reported habitual sleep 5 hours or less were 60% more likely to develop hypertension than peers sleeping 7 to 8 hours. Conversely, sleep duration was unrelated to outcomes in the older age strata (60–86 years). Several cohort studies

have subsequently replicated these null findings in the geriatric population.[8,11,12]

Women have been found to be more susceptible to the pressor effects of abnormal sleep. Estimates for both prevalent and incident hypertension derived from the Whitehall II study[13] were higher in middle-aged women who were sleeping 5 hours per night or less compared with those sleeping 7 hours, but not in men. Sex-specific associations have been confirmed and are further detailed in a transversal examination of the Western New York Health Study,[14] where a subanalysis of the female sample classified by menopausal status unveiled significantly higher odds only in premenopausal women.

Differential vulnerability to abnormal sleep length has also been reported across ethnicities. Event rates for hypertension were higher in Black subjects from the NHIS who were sleeping less than 6 hours per night or greater than 8 hours per night, compared with their White counterparts.[15] These data are in line with findings from the Coronary Artery Risk Development in Young Adults (CARDIA) study,[16] where objective sleep duration, as quantified from actigraphy, related to greater surges in BP in African Americans.

The moderating effect of demographic variables on the link between sleep duration and hypertension interestingly parallels the increased prevalence of this condition in women after 65 years old and in the African American population.[4]

When BP is treated as a continuous variable, again a U-shaped relationship with sleep hours can be described, although it is more robust for systolic values.[12,17] Abnormal sleep duration is also associated with altered diurnal BP rhythmicity. Both excess sleep and curtailed sleep have been linked with attenuated nocturnal dipping in BP,[17,18] which is a sensitive prognostic marker for cardiovascular disease.[19]

Coronary Heart Disease

Coronary heart disease (CHD), which comprises a spectrum of acute and chronic manifestations, remains the major cause of death worldwide,[20] with rising prevalence.[4] Abnormal sleep duration has been identified as a risk factor for CHD on the basis of epidemiologic studies, which show a cross-sectional relationship consistent with a U-shaped curve.[21–24] Weighted prevalence of total CHD was higher in respondents of the Behavioral Risk Factor Surveillance System (BRFSS) survey reporting either 6 hours per night or less (11.1%, 95% CI: 10.1–12.1) or 10 hours per night or more (14.8%, 12.0–17.6) than in the reference group sleeping 7 to 9 hours (7.9%, 7.3–8.5).[22] When the clinical presentations of CHD are considered separately, a heterogeneous pattern of risk emerges. Both sleep lengths of 6 or less hours per night and 9 or more hours per night were associated with heightened odds for history of myocardial infarction in a Finnish population[23] and in the NHIS cohort,[24] but only short sleepers had a significant adjusted prevalence of myocardial infarction using the 2007 to 2008 NHANES dataset.[21] Findings are discrepant for angina, although this condition seems more closely related to short sleep duration.[23,24]

Similarly to prevalence, incidence of fatal and nonfatal CHD events is greater with habitual sleep duration more than or less than 7 to 8 hours, as indicated by pooled relative disease risk of 1.48 (1.22–1.80) for short sleepers and 1.38 (1.15–1.66) for long sleepers.[25] This trend is in line with data on all-cause mortality,[26] which depict a curvilinear relationship between time asleep and death estimates, with best life expectancy achieved by those reporting sleeping habitually 7 to 8 hours per night.

In a longitudinal study comprising 71,617 female participants enrolled in the Nurses' Health Study,[27] multivariate-adjusted relative risks of CHD at 10-year follow-up were 1.39-fold higher in women reporting 5 hours per night or less and 1.37-fold higher in those sleeping 9 hours or more compared with those sleeping 8 hours per night. A similar pattern has been described for CHD deaths in a community-based Chinese cohort,[28] while likelihood of future fatal and nonfatal CHD was better predicted by the short sleep category in the Framingham Offspring Cohort.[29] Compared with 7 to 8 hours per night, self-reported sleep of 5 hours or less or 10 hours or more induced, respectively, a 25% and a 43% age- and race-adjusted raised risk for CHD in a large national cohort of postmenopausal women.[30] However, the estimates were markedly attenuated when controlling for behavioral, socioeconomic, and clinical covariates and were no longer of statistical significance. Comparable results were noted in a prospective investigation on a Dutch cohort.[31] Disparities in CHD risk have been evident in age- and sex-stratified analyses, although with divergent results.[32–35]

In addition to established coronary disease, sleep length has been examined in relationship with early indices of subclinical atherosclerotic disease, and findings are compatible with normal sleep duration being protective against later cardiovascular events.

Ultrasonographic measurement of carotid intima-media thickness (IMT) is often adopted as a noninvasive indicator of atherogenic vascular damage.[36] Data from the Study of Health in Pomerania[37] depict a J-shaped association between habitual hours of sleep and carotid wall thickening, with the lowest carotid IMT values detected in subjects sleeping 7 to 8 hours. A monotonic relationship was instead observed in the CARDIA study,[38] where actigraphy-derived sleep duration predicted carotid IMT in middle-aged men, but not in women, with each additional hour of sleep associated with a 0.026-mm decrease in IMT. A longitudinal examination sampling 495 individuals from the same cohort[39] confirmed the contribution of curtailed sleep to incident coronary risk. Using computed tomographic–assessed coronary artery calcification as an early predictor of CHD,[40] and accounting for conventional risk factors, risk of calcification at 5-year follow-up declined progressively as sleep time lengthened.

Cerebrovascular Disease

Cerebrovascular disease is among the leading causes of long-term disability[41] and is responsible for 16.4% of cardiovascular deaths.[4] As outlined recently in a meta-analysis by Ge and Guo,[42] enhanced cross-sectional and prospective vulnerability to cerebrovascular events is associated with both ends of the sleep duration distribution. Pooled ORs (95% CI) for prevalent stroke were 1.71 (1.39–2.02) for short sleep duration and 2.12 (1.51–2.73) for long sleep duration. The corresponding pooled HRs for incident stroke were 1.13 (1.02–1.25) and 1.40 (1.16–1.64). The concept of a U-shaped relationship is corroborated by results from large population-based studies including the BRFSS survey[22] and the NHIS.[24] There are also data reflecting a more robust association of stroke with excessive sleep.[35,43,44]

An early prospective investigation on how sleep pattern affects the likelihood of stroke was conducted using the NHANES I study population,[43] which comprised 7844 participants followed for 10 years. This analysis revealed that the independent relative risk of ischemic or hemorrhagic stroke was 1.5 times higher in individuals reporting greater than 8 hours per night than in those who were sleeping 6 to 8 hours.

Chen and colleagues[44] prospectively examined a cohort of 93,175 postmenopausal women and found both self-reported short (≤6 hours/night) and long sleep (≥9 hours/night) to be significant predictors of ischemic stroke (including fatal and nonfatal events) at 7.5-year follow-up in the age- and race-adjusted analysis. Although curtailed sleep was no longer an independent determinant in multivariate models, including socioeconomic, lifestyle, psychiatric and medical covariates

(HR: 1.14, 0.97–1.33), long sleep retained its predictive strength (HR: 1.70, 1.32–2.21). In addition, an association with short sleep was unmasked when the analysis was restricted to women without cardiovascular disease at baseline. Conversely, in a 4-year examination of a population of Japanese elderly hypertensives who underwent brain scans for detection of silent cerebral infarcts,[45] insufficient sleep predicted future stroke only in those with brain lesions at study entry.

Similarly to cardiovascular disorders, the impact of extreme sleep lengths on cerebrovascular disease risk appears to be modified by demographic characteristics. Among the 154,599 participants of the 2006 to 2011 NHIS study,[46] age-standardized prevalences of stroke were 2.78%, 1.99%, and 5.21% in respondents reporting sleeping less than or equal to 6, 7 to 8, and 9 or more hours per night, respectively. Risk of stroke remained more elevated in short and long sleepers in the pooled sample compared with the reference (7–8 hours/night) after controlling for pertinent covariates. Nonetheless, further stratification by age and gender revealed that the association with short sleep persisted in young women (18–44 years), while the association with long sleep was maintained in both male and female older adults (≥65 years). Notably, however, the increased crude hazard for incident stroke symptoms found in US employed individuals aged 45 years or older sleeping less than 6 hours per night[47] was abolished in adjusted models.

Putative Biological Mechanisms and Moderators

Observational findings from epidemiologic investigations are supplemented by experimental, laboratory-based evidence, which provide mechanistic insights into the biological substrate underlying the heightened cardiovascular risk associated with inadequate sleep.

A causative link between sleep deficiency and aberrant cardiovascular function is supported by multiple studies, which applied models of short-term, total sleep deprivation. Along with these traditional protocols, extended sleep restriction paradigms have been more recently implemented to better simulate the chronic, partial sleep loss commonly experienced in everyday life.

Acute surges in systolic and diastolic BP occur following 24 to 88 hours of sustained wakefulness.[48–53] In the absence of sizable increases in diurnal resting BP,[54–56] healthy individuals exposed to prolonged partial sleep curtailment exhibit elevations in nocturnal BP along with dampened nocturnal dipping[57] and an amplified morning surge.[58]

A sympathoexcitatory effect of sleep loss has been proposed to account for the rise in BP. Research on hemodynamics and neural circulatory control largely supports the enhanced release of plasma and urinary norepinephrine after sustained sleep restriction[54,59] but not in response to acute sleep loss.[49,50,60] Although results on heart rate are mixed, being either unaffected[48,49,54,55] or accelerated[50–52] after sleep loss, muscle sympathetic nerve activity has been consistently found to be inhibited.[48,49,60] An altered arterial baroreflex functioning in terms of resetting toward a higher BP level has thus been postulated, substantiated by findings of a rightward and downward shift in the operating point following sleep restriction.[48,60] Results on baroreflex sensitivity are less clear, showing an increase,[61] decrease,[62] or no change.[48] On the contrary, enhanced cardiac sympathetic drive as estimated from heart rate variability, a noninvasive index of cardiac autonomic modulation predictive of adverse events,[63] has been more consistently documented after total sleep loss[50,62] and after 5 days of sleep truncation.[54]

Electrocardiographic abnormalities in cardiac conduction and repolarization resembling a proarrhythmogenic profile have also been detected after acute experimental sleep deprivation.[64,65]

In addition, sleep debt provokes early deterioration of vascular structure and function that may promote cardiovascular risk. Exposure to one night of sleep deprivation increases arterial stiffness as estimated by brachial-ankle pulse-wave velocity.[53] Interestingly, these experimental data are in contrast with those gathered from population studies, which linked greater arterial stiffness to long sleep duration in men.[66,67] Impaired endothelial function reflects poor vascular health and is thought to be a precursor of atherosclerosis.[68] Individuals undergoing experimental sleep curtailment exhibit reduced endothelium-dependent vasodilation, indicated by diminished acetylcholine-induced cutaneous[50,55] and venous vasodilation[54] and decreased brachial flow-mediated vasodilation.[69] Sleep loss also damages the coronary microcirculation.[70] The concomitant enhanced release of cellular adhesion molecules and selectins from activated endothelial cells[50,71] further supports the concept of systemic endothelial dysfunction promoted by sleep deprivation. Findings of abbreviated prothrombin and thrombin times,[72] consistent with development of a prothrombotic state, have also been reported.

In addition to direct effects on cardiac and vascular regulation, sleep deficiency has been shown to adversely impact numerous physiologic functions that are implicated in increased cardiovascular risk.

There is substantial evidence that sleep loss impairs glucose homeostasis and insulin sensitivity.[59,73–75] Compared with 10 hours per night, 1 week of sleep restriction at 5 hours per night elicited a 20% decrease in insulin sensitivity.[73] Exposure to sleep truncation generated a positive energy balance leading ultimately to weight gain.[76–79] Current research indicates that the increase in body weight achieved with sleep restriction in the setting of ad libitum access to food is primarily driven by overeating, as results on energy expenditure are inconsistent. Likewise, the underlying molecular pathways accompanying excess food intake show discrepant responses in energy balance regulatory hormones such as leptin and ghrelin.[76,77] On the other hand, compelling epidemiologic data confirm the link between inadequate sleep and metabolic disorders, such as obesity and type 2 diabetes,[80,81] both major precursors of cardiovascular disease. Additional manifestations of endocrine derangements triggered by experimental sleep curtailment comprise reduced testosterone in men[48,55] and upregulation of the hypothalamic-pituitary-adrenal axis.[82,83] Enhanced secretion of inflammatory cytokines, such as C-reactive protein and interleukin-6, occurs in response to acute or cumulative sleep loss,[50,51,84,85] reflecting stimulation of proinflammatory pathways. Immune functions are also compromised under sleep debt conditions.[56,72]

An almost inevitable companion of sleep deprivation is circadian disruption, as demonstrated by distortion of diurnal rhythmicity of metabolic, cardiovascular, and immunologic function during experimental sleep manipulation.[57–59,82,84] Given that a 24-hour pattern of oscillation has been described in most physiologic processes,[86] it is not surprising that circadian misalignment may severely compromise health status. In this regard, hazards of shift work, in which circadian misalignment is often combined with chronic sleep debt, have been become increasingly apparent.[87]

It is noteworthy that experimental evidence corroborating harmful cardiovascular effects of excessive sleep duration is lacking, which contributes to making any causal association between long sleep and cardiovascular disease more elusive. Controversy has indeed been raised as to whether prolonged sleep duration is truly an independent risk predictor. It has been argued that excessive sleep duration may be simply an epiphenomenon of poor health, being secondary to undiagnosed illnesses or subclinical conditions. Cross-sectional data indeed support poor perceived health in long sleepers.[14,88] In addition, prolonged sleep is often reported in conjunction with a constellation of accepted cardiovascular risk factors, such as older age,[24,29,34] low socioeconomic status,[30,34] depressive mood,[7,12,24,30] hypnotic usage,[34] prevalent sleep disorders,[7] metabolic syndrome components,[22,24,34] and high-risk behaviors, such as smoking,[6,24] excess alcohol consumption,[6] and low physical activity.[6,24,32] However, consistent with a U-shaped relationship, these potential confounders are also prevalent in those who report insufficient sleep,[6,12,24,29,30,32,34] and therefore, could similarly bias the link between short sleep and cardiovascular risk.

In agreement with this hypothesis, as mentioned above, several studies have unmasked modifier effects exerted by gender, age, and ethnicity. Poor self-rated health,[88] insomnia,[30,89] sleep apnea,[90] and use of hypnotics/tranquilizers[91] have been found to moderate the association between sleep duration and cardiovascular outcomes.

Nevertheless, it should be noted that in numerous large cohort studies, sleep duration retained its predictive role after maximal adjustment,[7,22,24] although controlling for potential confounders and mediators generally attenuated the estimates. These findings still favor a pathogenic contribution of inadequate sleep to cardiovascular vulnerability.

It is important to acknowledge that although sleep duration is a relatively crude measure of a complex entity, such as sleep, other more refined indices of sleep quality and quantity, such as sleep efficiency, sleep fragmentation, or slow wave sleep, have been found to be significant predictors of cardiovascular risk, independent of sleep length.[16,92] Nevertheless, as these measures cannot be derived from questionnaires, but require technical instrumentations such as polysomnography or actigraphy, their suitability for epidemiologic research is limited.

SUMMARY

Observational and experimental data converge to indicate that inadequate sleep duration poses a substantial hazard for cardiovascular morbidity and mortality. Sleep deficiency seems to induce adverse, sustained, and systemic alterations that conceivably act in concert to ultimately predispose to cardiovascular disease. The concomitant occurrence of conventional risk factors in individuals exposed to chronic sleep debt is likely to further amplify the risk of poor outcomes. Conversely, although long sleepers exhibit a similar pattern of predominant risk factors, the putative pathophysiologic pathways leading to overt disease are still largely unknown. More mechanistic research is warranted to address this gap.

Given the pervasive and escalating prevalence of inadequate sleep and most sleep deficiency, the potential future burden on public health cannot be ignored. As sleep curtailment is largely voluntary and therefore modifiable, the cardiovascular complications may be preventable and plausibly reversible. Preventative strategies should therefore be undertaken to raise awareness of the possible deleterious sequelae in the general population, paralleled by interventional studies aimed at clarifying whether adherence to optimal sleep durations may improve cardiovascular risk profiles.

REFERENCES

1. Hirshkowitz M, Whiton K, Albert SM, et al. National Sleep Foundation's sleep time duration recommendations: methodology and results summary. Sleep Health 2015;1(1):40–3.
2. National Sleep Foundation. Sleep in America: bedroom poll 2012. Washington, DC: National Sleep Foundation; 2012.
3. Bin YS, Marshall NS, Glozier N. Secular trends in adult sleep duration: a systematic review. Sleep Med Rev 2012;16(3):223–30.
4. Go AS, Mozaffarian D, Roger VL, et al. Heart disease and stroke statistics–2013 update: a report from the American Heart Association. Circulation 2013;127(1):E6–245.
5. Merikanto I, Lahti T, Puolijoki H, et al. Associations of chronotype and sleep with cardiovascular diseases and type 2 diabetes. Chronobiol Int 2013;30(4):470–7.
6. Fang J, Wheaton AG, Keenan NL, et al. Association of sleep duration and hypertension among US adults varies by age and sex. Am J Hypertens 2012;25(3):335–41.
7. Gottlieb DJ, Redline S, Nieto FJ, et al. Association of usual sleep duration with hypertension: the Sleep Heart Health Study. Sleep 2006;29(8):1009–14.
8. Gangwisch JE, Feskanich D, Malaspina D, et al. Sleep duration and risk for hypertension in women: results from the Nurses Health Study. Am J Hypertens 2013;26(7):903–11.
9. Guo XF, Zheng LQ, Wang J, et al. Epidemiological evidence for the link between sleep duration and high blood pressure: a systematic review and meta-analysis. Sleep Med 2013;14(4):324–32.
10. Gangwisch JE, Heymsfield SB, Boden-Albala B, et al. Short sleep duration as a risk factor for hypertension: analyses of the first National Health and Nutrition Examination Survey. Hypertension 2006;47(5):833–9.
11. van den Berg JF, Tulen JH, Neven AK, et al. Sleep duration and hypertension are not associated in the elderly. Hypertension 2007;50(3):585–9.
12. Kim J, Jo I. Age-dependent association between sleep duration and hypertension in the adult Korean population. Am J Hypertens 2010;23(12):1286–91.
13. Cappuccio FP, Stranges S, Kandala NB, et al. Gender-specific associations of short sleep duration with prevalent and incident hypertension: the Whitehall II Study. Hypertension 2007;50(4):693–700.
14. Stranges S, Dorn JM, Cappuccio FP, et al. A population-based study of reduced sleep duration and hypertension: the strongest association may be in premenopausal women. J Hypertens 2010;28(5):896–902.
15. Pandey A, Williams N, Donat M, et al. Linking sleep to hypertension: greater risk for blacks. Int J Hypertens 2013;2013:436502.
16. Knutson KL, Van Cauter E, Rathouz PJ, et al. Association between sleep and blood pressure in midlife. The CARDIA Sleep Study. Arch Intern Med 2009;169(11):1055–61.
17. Ramos AR, Jin ZZ, Rundek T, et al. Relation between long sleep and left ventricular mass (from a multiethnic elderly cohort). Am J Cardiol 2013;112(4):599–603.
18. Friedman O, Shukla Y, Logan AG. Relationship between self-reported sleep duration and changes in circadian blood pressure. Am J Hypertens 2009;22(11):1205–11.
19. Yano Y, Kario K. Nocturnal blood pressure and cardiovascular disease: a review of recent advances. Hypertens Res 2012;35(7):695–701.
20. Lozano R, Naghavi M, Foreman K, et al. Global and regional mortality from 235 causes of death for 20 age groups in 1990 and 2010: a systematic analysis for the Global Burden of Disease Study 2010. Lancet 2012;380(9859):2095–128.
21. Aggarwal S, Loomba RS, Arora RR, et al. Associations between sleep duration and prevalence of cardiovascular events. Clin Cardiol 2013;36(11):671–6.
22. Liu Y, Wheaton AG, Chapman DP, et al. Sleep duration and chronic diseases among US adults age 45 years and older: evidence from the 2010 Behavioral Risk Factor Surveillance System. Sleep 2013;36(10):1421–7.
23. Partinen M, Putkonen PT, Kaprio J, et al. Sleep disorders in relation to coronary heart disease. Acta Med Scand Suppl 1982;660:69–83.
24. Sabanayagam C, Shankar A. Sleep duration and cardiovascular disease: results from the National Health Interview Survey. Sleep 2010;33(8):1037–42.
25. Cappuccio FP, Cooper D, D'Elia L, et al. Sleep duration predicts cardiovascular outcomes: a systematic review and meta-analysis of prospective studies. Eur Heart J 2011;32(12):1484–92.
26. Cappuccio FP, D'Elia L, Strazzullo P, et al. Sleep duration and all-cause mortality: a systematic review and meta-analysis of prospective studies. Sleep 2010;33(5):585–92.
27. Ayas NT, White DP, Manson JE, et al. A prospective study of sleep duration and coronary heart disease in women. Arch Intern Med 2003;163(2):205–9.

28. Shankar A, Koh WP, Yuan JM, et al. Sleep duration and coronary heart disease mortality among Chinese adults in Singapore: a population-based cohort study. Am J Epidemiol 2008;168(12):1367–73.

29. Liu J, Yuen J, Kang S. Sleep duration, C-reactive protein and risk of incident coronary heart disease–results from the Framingham Offspring Study. Nutr Metab Cardiovasc Dis 2014;24(6):600–5.

30. Sands-Lincoln M, Loucks EB, Lu B, et al. Sleep duration, insomnia, and coronary heart disease among postmenopausal women in the Women's Health Initiative. J Womens Health 2013;22(6):477–86.

31. Hoevenaar-Blom MP, Spijkerman AM, Kromhout D, et al. Sleep duration and sleep quality in relation to 12-year cardiovascular disease incidence: the MORGEN study. Sleep 2011;34(11):1487–92.

32. Meisinger C, Heier M, Lowel H, et al. Sleep duration and sleep complaints and risk of myocardial infarction in middle-aged men and women from the general population: the MONICA/KORA Augsburg cohort study. Sleep 2007;30(9):1121–7.

33. Amagai Y, Ishikawa S, Gotoh T, et al. Sleep duration and incidence of cardiovascular events in a Japanese population: the Jichi Medical School cohort study. J Epidemiol 2010;20(2):106–10.

34. Gangwisch JE, Heymsfield SB, Boden-Albala B, et al. Sleep duration associated with mortality in elderly, but not middle-aged, adults in a large US sample. Sleep 2008;31(8):1087–96.

35. Kronholm E, Laatikainen T, Peltonen M, et al. Self-reported sleep duration, all-cause mortality, cardiovascular mortality and morbidity in Finland. Sleep Med 2011;12(3):215–21.

36. Lorenz MW, Markus HS, Bots ML, et al. Prediction of clinical cardiovascular events with carotid intima-media thickness: a systematic review and meta-analysis. Circulation 2007;115(4):459–67.

37. Wolff B, Volzke H, Schwahn C, et al. Relation of self-reported sleep duration with carotid intima-media thickness in a general population sample. Atherosclerosis 2008;196(2):727–32.

38. Sands MR, Lauderdale DS, Liu K, et al. Short sleep duration is associated with carotid intima-media thickness among men in the Coronary Artery Risk Development in Young Adults (CARDIA) study. Stroke 2012;43(11):2858–64.

39. King CR, Knutson KL, Rathouz PJ, et al. Short sleep duration and incident coronary artery calcification. JAMA 2008;300(24):2859–66.

40. Polonsky TS, McClelland RL, Jorgensen NW, et al. Coronary artery calcium score and risk classification for coronary heart disease prediction. JAMA 2010;303(16):1610–6.

41. Center for Disease Control and Prevention. Prevalence and most common causes of disability among adults–United States, 2005. MMWR Morb Mortal Wkly Rep 2009;58:421–6.

42. Ge BH, Guo XM. Short and long sleep durations are both associated with increased risk of stroke: a meta-analysis of observational studies. Int J Stroke 2015;10(2):177–84.

43. Qureshi AI, Giles WH, Croft JB, et al. Habitual sleep patterns and risk for stroke and coronary heart disease: a 10-year follow-up from NHANES I. Neurology 1997;48(4):904–11.

44. Chen JC, Brunner RL, Ren H, et al. Sleep duration and risk of ischemic stroke in postmenopausal women. Stroke 2008;39(12):3185–92.

45. Eguchi K, Hoshide S, Ishikawa S, et al. Short sleep duration is an independent predictor of stroke events in elderly hypertensive patients. J Am Soc Hypertens 2010;4(5):255–62.

46. Fang J, Wheaton AG, Ayala C. Sleep duration and history of stroke among adults from the USA. J Sleep Res 2014;23(5):531–7.

47. Ruiter-Petrov ME, Letter AJ, Howard VJ, et al. Self-reported sleep duration in relation to incident stroke symptoms: nuances by body mass and race from the REGARDS study. J Stroke Cerebrovasc Dis 2014;23(2):e123–32.

48. Carter JR, Durocher JJ, Larson RA, et al. Sympathetic neural responses to 24-hour sleep deprivation in humans: sex differences. Am J Physiol Heart Circ Physiol 2012;302(10):H1991–7.

49. Kato M, Phillips BG, Sigurdsson G, et al. Effects of sleep deprivation on neural circulatory control. Hypertension 2000;35(5):1173–5.

50. Sauvet F, Leftheriotis G, Gomez-Merino D, et al. Effect of acute sleep deprivation on vascular function in healthy subjects. J Appl Physiol 2010;108(1):68–75.

51. Meier-Ewert HK, Ridker PM, Rifai N, et al. Effect of sleep loss on C-reactive protein, an inflammatory marker of cardiovascular risk. J Am Coll Cardiol 2004;43(4):678–83.

52. Lusardi P, Zoppi A, Preti P, et al. Effects of insufficient sleep on blood pressure in hypertensive patients: a 24-h study. Am J Hypertens 1999;12(1):63–8.

53. Sunbul M, Kanar BG, Durmus E, et al. Acute sleep deprivation is associated with increased arterial stiffness in healthy young adults. Sleep Breath 2014;18(1):215–20.

54. Dettoni JL, Consolim-Colombo FM, Drager LF, et al. Cardiovascular effects of partial sleep deprivation in healthy volunteers. J Appl Physiol 2012;113(2):232–6.

55. Sauvet F, Drogou C, Bougard C, et al. Vascular response to 1 week of sleep restriction in healthy subjects. A metabolic response? Int J Cardiol 2015;190:246–55.

56. van Leeuwen WMA, Lehto M, Karisola P, et al. Sleep restriction increases the risk of developing cardiovascular diseases by augmenting proinflammatory

responses through IL-17 and CRP. PLoS One 2009; 4(2):e4589.

57. Covassin N, Bukartyk J, Sahakyan K, et al. Experimental sleep restriction increases nocturnal blood pressure and attenuates blood pressure dipping in healthy individuals. J Am Coll Cardiol 2015; 65(Suppl 10):A1352.

58. Yang H, Haack M, Lamanna M, et al. Blunted nocturnal blood pressure dipping and exaggerated morning blood pressure surge in response to a novel repetitive sleep restriction challenge. FASEB J 2015;29(1 Suppl):957–8.

59. Nedeltcheva AV, Kessler L, Imperial J, et al. Exposure to recurrent sleep restriction in the setting of high caloric intake and physical inactivity results in increased insulin resistance and reduced glucose tolerance. J Clin Endocrinol Metab 2009;94(9): 3242–50.

60. Ogawa Y, Kanbayashi T, Saito Y, et al. Total sleep deprivation elevates blood pressure through arterial baroreflex resetting: a study with microneurographic technique. Sleep 2003;26(8):986–9.

61. Pagani M, Pizzinelli P, Pavy-Le Traon A, et al. Hemodynamic, autonomic and baroreflex changes after one night sleep deprivation in healthy volunteers. Auton Neurosci 2009;145(1–2):76–80.

62. Zhong X, Hilton HJ, Gates GJ, et al. Increased sympathetic and decreased parasympathetic cardiovascular modulation in normal humans with acute sleep deprivation. J Appl Physiol 2005;98(6):2024–32.

63. Thayer JF, Yamamoto SS, Brosschot JF. The relationship of autonomic imbalance, heart rate variability and cardiovascular disease risk factors. Int J Cardiol 2010;141(2):122–31.

64. Cakici M, Dogan A, Cetin M, et al. Negative effects of acute sleep deprivation on left ventricular functions and cardiac repolarization in healthy young adults. Pacing Clin Electrophysiol 2015; 38(6):713–22.

65. Ozer O, Ozbala B, Sari I, et al. Acute sleep deprivation is associated with increased QT dispersion in healthy young adults. Pacing Clin Electrophysiol 2008;31(8):979–84.

66. Yoshioka E, Saijo Y, Kita T, et al. Relation between self-reported sleep duration and arterial stiffness: a cross-sectional study of middle-aged Japanese civil servants. Sleep 2011;34(12):1681–6.

67. Tsai TC, Wu JS, Yang YC, et al. Long sleep duration associated with a higher risk of increased arterial stiffness in males. Sleep 2014;37(8):1315–20.

68. Verma S, Buchanan MR, Anderson TJ. Endothelial function testing as a biomarker of vascular disease. Circulation 2003;108(17):2054–9.

69. Calvin AD, Covassin N, Kremers WK, et al. Experimental sleep restriction causes endothelial dysfunction in healthy humans. J Am Heart Assoc 2014;3(6): e001143.

70. Sekine T, Daimon M, Hasegawa R, et al. The impact of sleep deprivation on the coronary circulation. Int J Cardiol 2010;144(2):266–7.

71. Frey DJ, Fleshner M, Wright KP. The effects of 40 hours of total sleep deprivation on inflammatory markers in healthy young adults. Brain Behav Immun 2007;21(8):1050–7.

72. Liu H, Wang GG, Luan GH, et al. Effects of sleep and sleep deprivation on blood cell count and hemostasis parameters in healthy humans. J Thromb Thrombolysis 2009;28(1):46–9.

73. Buxton OM, Pavlova M, Reid EW, et al. Sleep restriction for 1 week reduces insulin sensitivity in healthy men. Diabetes 2010;59(9):2126–33.

74. Reynolds AC, Dorrian J, Liu PY, et al. Impact of five nights of sleep restriction on glucose metabolism, leptin and testosterone in young adult men. PLoS One 2012;7(7):e41218.

75. van Leeuwen WMA, Hublin C, Sallinen M, et al. Prolonged sleep restriction affects glucose metabolism in healthy young men. Int J Endocrinol 2010;2010: 108641.

76. Bosy-Westphal A, Hinrichs S, Jauch-Chara K, et al. Influence of partial sleep deprivation on energy balance and insulin sensitivity in healthy women. Obes Facts 2008;1(5):266–73.

77. Markwald RR, Melanson EL, Smith MR, et al. Impact of insufficient sleep on total daily energy expenditure, food intake, and weight gain. Proc Natl Acad Sci U S A 2013;110(14):5695–700.

78. Nedeltcheva AV, Kilkus JM, Imperial J, et al. Sleep curtailment is accompanied by increased intake of calories from snacks. Am J Clin Nutr 2009;89(1): 126–33.

79. Calvin AD, Carter RE, Adachi T, et al. Effects of experimental sleep restriction on caloric intake and activity energy expenditure. Chest 2013; 144(1):79–86.

80. Cappuccio FP, D'Elia L, Strazzullo P, et al. Quantity and quality of sleep and incidence of type 2 diabetes: a systematic review and meta-analysis. Diabetes Care 2010;33(2):414–20.

81. Cappuccio FP, Taggart FM, Kandala NB, et al. Meta-analysis of short sleep duration and obesity in children and adults. Sleep 2008;31(5):619–26.

82. Guyon A, Balbo M, Morselli LL, et al. Adverse effects of two nights of sleep restriction on the hypothalamic-pituitary-adrenal axis in healthy men. J Clin Endocrinol Metab 2014;99(8):2861–8.

83. Minkel J, Moreta M, Muto J, et al. Sleep deprivation potentiates HPA axis stress reactivity in healthy adults. Health Psychol 2014;33(11):1430–4.

84. Haack M, Sanchez E, Mullington JM. Elevated inflammatory markers in response to prolonged sleep restriction are associated with increased pain experience in healthy volunteers. Sleep 2007; 30(9):1145–52.

85. Vgontzas AN, Zoumakis E, Bixler EO, et al. Adverse effects of modest sleep restriction on sleepiness, performance, and inflammatory cytokines. J Clin Endocr Metab 2004;89(5):2119–26.

86. Hastings MH, Reddy AB, Maywood ES. A clockwork web: circadian timing in brain and periphery, in health and disease. Nat Rev Neurosci 2003;4(8): 649–61.

87. Esquirol Y, Perret B, Ruidavets JB, et al. Shift work and cardiovascular risk factors: new knowledge from the past decade. Arch Cardiovasc Dis 2011; 104(12):636–68.

88. Kakizaki M, Kuriyama S, Nakaya N, et al. Long sleep duration and cause-specific mortality according to physical function and self-rated health: the Ohsaki Cohort Study. J Sleep Res 2013;22(2):209–16.

89. Vgontzas AN, Liao DP, Bixler EO, et al. Insomnia with objective short sleep duration is associated with a high risk for hypertension. Sleep 2009;32(4):491–7.

90. Priou P, Le Vaillant M, Meslier N, et al. Cumulative association of obstructive sleep apnea severity and short sleep duration with the risk for hypertension. PLoS One 2014;9(12):e115666.

91. Garde AH, Hansen AM, Holtermann A, et al. Sleep duration and ischemic heart disease and all-cause mortality: prospective cohort study on effects of tranquilizers/hypnotics and perceived stress. Scand J Work Environ Health 2013;39(6):550–8.

92. Fung MM, Peters K, Redline S, et al. Decreased slow wave sleep increases risk of developing hypertension in elderly men. Hypertension 2011;58(4): 596–603.

Sleep in the Pediatric Population

Jonathan P. Hintze, MD, Shalini Paruthi, MD*

KEYWORDS

- Restless legs syndrome • Narcolepsy • Parasomnia • Epilepsy • Headache • Pediatric • Sleep

KEY POINTS

- Pediatric sleep disorders are common and may have a significant impact on a child's daytime function and performance.
- Additionally having a co-morbid sleep disorder may worsen a neurologic disorder.
- Sleep disorders are well defined in the International Classification of Sleep Disorders, 3rd edition.
- The evaluation, diagnosis and treatments of common pediatric sleep disorders that frequently co-exist with neurologic disorders are reviewed here.

RESTLESS LEGS SYNDROME

Introduction

Restless legs syndrome (RLS) is a common neurologic sensorimotor disorder affecting 2% to 4% of the pediatric population.[1–3] It is characterized by the urge to move the legs or by unpleasant sensations. These urges are worst at night and improve with movement or distraction. Sleep disturbance is the most common complaint in pediatric RLS, and is present in approximately 85% of patients (International Classification of Sleep Disorders, Third Edition [ICSD-3][4]).

Impacts of RLS may include:

Poor mood, irritability
Increased risk of depression and anxiety
Decreased daytime function at school
Misdiagnosis of attention-deficit/hyperactivity disorder (ADHD)
Headaches[1,3–9]

Pathophysiology

Although not completely understood, dopamine has a prominent role in the pathophysiology of RLS. Inadequate dopamine production, use, and blockade are contributors. Iron is an essential cofactor for tyrosine hydroxylase, the enzyme of the rate-limiting step of dopamine synthesis. Low iron availability may reduce dopamine production and transport. Therefore, low iron status is a common cause or contributor to RLS. Of note, iron shows a diurnal pattern with a nadir in the late evening and early night, which may contribute to increased symptom severity at night.[10,11] Iron is also important in myelin synthesis, energy production, and other neurotransmitter systems that may play a role in RLS.[12–14] Antidopaminergic medications are also contributors to RLS, although they are uncommon in children.

Genetics

Multiple genomewide studies have reported gene variants associated with RLS.[15–20] Among children with RLS, at least 1 biological parent reported RLS symptoms in greater than 70% of families, with both parents affected in 16% of families.[1] Thus, individuals may have a genetic predisposition to RLS that combines with environmental factors, such as iron status, to determine clinical manifestations.

Diagnosis

The diagnosis of RLS is made by taking a specific history relevant to the diagnosis; a polysomnogram is not necessary to diagnose RLS. Special

Conflicts of interest: The authors have no commercial or financial conflicts of interest to disclose.
Department of Pediatrics, Saint Louis University School of Medicine, 1465 South Grand Boulevard, Glennon Hall 2712, St Louis, MO 63104, USA
* Corresponding author.
E-mail address: sparuthi@slu.edu

Sleep Med Clin 11 (2016) 91–103
http://dx.doi.org/10.1016/j.jsmc.2015.10.010

consideration should be given to possible descriptions of symptoms based on the patient's age. Physical examination is usually nonfocal.

ICSD-3 criteria for the diagnosis of RLS for adults and children are the same and all criteria should be met:

A. An urge to move the legs, usually accompanied by, or thought to be caused by, uncomfortable and unpleasant sensations in the legs. These symptoms must:
   1. Begin or worsen during periods of rest or inactivity, such as lying down or sitting
   2. Be partially or totally relieved by movement, such as walking or stretching, at least as long as the activity continues
   3. Occur exclusively or predominantly in the evening or night rather than during the day
B. The features listed earlier are not solely accounted for as symptoms of another medical or a behavioral condition (eg, leg cramps, positional discomfort, myalgia, venous stasis, leg edema, arthritis, habitual foot tapping).
C. The symptoms of RLS cause concern, distress, sleep disturbance, or impairment in mental, physical, social, occupational, educational, behavioral, or other important areas of functioning.

Young patients should be encouraged to use their own words and have described RLS as:

- Pain
- Growing pains
- Shark bites
- Soda in my legs
- Need to stretch
- Cannot get comfortable

The differential diagnosis of common mimics includes (from Ref.[21]):

- Positional discomfort
- Sore leg muscles
- Ligament sprain/tendon strain
- Positional ischemia (numbness)
- Dermatitis
- Bruises
- Leg cramps

Management

Management includes:

- Avoidance of exacerbating factors
- Iron supplementation when ferritin level is less than 75 μg/L
- Medications (off-label) that are approved for RLS in adults, including gabapentin, ropinirole, pramipexole, and rotigotine

- Nonpharmacologic treatments: massage, warm bath, socks warmed for 5 to 10 minutes in a clothes dryer, compression stockings, or soccer socks in the evenings, and so forth

Avoidance of exacerbating factors
Exacerbating factors may include[22]:

- Insufficient sleep for age
- Irregular sleep schedule
- Caffeine
- Nicotine
- Alcohol
- Medications (sedating antihistamines, serotonergic antidepressants, neuroleptics)

Serum ferritin and iron supplementation
Serum ferritin levels should be obtained on pediatric patients with RLS because more than 80% may have low levels.[4,23,24] These patients often have improvement or resolution of symptoms with oral iron therapy.[25–28] Serum ferritin results should be interpreted with caution because ferritin is an acute phase reactant and levels may remain increased for up to 4 weeks following a febrile illness.[29] Patients with serum ferritin levels less than 75 μg/L[30] should be treated with 2 to 4 mg/kg of elemental iron daily up to twice a day. Serum ferritin should be rechecked in 3 months, at which time symptoms are reassessed. Patients with ongoing iron therapy should continue to be monitored for iron overload, which is a rare but serious complication of iron therapy in individuals who carry hemochromatosis genes.[31]

Iron absorption is enhanced when taken with vitamin C (common in juices). Iron is more poorly absorbed when taken within 2 hours of calcium/dairy products and should be avoided.[22]

Side effects of iron supplementation may include:

- Dark green or black stools while taking iron
- Temporary brown or gray teeth discoloration (resolves by brushing teeth with baking soda toothpaste)
- Constipation/diarrhea
- Abdominal pain

Other medications
Because there are no RLS treatments specifically labeled by the US Food and Drug Administration (FDA) for pediatric use, caution is advised to select treatment medications for off-label use. Medications that have been shown to improve RLS severity include gabapentin[32,33] and dopaminergic medications, including ropinirole and pramipexole.[4,23,28,34–38] Medications that are FDA approved for RLS in adults are often efficacious in children at

significantly lower doses. It has been the authors' experience that, in appropriate children more than 2 years of age diagnosed with RLS, gabapentin at 50 to 100 mg (maximum of 5 mg/kg) approximately 2 to 3 hours before bedtime is a reasonable starting dose. Parents should be reminded of possible side effects, including excessive daytime sleepiness and aggressive behavior.

NARCOLEPSY
Introduction

Narcolepsy is a chronic condition of excessive daytime sleepiness that may be accompanied by cataplexy, hypnagogic/hypnopompic hallucinations, sleep paralysis, and/or highly fragmented overnight sleep. It is divided into 2 subgroups: type 1 (hypocretin deficiency, often cataplexy) and type 2 (without cataplexy). The prevalence of narcolepsy in all ages is estimated at between 0.025% and 0.40%.[39–42] Estimates about the age of onset vary, but in a retrospective study about 50% of adults with narcolepsy had the onset of symptoms in childhood[43]; there is a peak incidence around age 15 years. Another cohort showed that the mean age of onset is 9 years, with 8% diagnosed by age 5 years.[44]

Impact

Excessive daytime sleepiness is usually the first symptom of narcolepsy[45] and may be seen as the reemergence of naps in a child who had previously given up naps. Patients experience repeated daily episodes of an irrepressible need to sleep, which can be disabling. Children and adolescents with narcolepsy have significantly higher rates of behavioral problems and depression related to their disease.[46] Severe psychosocial and social problems are also common.[47] These patients often have significant weight gain not ascribable to inactivity or increased caloric intake, although the cause of this is not clear.[48–53]

Pathophysiology

Narcolepsy type 1 is caused by a deficiency of hypothalamic hypocretin (also known as orexin) signaling, likely secondary to selective loss of hypocretin-producing neurons.[54,55] Strong human leukocyte antigen (HLA) associations, specifically HLA DQB1*0602, and T-cell receptor polymorphisms suggest an autoimmune basis for the disease.[56–60] Furthermore, after a significant increase in the incidence of childhood narcolepsy after H1N1 vaccination with Pandemrix in 2009, a high frequency of antibodies to the hypocretin (orexin) receptor 2 were found that were cross reactive with the influenza nucleoprotein.[61–63] This finding further suggests an autoimmune origin.

Narcolepsy type 2 is likely a heterogeneous disorder with multiple causes. Some cases likely have the same cause as type 1, but the patients do not experience cataplexy and have not had a cerebrospinal fluid (CSF) hypocretin-1 level performed or the level is higher than 110 pg/mL. In the postmortem examination in a patient with narcolepsy without cataplexy the number of hypocretin cells was decreased, but not to the degree of patients with narcolepsy with cataplexy.[64]

Diagnosis

The ICSD-3 diagnostic criteria are the same for adults and children, as listed later. Physical examination may reveal a sleepy child in the office, precocious puberty features, cataplexy that can be induced with cartoons, absent tendon reflexes during an episode of cataplexy, or a normal physical examination.

Narcolepsy type 1
  Criteria A and B must be met:
  A. The patient has daily periods of irrepressible need to sleep or daytime lapses into sleep occurring for at least 3 months.
  B. The presence of 1 or both of the following:
     1. Cataplexy and a mean sleep latency of less than or equal to 8 minutes and 2 or more sleep-onset rapid eye movement periods (SOREMPs) on a multiple sleep latency test (MSLT) performed according to standard techniques. A SOREMP (within 15 minutes of sleep onset) on the preceding nocturnal polysomnogram may replace 1 of the SOREMPs on the MSLT.
     2. CSF hypocretin-1 concentration, measured by immunoreactivity, is either less than or equal to 110 pg/mL or less than one-third of mean values obtained in normal subjects with the same standardized assay.

Narcolepsy type 2
  Criteria A to E must be met
  A. The patient has daily periods of irrepressible need to sleep or daytime lapses into sleep occurring for at least 3 months.
  B. A mean sleep latency of less than or equal to 8 minutes and 2 or more SOREMPs are found on an MSLT performed according to standard techniques. A SOREMP (within 15 minutes of sleep onset) on the preceding nocturnal polysomnogram may replace 1 of the SOREMPs on the MSLT.

C. Cataplexy is absent.
D. Either CSF hypocretin-1 concentration has not been measured or CSF hypocretin-1 concentration measured by immunoreactivity is either greater than 110 pg/mL or greater than one-third of mean values obtained in normal subjects with the same standardized assay.
E. The hypersomnolence and/or MSLT findings are not better explained by other causes, such as insufficient sleep, obstructive sleep apnea (OSA), delayed sleep phase disorder, or the effect of medication or substances or their withdrawal.

Diagnostic considerations

Diagnosis is based on clinical history consistent with excessive sleepiness (not of other causes) and an MSLT with mean sleep latency of less than 8 minutes and containing 2 SOREMPs. If the MSLT is equivocal or shows a mean sleep latency of less than 8 minutes without SOREMPs in a child highly suspected for narcolepsy, HLA typing for HLA DQB1*0602 can be considered. Patients who are negative for HLA DQB1*0602 are unlikely to have low CSF hypocretin-1 levels. CSF hypocretin-1 measurement is available in select biochemical laboratories. In addition, lumbar puncture is not warranted in patients with typical narcolepsy clinical findings and a positive MSLT. The value of MSLT in children who physiologically still nap (typically <7 years of age) is not well established. Therefore, additional methods, such as sleep diaries, sleepiness surveys/questionnaires, actigraphy, or HLA typing, may be useful in clarifying the diagnosis.[65] In addition, because narcolepsy is especially rare in preschool children or early school children, consider imaging by computed tomography or MRI to assess for the presence of brain tumors or structural abnormalities.

Cataplexy

Cataplexy may be diagnosed in patients with at least 2 episodes of brief, sudden loss of muscle tone with retained consciousness. Patients can see and hear, but they are temporarily overcome by muscle weakness. These symptoms are often precipitated by strong, usually positive, emotions, with nearly all patients reporting some episodes precipitated by laughter. In young children, anticipation of a reward is a common precipitant. Transient reversible loss of deep tendon reflexes during an attack is a strong diagnostic finding. In some children, cataplexy is not clearly associated with an emotion and is represented only by facial hypotonia (droopy eyelids, mouth opening, and protruded tongue) or gait instability.[66] It is helpful for parents to bring in home videos on smartphones or tablets for review.

Hypnagogic hallucinations

Hypnagogic hallucinations may involve visual or auditory imagery that young children are unable to distinguish from reality, as if they are dreaming while awake. Hallucinations commonly involve people, animals, or shapes that are not present. They can usually be distinguished from schizophrenia because they only occur at sleep-wake transitions and not otherwise.[67] Also, the voices do not provide specific instruction.

Sleep paralysis

Sleep paralysis is the inability to move during wake just before sleep or just after awakening, although respiratory and extraocular movements are preserved. Episodes may be interrupted if the child is touched or spoken to by a parent.[46] Although a common feature of narcolepsy, this may occur in isolation as a benign condition.

Other common features

- Difficulty with sleep maintenance at night[66]
- Excessive sleeping at night in young children[68]
- Panic attacks or social phobias
- Precocious puberty
- Poor school performance

Differential Diagnosis

Differential diagnosis for excessive daytime sleepiness

- Insufficient sleep syndrome (most common)
- Substance abuse
- Medication side effect
- OSA
- Idiopathic hypersomnia

Differential diagnosis for cataplexy

- Hypotension
- Transient ischemic attacks
- Drop attacks
- Akinetic seizures
- Neuromuscular disorder
- Psychiatric disorder
- Other medical disorders, most commonly including Niemann-Pick disease type C, Prader-Willi syndrome

Management

It is highly recommended that children keep up with normal, and perhaps slightly increased, physical activity, such as through organized physical activities. Scheduled short naps (up to 30–60 minutes) may also be beneficial when placed strategically throughout the day, such as 1 nap in school, and 1 after school. Limited driving may be considered on a strict, case-by-case basis in appropriate situations. Up to 72% of adults have reported falling asleep while driving and up to 28% reported cataplexy when driving.[69,70]

Nonpharmacologic treatment considerations in children with narcolepsy

> Regular sleep-wake schedules
> Planned naps
> Exercise regularly/engage in after-school sports
> Sit in the first row in the classroom
> Discuss safety precautions: children should avoid activities that may trigger cataplexy and injury, such as climbing monkey bars or cooking
> Screen for and treat coexisting depression
> Assist the child to develop coping strategies
> Screen for and treat precocious puberty
> Limited, well-supervised driving
> Avoid alcohol
> Vocational guidance to assist in choice of a profession

Pharmacotherapy in narcolepsy is targeted at symptomatic relief in order to restore a normal or improved level of alertness and function. Several best-practice recommendations have been published.[71–74] Nearly all medications discussed later (except methylphenidate and amphetamines such as Dexedrine, Dextrostat, and Adderall) are off-label for treatment of narcolepsy in children. Stimulants are not recommended in children less than the age of 6 years and in children with known structural cardiac defects. It is also important to review possible side effects with caregivers and children, and to review with parents and children the black box warning for increased suicidality for any antidepressants used in children.

Pharmacology treatments: stimulants for daytime sleepiness (some listed medications are off-label treatments)

- Methylphenidate hydrochloride (Ritalin, Ritalin SR, Ritalin LA, Methylin [liquid], Concerta, Metadate CD, Metadate ER, Daytrana [skin patch]) is a commonly chosen initial treatment because many providers are familiar with it for treatment of ADHD. Recommended dosing is similar for ADHD and narcolepsy. Common side effects include loss of appetite, nervousness, tics, headaches, and sleep-onset insomnia.

- Dextroamphetamine/methamphetamine (Focalin, Focalin XR, Dexedrine, Dextrostat Desoxyn, Adderall, Adderall XR) should be used cautiously. Side effects include insomnia, irritability, hypertension, and psychotic reactions. Patients are at risk for tolerance and dependence.
- Lisdexamfetamine (Vyvanse) is a long-acting stimulant prodrug primarily used for ADHD and may be useful in pediatric narcolepsy.
- Modafinil and armodafinil (Provigil and Nuvigil) are FDA approved for sleepiness in patients more than 16 years of age.[75–79] Common side effects include headache, irritability, and loss of appetite.[78] Because these agents induce cytochrome P450, sexually active young women who are on birth control pills should use an alternate barrier method. Modafinil has also been implicated in Stevens-Johnson syndrome, although this is uncommon.[80]
- Sodium oxybate (Xyrem) may be considered in rare cases in children with narcolepsy with cataplexy.[75,79,81,82] The most common side effects are headache, dizziness, depression, sleepwalking, enuresis, and terminal insomnia. Alcohol is strictly contraindicated because of the risk of respiratory depression, hypotension, and profound sedation. Providers and patients must enroll in the XYREM REMS Program if a patient is prescribed sodium oxybate.

Pharmacology treatment (off-label treatments): cataplexy that is bothersome to the child

- In some children, cataplexy may improve with methylphenidate treatment.
- Selective serotonin reuptake inhibitors, such as fluoxetine, and serotonin and norepinephrine reuptake inhibitors, such as venlafaxine, are all used off-label for treatment of cataplexy, and may also be useful for hypnagogic hallucinations and sleep paralysis. It is important to review the black box warning for increased suicidality for any antidepressants with parents and children.
- Tricyclic antidepressants are another second-line treatment of cataplexy. It is important to review the black box warning for increased suicidality for any antidepressants with parents and children.
- Sodium oxybate may also be considered.

Pharmacology treatment (off-label treatment): other medications

- Intravenous immunoglobulin has been reported with mixed efficacy.[83–91]

- Pitolisant, an H3 receptor inverse agonist, has shown limited positive preliminary results in adults and adolescents.[92,93]
- Intranasal hypocretin has undergone preliminary studies with positive effects, although additional studies are needed.[94,95]

PARASOMNIAS
Introduction

Parasomnias are physical events occurring either during sleep or at the sleep-wake transition. Childhood parasomnias are common, with a prevalence approaching 90%.[96] The most common, in order of prevalence, are somniloquy (sleep talking), bruxism, sleep terrors, enuresis, and somnambulism (sleepwalking). In the interest of brevity, this section focuses on sleepwalking, sleep terrors, and nightmares.

Sleepwalking and sleep terrors are both disorders of arousal from non–rapid eye movement (NREM) sleep. In contrast, nightmares are a rapid eye movement (REM) sleep parasomnia. Because REM is most abundant during the final third of a night's sleep, nightmares are most common in the early morning hours, whereas sleepwalking and sleep terrors are more frequent earlier in sleep.[97]

Causes

Many priming factors for disorders of arousal have been identified:

- Sleep deprivation
- Physical or emotional stress
- OSA
- RLS
- Phone calls, other noises
- Sleeping in unfamiliar surroundings
- Febrile illness
- Other disorders causing frequent arousals

Sleepwalking (International Classification of Sleep Disorders, 3rd Edition)

Sleepwalking description

Sleepwalking typically begins as confusional arousal, with the patient sitting up in bed. However, it might also begin with the individual immediately leaving the bed and walking or running. Behaviors are varied, and range from simple, non–goal-directed activities to complex tasks. Children may show bizarre behaviors, such as urinating in inappropriate locations or leaving the house. The sleepwalking individual may appear to be awake and responsive, but is disoriented and has diminished mentation.[98,99]

Sleepwalking may have a genetic component. The rate of childhood sleepwalking increases in relation to the number of affected parents: 22% when neither parent has the disorder, 45% if 1 parent is affected, and 60% when both are affected.[100]

Sleepwalking diagnosis

The diagnosis is made by clinical history provided by parents/caregivers. The children have no recollection of the sleepwalking. The clinical history must meet criteria for disorders of arousal and for sleepwalking specifically, as per the ICSD-3. Physical examination is usually nonfocal, although the child may have signs of OSA in the context of appropriate clinical history.

General diagnostic criteria for disorders of arousal

Criteria A to E must be met
A. Recurrent episodes of incomplete awakening from sleep.
B. Inappropriate or absent responsiveness to efforts of others to intervene or redirect the person during the episode.
C. Limited (eg, a single visual scene) or no associated cognition or dream imagery.
D. Partial or complete amnesia for the episode.
E. The disturbance is not better explained by another sleep disorder, mental disorder, medical condition, medication, or substance use.

Additional diagnostic criteria for sleepwalking

Criteria A and B must be met
A. The disorder meets general criteria for NREM disorders of arousal.
B. The arousals are associated with ambulation and other complex behaviors out of bed.

Sleepwalking management

Management should focus on creating a safe environment for the child and uncovering any underlying sleep disorder. Safety measures include:
- Alarms or bells on the child's door to alert parents
- Door and window alarms (purchase at home-improvement stores)
- Removal of sharp or breakable objects from the child's room or common pathways
- Have the child sleep on the floor on a mattress
- Have the child sleep on the ground floor
- Lock up items that could become potentially dangerous to the child (eg, keys, guns, knives)
- Screen for OSA and RLS. Treatment of these disorders may eliminate the increased

frequency of arousals that trigger NREM parasomnias

- Take sleepwalking seriously; children have been seriously harmed when leaving the home asleep, such as freezing to death, being hit by vehicles, or drowning

If sleepwalking persists in the absence of OSA or RLS, or does not improve with treatment of OSA or RLS, with adequate age-appropriate sleep opportunity, then a low dose of imipramine or clonazepam (clonazepam 0.125–0.5 mg at bedtime) given for 3 to 6 months, with slow tapering, may be helpful.[101]

Sleep Terrors

Sleep terrors description
Sleep terrors (night terrors, or pavor nocturnus) are arousals typically involving shrieking and behavioral manifestations of intense fear. These arousals are usually seen between the ages of 2 and 12 years. A family history of sleep terrors is common. Episodes can be distressing to parents and may prompt emergency department evaluation.

Sleep terrors diagnosis
The diagnosis of sleep terrors is made by the General Diagnostic Criteria for Disorders of Arousal outlined earlier, along with the following additional criteria. It is helpful when parents are able to bring videos recorded on smartphones or tablets. Physical examination is usually nonfocal, although the child may have signs of OSA in the context of appropriate clinical history.

A. The arousals are characterized by episodes of abrupt terror, typically beginning with an alarming vocalization, such as a frightening scream.
B. There is intense fear and signs of autonomic arousal, including mydriasis, tachycardia, tachypnea, and diaphoresis, during an episode.

Sleep terrors management
Similar to sleepwalking, history taking should focus on uncovering other sleep disorders, such as OSA or RLS. Recurrent arousals from one of these disorders may be associated with increased night terrors. Once underlying sleep disorders have been treated, management should focus on reassuring families, because sleep terrors are self-limited and typically resolve after puberty, possibly because of the decrease in slow-wave sleep at that age.

If a child has nightly episodes, scheduled awakenings 15 to 30 minutes before the time of usual episode occurrence may be tried. This approach can be continued for 2 to 4 weeks and repeated if episodes recur. If sleep terrors persist in the absence of OSA or RLS, or do not improve with treatment of OSA or RLS, with adequate age-appropriate sleep opportunity, then a low dose of imipramine or clonazepam (clonazepam 0.125–0.5 mg at bedtime) given for 3 to 6 months, with slow tapering, may be helpful.[101]

Nightmare Disorder

Nightmare description
Nightmares are disturbing dreams usually occurring during REM sleep and resulting in awakening. They are accompanied by postawakening anxiety and difficulty returning to sleep. They may be particularly distressing to young children who are unable to distinguish them from reality.

Nightmares can be distinguished from night terrors by the following typical characteristics:

Nightmare	Night Terror
Second half of night	First half of night
Child recalls event	Child confused during event, no recollection afterward
Markedly delayed return to sleep	Able to return to sleep
Typically arise from REM sleep	Typically arise from NREM sleep

Nightmare disorder diagnosis is as per the ICSD-3. Because childhood nightmares often resolve spontaneously, the diagnosis should be given only if there is persistent distress or impairment. Physical examination is usually nonfocal, although the child may have signs of OSA in the context of appropriate clinical history.

Criteria A to C must be met
A. Repeated occurrences of extended, extremely dysphoric, and well-remembered dreams that usually involve threats to survival, security, or physical integrity.
B. On awakening from the dysphoric dreams, the person rapidly becomes oriented and alert.
C. The dream experience, or the sleep disturbance produced by awakening from it, causes clinically significant distress or impairment in social, occupational, or other important areas of functioning as indicated by the report of at least 1 of the following:
1. Mood disturbance (eg, persistence of nightmare affect, anxiety, dysphoria)

2. Sleep resistance (eg, bedtime anxiety, fear of sleep/subsequent nightmares)
3. Cognitive impairments (eg, intrusive nightmare imagery, impaired concentration or memory)
4. Negative impact on caregiver or family functioning (eg, nighttime disruption)
5. Behavioral problems (eg, bedtime avoidance, fear of the dark)
6. Daytime sleepiness
7. Fatigue or low energy
8. Impaired occupational or educational function
9. Impaired interpersonal/social function

Nightmare management

Management of frequent nightmares can include the following[102]:

- Avoiding television for 2 to 3 hours before bedtime[97]
- A dim night-light in the room
- Rescripting techniques/imagery rehearsal: teaching the child to have a new, pleasant alternative ending to the nightmare; 10 to 15 minutes every night before lights out for 28 nights
- Writing down the content of the dream or drawing pictures of them, which may make them less scary
- In difficult cases, referral to a developmental-behavioral pediatrician for relaxation strategies, desensitization, or hypnotherapy[103]
- Review history for causes of arousals from sleep, including environmental factors and medical disorders of OSA and RLS

SLEEP AND EPILEPSY
Introduction

Several types of epilepsy tend to manifest only or predominantly during sleep. These types include nocturnal frontal lobe epilepsy, benign epilepsy of childhood with centrotemporal spikes, benign epilepsy with occipital paroxysms, juvenile myoclonic epilepsy, and continuous spike waves during NREM sleep. Patients with these and other types of epilepsy often have coexisting sleep-related complaints, the most common being excessive daytime sleepiness or insomnia.[104] In contrast, sleep deprivation alone has long been recognized as a seizure precipitant,[105] as well as untreated OSA. The interface of sleep and epilepsy is discussed here, without discussing specific types of epilepsy.

Interactions Between Sleep and Epilepsy

Children with epilepsy frequently have poor sleep quality and are anxious about sleep. Nighttime seizures can cause brief arousals in sleep, leading to sleep fragmentation and poor daytime function. Epilepsy may also reduce the total amount of sleep significantly, which has a significant negative impact on seizure control.[106–108] In addition, nocturnal seizures, polytherapy, developmental delay, and refractory epilepsy are associated with poor sleep habits and sleep disorders.[109–111] Of note, OSA, RLS, and periodic limb movements are particularly common in children with epilepsy.[112–117] Treating OSA, and likely other sleep disorders, improves seizure control and reduces interictal epileptogenic activity.[112,115,116,118]

Antiepileptic Drugs and Sleep

Certain antiepileptic drugs tend to affect sleep and daytime sleepiness. For examples, barbiturates can cause daytime sleepiness, whereas phenytoin causes insomnia. Benzodiazepines not only cause sedation but may cause some degree of respiratory depression and decreased muscle tone at night, which may cause or worsen OSA. In addition, valproate may cause excessive weight gain and lead to development of OSA.

The Role of Melatonin

Melatonin is a hormone secreted by the pineal gland and is responsible for normal circadian rhythm. It is also thought to have sedative, anxiolytic, and anticonvulsant properties.[119] Individuals with intractable epilepsy often have depressed baseline levels of melatonin.[120–122] Supplemental melatonin therapy may help control seizures in some patients, as well as improve sleep efficiency and decrease sleep disruption.[122] However, in rare cases, melatonin can lower the seizure threshold, with children having more seizures when on melatonin.

Screening for Sleep Disturbance in Children with Epilepsy

Children with epilepsy should routinely be screened for sleep disturbances. Screening questions should include the following aspects:

- Difficulty falling asleep
- Waking during the night
- Breathing problems while asleep
- Unusual behaviors/parasomnias at night
- Twitching around the mouth while sleeping
- Large movements or jerking during the night
- Difficulty waking in the morning
- Being sleepy or tired during the day

Diagnosis of nighttime epilepsy requires coordination of care between the neurologist and sleep team. Polysomnograms can be requested to have an extended electroencephalogram (EEG) montage, capturing the same 16 leads as performed on routine EEG. Because video recordings are part of a polysomnogram, any unusual activity or behaviors may be captured. The polysomnogram is also helpful to evaluate for the presence of OSA. Physical examination is usually nonfocal, although the child may have signs of OSA in the context of appropriate clinical history.

Treatment typically decreases the unusual behaviors/activities that initially brought the child to the caregiver's attention.

SLEEP AND HEADACHES
Introduction

Headache is a common complaint in children, and has a strong relationship with sleep.[123] Inadequate sleep duration and poor sleep quality are common headache triggers.[124] In contrast, sleep can relieve or even terminate headaches in children.[125]

Children with headaches have higher rates of several sleep disorders, including OSA, narcolepsy, insomnia, parasomnias, and restless sleep (some of these are likely with RLS).[126–128] Sleep hygiene alone has been shown to improve both headache control and sleep in children.[129]

Sleep and headaches not only have significant clinical overlap but share common anatomic and physiologic pathways.

OSA can cause secondary morning headaches that may completely resolve with treatment. These headaches seem to be caused by generalized intracranial and extracranial vasodilation from hypoxemia and hypercapnia, and subsequent activation of trigeminal nociceptors.[130]

Sleep Duration in Children

Typical sleep needs in children (total per 24 hours)

- Toddlers: 11 to 14 hours
- School age (kindergarten to eighth grade): approximately 10 hours
- High school age: approximately 9 hours

SUMMARY

Children who present in the neurologists' office often have overlap of sleep problems in addition to their neurologic problems. Many of these children present with persistent headaches, seizures, neuromuscular disorders, pain syndrome, cognitive dysfunction, developmental delays, mood disorders, and inattention disorders. In addition, children may present on the autism spectrum, following brain injury, or with learning difficulties to the neurology clinic. Screening for sleep disorders with appropriate questions assists clinicians to choose the most appropriate testing and then treatment. Individualized therapy for common sleep disorders, such as OSA and RLS, is likely to improve concurrent neurologic disorders.

REFERENCES

1. Picchietti D, Allen RP, Walters AS, et al. Restless legs syndrome: prevalence and impact in children and adolescents—the Peds REST study. Pediatrics 2007;120:253–66.
2. Turkdogan D, Bekiroglu N, Zaimoglu S. A prevalence study of restless legs syndrome in Turkish children and adolescents. Sleep Med 2011;12:315–21.
3. Yilmaz K, Kilincaslan A, Aydin N, et al. Prevalence and correlates of restless legs syndrome in adolescents. Dev Med Child Neurol 2011;53:40–7.
4. Picchietti D, Stevens HE. Early manifestations of restless legs syndrome in childhood and adolescence. Sleep Med 2008;9:770–81.
5. Arbuckle R, Abetz L, Durmer JS, et al. Development of the Pediatric Restless Legs Syndrome Severity Scale (P-RLS-SS): a patient-reported outcome measure of pediatric RLS symptoms and impact. Sleep Med 2010;11:897–906.
6. Oner P, Dirik EB, Taner Y, et al. Association between low serum ferritin and restless legs syndrome in patients with attention deficit hyperactivity disorder. Tohoku J Exp Med 2007;213(3):269–76.
7. Silvestri R, Gagliano A, Arico I, et al. Sleep disorders in children with attention-deficit/hyperactivity disorder (ADHD) recorded overnight by video-polysomnography. Sleep Med 2009;10(10):1132–8.
8. Wagner ML, Walters AS, Fisher BC. Symptoms of attention-deficit/hyperactivity disorder in adults with restless legs syndrome. Sleep 2004;27(8):1499–504.
9. Wiggs L, Montgomery P, Stores G. Actigraphic and parent reports of sleep patterns and sleep disorders in children with subtypes of attention-deficit hyperactivity disorder. Sleep 2005;28(11):1437–45.
10. Trotti LM, Bhadriraju S, Rye DB. An update on the pathophysiology and genetics of restless legs syndrome. Curr Neurol Neurosci Rep 2008;8(4):281–7.
11. Earley CJ, Allen RP, Beard JL, et al. Insight into the pathophysiology of restless legs syndrome. J Neurosci Res 2000;62(5):623–8.
12. Allen R. Dopamine and iron in the pathophysiology of restless legs syndrome (RLS). Sleep Med 2004;5(4):385–91.
13. Beard JL, Connor JR. Iron status and neural functioning. Annu Rev Nutr 2003;23:41–58.
14. Burhans MS, Dailey C, Beard Z, et al. Iron deficiency: differential effects on monoamine transporters. Nutr Neurosci 2005;8(1):31–8.

15. Kemlink D, Polo O, Frauscher B, et al. Replication of restless legs syndrome loci in three European populations. J Med Genet 2009;46(5):315–8.

16. Schormair B, Kemlink D, Roeske D, et al. PTPRD (protein tyrosine phosphatase receptor type delta) is associated with restless legs syndrome. Nat Genet 2008;40(8):946–8.

17. Stefansson H, Rye DB, Hicks A, et al. A genetic risk factor for periodic limb movements in sleep. N Engl J Med 2007;357(7):639–47.

18. Trenkwalder C, Hogl B, Winkelmann J. Recent advances in the diagnosis, genetics and treatment of restless legs syndrome. J Neurol 2009;256: 539–53.

19. Vilarino-Guell C, Farrer MJ, Lin SC. A genetic risk factor for periodic limb movements in sleep. N Engl J Med 2008;358(4):425–7.

20. Winkelmann J, Schormair B, Lichtner P, et al. Genome-wide association study of restless legs syndrome identifies common variants in three genomic regions. Nat Genet 2007;39(8):1000–6.

21. Picchietti DL, Bruni O, de Weerd A, et al, International Restless Legs Syndrome Study Group. Pediatric restless legs syndrome diagnostic criteria: an update by the International Restless Legs Syndrome Study Group. Sleep Med 2013;14(12): 1253–9.

22. Picchietti MA, Picchietti DL. Advances in pediatric restless legs syndrome: iron, genetics, diagnosis and treatment. Sleep Med 2010;11:643–51.

23. Kotagal S, Silber MH. Childhood-onset restless legs syndrome. Ann Neurol 2004;56(6):803–7.

24. Kotagal S, Chopra A. Pediatric sleep-wake disorders. Neurol Clin 2012;30(4):1193–212.

25. Banno K, Koike S, Yamamoto K. Restless legs syndrome in a 5-year-old boy with low body stores of iron. Sleep Biol Rhythms 2009;7(1):52–4.

26. Kryger MH, Otake K, Foerster J. Low body stores of iron and restless legs syndrome: a correctable cause of insomnia in adolescents and teenagers. Sleep Med 2002;3(2):127–32.

27. Mohri I, Kato-Nishimura K, Tachibana N, et al. Restless legs syndrome (RLS): an unrecognized cause for bedtime problems and insomnia in children. Sleep Med 2008;9(6):701–2.

28. Starn AL, Udall JN Jr. Iron deficiency anemia, pica, and restless legs syndrome in a teenage girl. Clin Pediatr (Phila) 2008;47(1):83–5.

29. Eskeland B, Baerheim A, Ulvik R, et al. Influence of mild infections on iron status parameters in women of reproductive age. Scand J Prim Health Care 2002;20(1):50–6.

30. Wang J, O'Reilly B, Venkataraman R, et al. Efficacy of oral iron in patients with restless legs syndrome and a low-normal ferritin: a randomized, double-blind, placebo-controlled study. Sleep Med 2009; 10(9):973–5.

31. Barton JC, Wooten VD, Acton RT. Hemochromatosis and iron therapy of restless legs syndrome. Sleep Med 2001;2(3):249–51.

32. Garcia-Borreguero D, Larrosa O, de la Llave Y, et al. Treatment of restless legs syndrome with gabapentin: a double-blind, cross-over study. Neurology 2002;59(10):1573–9.

33. Happe S, Sauter C, Klosch G, et al. Gabapentin versus ropinirole in the treatment of idiopathic restless legs syndrome. Neuropsychobiology 2003; 48(2):82–6.

34. Cortese S, Konofal E, Lecendreux M. Effectiveness of ropinirole for RLS and depressive symptoms in an 11-year-old girl. Sleep Med 2009; 10(2):259–61.

35. Konofal E, Arnulf I, Lecendreux M, et al. Ropinirole in a child with attention-deficit hyperactivity disorder and restless legs syndrome. Pediatr Neurol 2005;32:350–1.

36. Walters AS, Mandelbaum DE, Lewin DS, et al. Dopaminergic therapy in children with restless legs/periodic limb movements in sleep and ADHD. Dopaminergic Therapy Study Group. Pediatr Neurol 2000;22(3):182–6.

37. Walters AS, Silvestri R, Zucconi M, et al. Review of the possible relationship and hypothetical links between attention deficit hyperactivity disorder (ADHD) and simple sleep related movement disorders, parasomnias, hypersomnias and circadian rhythm disorders. J Clin Sleep Med 2008;4:591–600.

38. Muhle H, Neumann A, Lohmann-Hedrich K, et al. Childhood-onset restless legs syndrome: clinical and genetic features of 22 families. Mov Disord 2008;23(8):1113–21; quiz 1203.

39. Dauvilliers Y, Montplaisir J, Molinari N, et al. Age at onset of narcolepsy in two large populations of patients in France and Quebec. Neurology 2001;57: 2029–33.

40. Ohayon MM, Priest RG, Zulley J, et al. Prevalence of narcolepsy symptomatology and diagnosis in the European general population. Neurology 2002;58:1826–33.

41. Silber MH, Krahn LE, Olson E, et al. The epidemiology of narcolepsy in Olmsted County, Minnesota: a population-based study. Sleep 2002;25:197–202.

42. Silber MH, Becker PM, Earley C, et al. Willis-Ekbom Disease Foundation revised consensus statement on the management of restless legs syndrome. Mayo Clin Proc 2013;88:977–86.

43. Morish E, King MA, Smith IE, et al. Factors associated with a delay in the diagnosis of narcolepsy. Sleep Med 2004;5:37–41.

44. Challamel MJ, Mazzola ME, Nevsimalova S, et al. Narcolepsy in children. Sleep 1994;17(Suppl 8): S17–20.

45. Peterson PC, Husain AM. Pediatric narcolepsy. Brain Dev 2008;30:609–23.

46. Stores G, Montgomery P, Wiggs L. The psychosocial problems of children with narcolepsy and those with excessive daytime sleepiness of uncertain origin. Pediatrics 2006;118:1116–23.

47. Dorris L, Zuberi SM, Scott N, et al. Psychosocial and intellectual functioning in childhood narcolepsy. Dev Neurorehabil 2008;11:187–94.

48. Chabas D, Foulon C, Gonzales J, et al. Eating disorder and metabolism in narcoleptic patients. Sleep 2007;30:1267–73.

49. Dahmen N, Bierbrauer J, Kasten M. Increased prevalence of obesity in narcoleptic patients and relatives. Eur Arch Psychiatry Clin Neurosci 2001; 251:85–9.

50. Inocente CO, Lavault S, Lecendreux M, et al. Impact of obesity in children with narcolepsy. CNS Neurosci Ther 2013;19:521–8.

51. Kok SW, Overeem S, Visscher TL, et al. Hypocretin deficiency in narcoleptic humans is associated with abdominal obesity. Obes Res 2003;11:1147–54.

52. Kotagal S, Krahn LE, Slocumb N. A putative link between childhood narcolepsy and obesity. Sleep Med 2004;5:147–50.

53. Schuld A, Beitinger PA, Dalal M, et al. Increased body mass index (BMI) in male narcoleptic patients, but not in HLA-DR2-positive healthy male volunteers. Sleep Med 2002;3:335–9.

54. Nishino S, Ripley B, Overeem S, et al. Hypocretin (orexin) deficiency in human narcolepsy. Lancet 2000;355:39–40.

55. Peyron C, Faraco J, Rogers W, et al. A mutation in a case of early onset narcolepsy and a generalized absence of hypocretin peptides in human narcoleptic brains. Nat Med 2000;6:991–7.

56. De la Herrán-Arita AK, Kornum BR, Mahlios J, et al. CD4+ T cell autoimmunity to hypocretin/orexin and cross-reactivity to a 2009 H1N1 influenza A epitope in narcolepsy. Sci Transl Med 2013;5:216ra176.

57. Faraco J, Lin L, Kornum BR, et al. ImmunoChip study implicates antigen presentation to T cells in narcolepsy. PLoS Genet 2013;9(2):e1003270.

58. Nishino S, Ripley B, Overeem S, et al. Low cerebrospinal fluid hypocretin (Orexin) and altered energy homeostasis in human narcolepsy. Ann Neurol 2001;50(3):381–8.

59. Nittur N, Konofal E, Dauvilliers Y, et al. Mazindol in narcolepsy and idiopathic and symptomatic hypersomnia refractory to stimulants: a long-term chart review. Sleep Med 2013;14(1):30–6.

60. van der Heide A, Verduijn W, Haasnoot GW, et al. HLA dosage effect in narcolepsy with cataplexy. Immunogenetics 2015;67:1–6.

61. Ahmed SS, Volkmuth W, Duca J, et al. Antibodies to influenza nucleoprotein cross-react with human hypocretin receptor 2. Sci Transl Med 2015;7(294): 294ra105.

62. American Academy of Sleep Medicine. International classification of sleep disorders. 3rd edition. Darien (IL): American Academy of Sleep Medicine; 2014.

63. Johansen K. The roles of influenza virus antigens and the AS03 adjuvant in the 2009 pandemic vaccine associated with narcolepsy needs further investigation. Dev Med Child Neurol 2014;56: 1041–2.

64. Thannickal TC, Nienhuis R, Siegel JM. Localized loss of hypocretin (orexin) cells in narcolepsy without cataplexy. Sleep 2009;32(8):993.

65. Nevsimalova S. The diagnosis and treatment of pediatric narcolepsy. Curr Neurol Neurosci Rep 2014; 14(8):1–10.

66. Serra L, Montagna P, Mignot E, et al. Cataplexy features in childhood narcolepsy. Mov Disord 2008;23: 858–65.

67. Droogleever-Fortuyn H, Lappenschaar M, Nienhuis F, et al. Hypnagogic hallucinations and "psychotic" symptoms in narcolepsy: a comparison with control subjects and schizophrenic patients. Sleep 2009;32(Suppl):A244–5.

68. Vernet C, Arnulf A. Narcolepsy with long sleep time: a specific entity? Sleep 2009;32:1229–35.

69. Broughton R, Ghanem Q, Hishikawa Y, et al. Life effects of narcolepsy in 180 patients from North-America, Asia, and Europe compared to matched controls. Can J Neurol Sci 1981;8(4): 299–304.

70. Randomized trial of modafinil as a treatment for the excessive daytime somnolence of narcolepsy: US Modafinil in Narcolepsy Multicenter Study Group. Neurology 2000;54(5):1166–75.

71. Guilleminault C, Cao M. Narcolepsy: diagnosis and management. In: Kryger MH, Roth T, Dement WC, editors. Principles and practice of sleep medicine. 5th edition. St Louis (MO): Elsevier; 2011. p. 957–68.

72. Lecendreux M. Pharmacological management of narcolepsy and cataplexy in pediatric patients. Pediatr Drugs 2014;16(5):363–72.

73. Lecendreux M. Pediatric narcolepsy: clinical and therapeutical approaches. Handb Clin Neurol 2013;112:839–45.

74. Mignot EJ. A practical guide to the therapy of narcolepsy and hypersomnia syndromes. Neurotherapeutics 2012;9(4):739–52.

75. Billiard M, Bassetti C, Dauvilliers Y, et al. EFNS guidelines on management of narcolepsy. Eur J Neurol 2006;13(10):1035–48.

76. Harsh JR, Hayduk R, Rosenberg R, et al. The efficacy and safety of armodafinil as treatment for adults with excessive sleepiness associated with narcolepsy. Curr Med Res Opin 2006;22(4): 761–74.

77. Ivanenko A, Tauman R, Gozal D. Modafinil in the treatment of excessive daytime sleepiness in children. Sleep Med 2003;4(6):579–82.

78. Lecendreux M, Bruni O, Franco P, et al. Clinical experience suggests that modafinil is an effective and safe treatment for paediatric narcolepsy. J Sleep Res 2012;21(4):481–3.

79. Morgenthaler TI, Kapur VK, Brown T, et al. Practice parameters for the treatment of narcolepsy and other hypersomnias of central origin. Sleep 2007; 30(12):1705–11.

80. Rugino T. A review of modafinil film-coated tablets for attention-deficit/hyperactivity disorder in children and adolescents. Neuropsychiatr Dis Treat 2007;3(3):293–301.

81. Aran A, Einen M, Lin L, et al. Clinical and therapeutic aspects of childhood narcolepsy-cataplexy: a retrospective study of 51 children. Sleep 2010; 33(11):1457–64.

82. Murali H, Kotagal S. Off-label treatment of severe childhood narcolepsy-cataplexy with sodium oxybate. Sleep 2006;29(8):1025–9.

83. Dauvilliers Y, Abril B, Mas E, et al. Normalization of hypocretin-1 in narcolepsy after intravenous immunoglobulin treatment. Neurology 2009;73(16):1333–4.

84. Fronczek R, Verschuuren J, Lammers GJ. Response to intravenous immunoglobulins and placebo in a patient with narcolepsy with cataplexy. J Neurol 2007;254(11):1607–8.

85. Garcia-Borreguero D, Stillman P, Benes H, et al. Algorithms for the diagnosis and treatment of restless legs syndrome in primary care. BMC Neurol 2011; 11:28.

86. Knudsen S, Biering-Sorensen B, Kornum BR, et al. Early IVIG treatment has no effect on post-H1N1 narcolepsy phenotype or hypocretin deficiency. Neurology 2012;79(1):102–3.

87. Knudsen S, Mikkelsen JD, Bang B, et al. Intravenous immunoglobulin treatment and screening for hypocretin neuron-specific autoantibodies in recent onset childhood narcolepsy with cataplexy. Neuropediatrics 2010;41(5):217–22.

88. Lecendreux M, Maret S, Bassetti C, et al. Clinical efficacy of high-dose intravenous immunoglobulins near the onset of narcolepsy in a 10-year-old boy. J Sleep Res 2003;12(4):347–8.

89. Leon-Munoz L, de la Calzada MD, Guitart M. Accident prevalence in a group of patients with the narcolepsy-cataplexy syndrome. Rev Neurol 2000;30(6):596–8.

90. Plazzi G, Poli F, Franceschini C, et al. Intravenous high-dose immunoglobulin treatment in recent onset childhood narcolepsy with cataplexy. J Neurol 2008;255(10):1549–54.

91. Valko PO, Khatami R, Baumann CR, et al. No persistent effect of intravenous immunoglobulins in patients with narcolepsy with cataplexy. J Neurol 2008;255(12):1900–3.

92. Dauvilliers Y, Bassetti C, Lammers GJ, et al. Pitolisant versus placebo or modafinil in patients with narcolepsy: a double-blind, randomised trial. Lancet Neurol 2013;12(11):1068–75.

93. Inocente C, Arnulf I, Bastuji H, et al. Pitolisant, an inverse agonist of the histamine H3 receptor: an alternative stimulant for narcolepsy-cataplexy in teenagers with refractory sleepiness. Clin Neuropharmacol 2012;35(2):55–60.

94. Baier PC, Hallschmid M, Seeck-Hirschner M, et al. Effects of intranasal hypocretin-1 (orexin A) on sleep in narcolepsy with cataplexy. Sleep Med 2011;12(10):941–6.

95. Weinhold SL, Seeck-Hirschner M, Nowak A, et al. The effect of intranasal orexin-A (hypocretin-1) on sleep, wakefulness and attention in narcolepsy with cataplexy. Behav Brain Res 2014;262:8–13.

96. Petit D, Touchette E, Tremblay RE, et al. Dyssomnias and parasomnias in early childhood. Pediatrics 2007;119:e1016–25.

97. Kotagal S. Parasomnias in childhood. Sleep Med Rev 2009;13:157–68.

98. Bhargava S. Diagnosis and management of common sleep problems in children. Pediatr Rev 2011;32:91–9.

99. Bille B. Migraine in childhood and its prognosis. Cephalalgia 1981;1:71–5.

100. Petit D, Pennestri MH, Paquet J, et al. Childhood sleepwalking and sleep terrors: a longitudinal study of prevalence and familial aggregation. JAMA Pediatr 2015;169(7):653–8.

101. Provini F, Tinuper P, Bisulli F, et al. Arousal disorders. Sleep Med 2011;12(Suppl 2):S22–6.

102. Sadeh A. Cognitive behavioral treatment for childhood sleep disorders. Clin Psychol Rev 2005;25: L612–28.

103. Hauri PJ, Silber MH, Boeve BF. The treatment of parasomnias with hypnosis: a 5-year follow up study. J Clin Sleep Med 2007;3:369–73.

104. Stores G. Sleep disturbance in childhood epilepsy: clinical implications, assessment and treatment. Arch Dis Child 2013;98:548–51.

105. Foldvary-Schaefer N, Grigg-Damberger M. Sleep and epilepsy: what we know, don't know, and need to know. J Clin Neurophysiol 2006; 23(1):4–20.

106. Becker DA, Fennell EB, Carney PR. Sleep disturbance in children with epilepsy. Epilepsy Behav 2003;4:651–8.

107. Cortesi F, Giannotti F, Ottaviano S. Sleep problems and daytime behaviour in childhood idiopathic epilepsy. Epilepsia 1999;40:1557–65.

108. Stores G, Wiggs L, Campling G. Sleep disorders and their relationship to psychological disturbance in children with epilepsy. Child Care Health Dev 1998;24:5–19.

109. Batista BH, Nunes ML. Evaluation of sleep habits in children with epilepsy. Epilepsy Behav 2007;11: 60–4.

110. Wirrel E, Blackman M, Barlow K, et al. Sleep disturbances in children with epilepsy compared with their nearest-aged siblings. Dev Med Child Neurol 2005;47:754–9.

111. Wise MS. Childhood narcolepsy. Neurology 1998; 50(Suppl 1):S37–42.

112. Foldvary-Schaefer N. Obstructive sleep apnoea in patients with epilepsy: does treatment affect seizure control? Sleep Med 2004;4:483–4.

113. Jain SV, Simakajornboon S, Shapiro SM, et al. Obstructive sleep apnea in children with epilepsy: prospective pilot trial. Acta Neurol Scand 2012; 125(1):e3–6.

114. Kaleyias J, Cruz M, Goraya JS, et al. Spectrum of polysomnographic abnormalities in children with epilepsy. Pediatr Neurol 2008;39:170–6.

115. Miano S, Paolino MC, Peraita-Adrados R, et al. Prevalence of EEG paroxysmal activity in a population of children with obstructive sleep apnoea syndrome. Sleep 2009;32:522–9.

116. Oliveira AJ, Zamagni M, Dolso P, et al. Respiratory disorders during sleep in patients with epilepsy: effect of ventilatory therapy on EEG interictal epileptiform discharges. Clin Neurophysiol 2000; 111(Suppl 2):S141–5.

117. Tezer FI, Rémi J, Noachtar S. Ictal apnoea of epileptic origin. Neurology 2009;72:855–7.

118. Vendrame M, Auerbach S, Loddenkemper T, et al. Effect of continuous positive airway pressure treatment on seizure control in patients with obstructive sleep apnea and epilepsy. Epilepsia 2011;52(11): e168–71.

119. Parisi P, Bruni O, Pia Villa M, et al. The relationship between sleep and epilepsy: the effect on cognitive functioning in children. Dev Med Child Neurol 2010;52(9):805–10.

120. Bazil CW, Short D, Crispin D, et al. Patients with intractable epilepsy have low melatonin, which increases following seizures. Neurology 2000;55: 1746–8.

121. Coppola G, Iervolino G, Mastrosimone M, et al. Melatonin in wake-sleep disorders in children, adolescents and young adults with mental retardation with or without epilepsy: a double-blind, cross-over, placebo-controlled trial. Brain Dev 2004;26: 373–6.

122. Fenoglio-Simeone K, Mazarati A, Sefidvash-Hockley S, et al. Anticonvulsant effects of the selective melatonin receptor agonist ramelteon. Epilepsy Behav 2009;16:52–7.

123. Bruni O, Russo PM, Ferri R, et al. Relationships between headache and sleep in a non-clinical population of children and adolescents. Sleep Med 2008;9(5):542–8.

124. Sahota PK, Dexter JD. Sleep and headache syndromes: a clinical review. Headache 1990;30:80–4.

125. Aaltonen K, Hamalainen ML, Hoppu K. Migraine attacks and sleep in children. Cephalalgia 2000;20: 580–4.

126. Bruni O, Fabrizi P, Ottaviano S, et al. Prevalence of sleep disorders in childhood and adolescence with headache: a case-control study. Cephalalgia 1997; 17:492–8.

127. Luc ME, Gupta A, Birnberg JM, et al. Characterization of symptoms of sleep disorders in children with headache. Pediatr Neurol 2006;34(1):7–12.

128. Miller VA, Palermo TM, Powers SW, et al. Migraine headaches and sleep disturbances in children. Headache 2003;43:362–8.

129. Bruni O, Galli F, Guidetti V. Sleep hygiene and migraine in children and adolescents. Cephalalgia 1999;S25:57–9.

130. Brennan KC, Charles A. Sleep and headache. Semin Neurol 2009;29(4).

Sleep Neurobiology and Critical Care Illness

Xavier Drouot, MD, PhD[a,b,c],*, Solene Quentin, MD[a,b,c]

KEYWORDS

• Sleep alterations • Neurobiology • Sleep EEG pattern • Sleep organization • Circadian rhythms

KEY POINTS

• Intensive care unit (ICU) patients experience severe sleep alterations, with reductions in several sleep stages, marked sleep fragmentation, low sleep continuity, and circadian rhythm disorganization.

• The numerous sources of these sleep alterations are associated with disruptions of sleep neurobiological processes and sleep dynamics that can alter sleep restorative functions.

• Understanding the neurobiology of sleep in the ICU is a major challenge for future sleep studies in critically ill patients.

INTRODUCTION

That critical illnesses and environmental factors in intensive care units (ICUs) are associated with sleep disturbances was recognized shortly after the first ICUs were created. Many studies documented objective lack of restorative sleep.[1–4] Sleep alterations in critically ill patients differ from sleep changes observed in ambulatory patients (such as patients with sleep apnea syndrome) in pathophysiology as well as the consequences of sleep loss.

The literature regarding consequences of sleep deprivation on health is growing rapidly but ICU patients are unlikely to avoid the biological and neurobehavioral repercussions of sleep loss. To appreciate all of the phenomena triggered by sleep loss in the ICU, it is important to understand the neurobiology of healthy sleep and the specific neurobiological derangements of sleep in critically ill patients.

NEUROBIOLOGY OF THE NORMAL SLEEP CYCLE

In human beings, sleep is composed of non–rapid eye movement (NREM) sleep, which can be light NREM (stages 1 and 2) or deep sleep (stages 3 and 4). The distinction between wake and NREM sleep is made by visual analysis of a 30-second portion of an electroencephalogram (EEG): during waking, the EEG shows a mix of fast oscillations (>16 Hz) and alpha rhythm (8–12 Hz) of low amplitudes (<10 μV). During light NREM sleep (stages 1 and 2), the background EEG is characterized by slow theta oscillations (frequency between 4 and 7 Hz) and sleep spindle and K complexes. These latter regularly occur and provide the landmark of stage 2. During deep NREM sleep (also called slow wave sleep; stages 3 and 4), the EEG shows slow waves (0.5–2 Hz) of high amplitude (>75 μV). Rapid eye movement (REM) sleep is a particular sleep stage in which the EEG shows theta and

This article originally appeared in Critical Care Clinics, Volume 31, Issue 3, July 2015.
Funding sources: None.
Conflicts of interest: None.
[a] CHU de Poitiers, Department of Clinical Neurophysiology, Hôpital Jean Bernard, 2 rue de la Milétrie, Poitiers 86000, France; [b] Univ Poitiers, University of Medicine and Pharmacy, 6 rue de la Milétrie, Poitiers 86000, France; [c] INSERM, CIC 1402, Equipe Alive, CHU de Poitiers, Cours Est J. Bernard, Poitiers 86000, France
* Corresponding author. CHU de Poitiers, Department of Clinical Neurophysiology, Hôpital Jean Bernard, 2 rue de la Milétrie, Poitiers 86000, France.
E-mail address: xavier.drouot@chu-poitiers.fr

Sleep Med Clin 11 (2016) 105–113
http://dx.doi.org/10.1016/j.jsmc.2015.10.001
1556-407X/16/$ – see front matter © 2016 Elsevier Inc. All rights reserved.

alpha rhythms. Identification of REM sleep is based on the presence of rapid eye movements identified on electro-oculograms and complete chin muscle atonia. During REM sleep, the brain is highly active, and most dreams and nightmares occur during this stage.

Human sleep is monophasic, and is programmed to occur during nighttime. The sleep-wake cycle is accurately organized and controlled. A sleep deficit elicits a compensatory increase in the intensity and duration of sleep, and excessive sleep reduces sleep propensity. This process could be represented as a sleep-pressure regulation, which would maintain this pressure between an upper and a lower limit. Sleep homeostasis can be represented by the interaction of 2 main physiologic processes. The first process is known as process S, which increases during waking and declines during sleep. Electroencephalographic slow wave activity (SWA) corresponds with an indicator of sleep homeostasis and the level of SWA is determined by the duration of prior sleep and waking. The timing and propensity to fall asleep are also modulated by a circadian process. This second process is driven by the internal clock. This circadian rhythm is sensible to external factors that help to keep the sleep-wake cycle synchronized with night-day alternation. The main external synchronizing factors are light, physical activities, meals, and social interactions.

The quantity of sleep is acutely regulated, and sleep deprivation has many neurobiological consequences. On the day following 1 night without sleep, brain performances are severely decreased. The most visible behavior is an increased tendency to fall asleep, even when the person fights to remain awake. The night following the sleep deprivation is modified and a sleep rebound usually occurs. This sleep rebound triggers a lengthening of nighttime sleep, an increase in slow wave sleep, and an increase in REM sleep.

METHODS FOR SLEEP STUDY IN INTENSIVE CARE UNIT PATIENTS

Sleep can be assessed in terms of quantity (total sleep time and time spent in each sleep stage), quality (fragmentation, sleep EEG patterns), and distribution over the 24-hour cycle.

Full polysomnography (PSG) is the only reliable tool for measuring sleep, especially in patients with marked sleep disturbances. Accurate sleep scoring requires the recording of at least 3 EEG signals (preferentially F4-A1, C4-A1, O2-A1), 2 electro-oculography signals, and a submental electromyography (EMG) signal. Additional signals are usually recorded, such as nasal and oral airflow, thoracic and abdominal belts, electrocardiogram, and pulse oximetry. Sound and light levels should be measured, although these data are not obtained routinely.

SLEEP ELECTROENCEPHALOGRAM PATTERNS IN THE INTENSIVE CARE UNIT

Sleep scoring using either the system of Rechtschaffen and Kales[5] or the recently modified rules[6] poses a specific problem in critical care patients. A variable portion of the brains of critically ill patients does not generate the usual sleep EEG patterns and habitual markers of sleep.[7–11] The presence of theta and delta EEG activities during wakefulness, rapid fluctuations between EEG features of wake and NREM sleep, rapid eye movements during stage 2, and low-amplitude fast frequencies caused by sedation and delta burst arousal pattern are often observed.[8,12,13] In a study in conscious patients (Glasgow score >8) without neurologic disease who required mechanical ventilation for lung injury, 12 of 20 patients had abnormal sleep patterns[8]; among them, 7 patients showed EEG features of coma with reactive theta-delta activity and 5 had atypical sleep with virtually no stage 2 sleep and the presence of pathologic wakefulness (a combination of EEG features of slow wave sleep and behavioral correlates of wakefulness such as saccadic eye movements and sustained EMG activity). These 5 patients had worse acute physiology scores and received a higher mean benzodiazepine dose than the patients with disrupted but recognizable sleep patterns. In a similar group of 22 patients without sedation or neurologic disease,[9] only 17 patients (77.3%) had PSG recordings that could be scored. The remaining 5 patients had an EEG pattern of low-voltage mixed-frequency waves and variable amounts of theta-delta activity; all 5 developed sepsis during the study period, suggesting that sleep abnormalities were related to sepsis encephalopathy.[9]

In a recent study, Watson and colleagues[13] found major dissociations between EEG patterns and behavior in a group of 37 ICU patients. These dissociations consisted of abnormally slow EEG frequency in the theta range (3–7 Hz), a frequency that normally indicates sleep, or even delta range in some awake patients; In contrast, they observed low-amplitude, high-frequency beta EEG activity in patients who were in coma. Some patients who were awake and interactive with research personnel showed predominately theta activity (3–7 Hz), a frequency that normally indicates sleep. One patient, awake and able to follow simple instructions, was documented to have important delta activity, a finding that is normally associated with slow wave sleep. In contrast, unresponsive comatose patients were noted to have alpha activity present on PSG, which is an EEG frequency typically seen in the wake state. These observations led Cooper and colleagues[8] to propose new sleep states called pathologic wakefulness and atypical sleep.

Atypical Sleep and Pathologic Wakefulness

Several teams have deal in depth with the concept of atypical sleep and pathologic wakefulness. Drouot and colleagues[11] proposed a new classification based on the reports of Cooper and colleagues.[8] Drouot and colleagues'[11] study focused on ICU patients admitted for respiratory failure, treated with noninvasive ventilation, and who were not sedated nor taking drugs interfering with sleep physiology. The investigators proposed that atypical sleep and pathologic wake have to be used when patients clearly show alternation between 2 distinct vigilance states. Atypical sleep was defined as non-REM sleep without spindle or K complexes. In contrast, pathologic wakefulness was defined by the association of a global slowing of EEG frequencies (with a peak frequency $\leq$7 Hz) and an impaired EEG reactivity.[11] Watson and colleagues[13] emphasized Drouot and colleagues'[11] new classification by extending their findings in patients with higher severity of illness and receiving sedation. Investigators also incorporate the judicious EEG classification for coma developed by Young and colleagues.[14] In a similar way, Watson and colleagues[13] proposed a new algorithm that includes, as a first step, a comparison between patients' behavior and EEG patterns.

Pathophysiology of Atypical Sleep and Pathologic Wakefulness

Several factors may explain the EEG abnormalities seen in patients with atypical sleep. The first factor could be hypercapnia. In the Drouot and colleagues[11] study, several patients had hypercapnic respiratory failure, which is known to induce various abnormalities in brain function, ranging from mild hypovigilance to encephalopathy.[15–18] Similar EEG alterations have been reported in healthy awake individuals during hypercapnia.[19] However, arterial Pco_2 values did not differ between the group with atypical sleep/pathologic wakefulness and the group with normal sleep, suggesting that other factors could be involved in atypical sleep.[11] Sleep deprivation per se is known to alter EEG patterns during prolonged wakefulness and also during the subsequent recovery sleep. Sleep deprivation experiments showed

linear decreases in alpha activity and increases in theta and delta activities on wakefulness EEGs.[20] The background EEG activity alterations in patients with atypical sleep/pathologic wakefulness were similar to those reported in healthy individuals subjected to sleep deprivation for 24 hours.[21,22] Recovery sleep following sleep deprivation is characterized by significantly decreased spindle[23] and K-complex densities.[24] Because ICU patients are exposed to sleep deprivation for several consecutive days or weeks,[25,26] atypical sleep may constitute a compensatory mechanism in which deep sleep predominates over light (stage 2) sleep to maximize sleep debt recovery. The association of hypercapnia and sleep deprivation in the genesis of atypical sleep has been suggested because spindle density (a marker of atypical sleep) decreases with increase of both SWA and arterial CO_2 levels.[27] Some patients with atypical sleep (with no spindle or very low spindle density) showed normal levels of arterial Pco_2. These patterns could have turned into atypical sleep because of a severe sleep deprivation.[27] However, whether hypercapnia inhibits spindle circuitry and K-complex generators or favor sleep stage associated with low spindle densities, such as slow waves sleep,[28] remains unknown.

Rapid Eye Movement Sleep in the Intensive Care Unit

Most of studies have reported that REM is commonly lacking in ICU patients.[3] However, REM sleep scoring can be difficult when submental muscle atonia, a hallmark of REM sleep, is lacking. REM sleep without atonia and dissociated REM sleep seems uncommon in ICU patients,[29] but these conditions have not been extensively studied. Whether loss of muscle atonia is related to pre-existing disease, medications, or the ICU environment remains to be established.[29] A study of ICU patients with Guillain-Barré syndrome showed a higher incidence of REM sleep abnormalities (including loss of atonia, short REM latency, and daytime REM sleep episodes) compared with ICU patients with paraplegia.[30]

Furthermore, hypercapnia can also produce a REM deficit. The amount of REM sleep was decreased in patients with hypercapnic respiratory failure.[31] However, contrasting results have been reported in experiments in rodents, which showed that hypercapnia increased the amount of REM sleep.[32]

In addition, most studies are transversal experiments and have performed a single PSG at a defined time during an ICU stay. Few studies have been published with longitudinal and repeated PSG, so the initial course of REM deprivation, and the presence and the timing of a potential REM rebound, are unknown, at least in medical ICUs. Some rare reports performed in surgical ICUs have shown an initial, severe REM sleep deficit, followed by an important rebound of REM sleep in the first week after surgery.[33–36]

SLEEP ORGANIZATION IN THE INTENSIVE CARE UNIT
Sleep Architecture

As mentioned in earlier, better analysis of sleep quantity and quality disturbances in ICU patients requires prolonged PSG that lasts at least 16 to 24 hours. Severe sleep-wake disorganization is a major characteristic of sleep in ICU patients. Loss of light/dark circadian synchronization and the prolonged inactive decubitus favor daytime sleep. Studies using long-duration recordings consistently showed abnormal sleep distribution over the 24-hour cycle, with as much as 50% of sleep occurring during the day.[8,9,25,37,38] All the studies found considerable interindividual variability in TST. For instance, TST ranged from 1.7 to 19.4 hours in one study.[9] Nevertheless, the results indicate that quantitative sleep deprivation is not consistently present.

Sleep stage distribution is substantially altered in ICU patients. Sleep stage 1, which normally constitutes less than 5% of TST, accounts for up to 60% of TST in critically ill patients.[8,9,25,33,34] Marked deficits in slow wave sleep (sleep stages 3 and 4) were documented in medical ICU patients and postsurgical patients.[25,33–36] REM sleep is often reduced or abolished,[8,25,39] especially during the first night following surgery.[33–36] Data on sleep stage 2 are conflicting. Sleep stage 2 was normal or increased in some studies[25,34,35,40] and decreased in other studies.[9,36,39] The discrepancies across studies preclude general conclusions.

In addition, differences in the time point of sleep recording may contribute to interindividual variability of sleep parameters. Surgical ICU patients best illustrate this fact because PSG can be performed at baseline (before surgery) and after anesthesia using a standardized regimen. The results showed marked reduction or elimination of slow wave sleep and REM sleep during the first 2 postoperative nights, with a significant rebound of REM sleep in the third or fourth postoperative night,[33–36,41] contrasting with little[35] or no rebound of slow wave sleep.[34,36] These results also highlight the need for longitudinal studies describing changes in sleep over time according to the reason for ICU admission and to disease severity.

Sleep Fragmentation

Concomitantly with sleep stage disorganization, ICU patients experience severe sleep fragmentation with arousals or awakenings. Studies of mechanically ventilated patients showed up to 79 arousals and awakenings per hour of sleep, leading to interruption of sleep every 46 seconds.[8,25,42]

Sleep Continuity

Based on Bonnet's[43] sleep continuity theory, which posits that at least 10 minutes of uninterrupted sleep are needed to serve a recuperative function, several investigators have deemed quantification of sleep continuity to be of interest. Recently, Drouot and colleagues[44] showed that, in nonsedated patients admitted for hypercapnic respiratory failure treated with noninvasive ventilation (NIV), the percentage of TST spent in short naps (ie, sleep episodes lasting between 10 and 30 minutes) was higher and the percentage of sleep time spent in sleep bouts (ie, sleep episodes lasting <10 minutes) was lower in patients with successful NIV compared with patients with NIV failure. Usual sleep quantification, such as TST, sleep stages composition, and sleep fragmentation, were not different between patients with good outcome compared with patients with poor outcome.

CIRCADIAN RHYTHMS AND MELATONIN IN INTENSIVE CARE UNIT PATIENTS

Not only sleep is disturbed, but more generally circadian rhythm. The latter can be assessed indirectly by measuring the oscillations in core body temperature, or directly by melatonin and melatonin metabolite assays.

In a study of 15 ICU patients, the circadian rhythm of core body temperature persisted, but the time of the acrophase showed marked intraindividual variability with shifts of several hours from day to day.[45] In a recent study, Gazendam and colleagues[46] found that acrophases were shifted (advanced or delayed) in 81% of patients, but that this shift was stable across days in each individual. In contrast, in a large cohort of 137 patients investigated after thoracic or vascular surgery, core body temperature showed no circadian rhythmicity in most patients during the first 3 postoperative days.[47]

The circadian rhythm generator, located in the suprachiasmatic nucleus, triggers melatonin production and release by the pineal gland. Melatonin levels start to increase around bedtime and peak at about 3 AM. The onset of melatonin secretion is a robust marker of circadian rhythms.[48] It can be investigated either by assaying serum melatonin concentrations or by determining the urinary 6-sulfatoxymelatonin (6-SMT) level, a surrogate marker for plasma melatonin in healthy subjects. Following the first report by Shilo and colleagues[49] of altered 6-SMT rhythm in ICU patients, several groups investigated melatonin production. One study showed striking abnormalities in urinary 6-SMT excretion in 16 of 17 ICU patients with sepsis, contrasting with normal excretion in 6 of 7 ICU patients without sepsis and in 18 of 23 controls.[50] In another study, the circadian rhythm of urinary 6-SMT concentration was altered in 12 of 16 ICU patients, and 6-SMT excretion was lower during periods with ventilation than during periods of spontaneous breathing.[51] In a recent study, a circadian rhythm of 6-SMT excretion was present in most (81%) patients, but only 4 subjects had normal timing, the others being phase delayed.[52] In addition, the circadian melatonin rhythm was altered in 7 of 8 ICU patients, with no correlation between melatonin levels and levels of sedation.[53]

Factors Interfering with Circadian Rhythms and Melatonin

Melatonin secretion can be influenced by numerous factors,[48] such as age, benzodiazepines, adrenergic compounds, β-blockers, opiates, light exposure, sedation, mechanical ventilation,[51] and sepsis.[50] The contribution of each of these factors in the melatonin release disturbances documented in ICU patients remains unclear.[54]

FACTORS RESPONSIBLE FOR SLEEP DISRUPTION IN THE INTENSIVE CARE UNIT

Numerous factors contribute to sleep disruption in ICU. Some of them are not specific to the ICU (eg, noise and light), although they are intense and frequent in the ICU. Some other conditions are more specifically met in the ICU and interfere with sleep neurobiology, such as continuous lighting, continuous bed rest, and sedation.

The Intensive Care Unit Environment

The level of noise is more than the World Health Organization recommendations in many ICUs,[55] making sleep difficult, and it was rated by patients as one of most sleep disruptive factors.[55,56] In a study involving completion of a questionnaire by patients recently discharged from the ICU, patients reported that vital sign assessments and phlebotomy were more disruptive than noise.[57] In a subsequent study using PSG and synchronized recordings of environmental noise in 22 ICU patients, episodes of noise were related to only 11.5% of all arousals and 17% of all awakenings.[9] Similarly, in another study, noise and patient-care activities explained only 30% of all arousals and awakenings; no causative factors were identified in the other cases.[25] However, because of the large number of peak sounds in the ICU (36.5 per hour of sleep in one study),[25] as well as the large number of arousals and awakenings in ICU patients (from 22 to 79 per hour of sleep),[8,25,42] a causal relationship between noise and arousal/awakening is difficult to ascertain.

Light Exposure

Continuous light exposure and the disappearance of the natural day-night rhythm in the ICU may alter the circadian clock. Nocturnal light intensities vary across ICUs but can exceed 1000 lux.[58,59] Because 100 lux is sufficient to affect melatonin secretion, nocturnal light exposure may modify circadian rhythms. In one recent study, light exposure at night was appropriate (median, <2 lux) but low during the day (median, 74 lux), further reducing day-night contrast.[40]

Loss of Physical Activity

Physical activity is a powerful zeitgeber (time cue), and greater diurnal activity is associated with larger variations in body temperature oscillations.[60] In bed rest experiments in which healthy individuals were asked to stay in bed for 36 hours, daytime naps were common, and sleep-onset REM occurred in up to 43% of naps and 80% of individuals.[61] In an elegant study[25] in which healthy volunteers stayed in bed in an ICU, most of the volunteers lost their circadian organization of sleep and slept during the day, suggesting that loss of activity per se may disrupt circadian rhythms and the sleep-wake cycle.

Effects of Drugs on Sleep

Many drugs used for light sedation or analgesia in the ICU influence sleep in healthy individuals and therefore could be causes of sleep disturbances.[62] Benzodiazepines are used to shorten sleep latency and facilitate sleep continuity. In healthy individuals, benzodiazepines lengthen sleep stage 2, increase TST, and decrease both slow wave sleep duration and REM sleep.[63,64] Tricyclic antidepressants and serotonin reuptake inhibitors increase slow wave sleep and block REM sleep.[65] In addition, tricyclic antidepressants and serotonin reuptake inhibitors may disrupt REM muscle atonia,[66] making this sleep stage difficult to recognize. Antipsychotics induce various sleep changes. Although haloperidol does not modify sleep architecture, olanzapine increases TST, slow wave sleep, and REM sleep, and risperidone only decreases REM sleep.[67] Anticonvulsants may alter the sleep architecture.[68–70] It should be emphasized that all neurotropic molecules may affect EEG patterns during sleep and wakefulness. Opioids reduce slow wave sleep and REM sleep.[71] In addition, abrupt drug discontinuation may elicit withdrawal reactions such as insomnia after discontinuation of sedatives.[72]

Sedation and Sleep Function

Some experiments suggested that propofol may subserve a function that overlaps with sleep function. In an elegant study, Tung and colleagues[73] showed that rats sedated with propofol during their habitual sleep period did not show signs of sleep deprivation (such as sleep rebound) in the following hours. In a second experiment, the restorative effect of natural sleep and 6-hour propofol anesthesia were compared in sleep-deprived rats. No differences were found between natural sleep and anesthesia regarding delta power, REM sleep, or NREM sleep, suggesting that sleep and anesthesia provided similar recovery from sleep deprivation.[74]

However, although propofol may mimic some NREM sleep functions, this does not extend to all sleep functions because propofol consistently suppresses REM sleep in humans.[75]

CONSEQUENCES OF SLEEP DISRUPTIONS ON SLEEP NEUROBIOLOGY
Prolonged Sleep Privation

Regarding the severity of sleep disruptions in the ICU, it is important to note that the sleep regimens imposed on ICU patients is different from those experienced by ambulatory patients, such as patients with sleep apnea syndrome. The critical illness and the environment trigger a severe state of prolonged sleep deprivation. Studies conducted in healthy volunteers have shown that chronic restriction to 4 hours of sleep per night produced a cumulative cognitive performance deficit.[76]

Biological Effect of Sleep Deprivation

The immune system has long been regarded as vulnerable to sleep deprivation. Numerous studies have established that sleep deprivation impairs cellular and humoral immune responses and alters cytokine production.[77] Sleep deprivation was followed by decreases in natural killer (NK) cell and lymphocyte counts in some studies[78] and by increases in others.[79] Counts of T-helper cells and NK cells decreased after 1 night, but increased

after 2 nights without sleep.[78] Sleep restriction (4 hours of sleep for 6 nights) in healthy volunteers was followed by a blunted response to immunization after influenza vaccination.[80] These data suggest that sleep loss in ICU patients may decrease the strength of immune responses.

Sleep and Sepsis

There have been few studies of the relationship between sleep deprivation and sepsis. In rodents, Friese and colleagues[81] reported that the experimental fragmentation of sleep after sepsis was associated with an increased mortality. These data suggest that loss of natural increase of sleep triggered by severe infection could be detrimental to health. Whether this is also the case in humans remains to be investigated.

Neurophysiologic Consequences of Sleep Loss

Sleep deprivation may affect pulmonary mechanics and respiratory muscles. In several studies, sleep deprivation for 24 hours reduced both hypercapnic and hypoxic ventilatory responses by 19% in healthy individuals.[82–84] Inspiratory muscle endurance and maximal voluntary ventilation were decreased after 30 hours without sleep.[85] All these data were obtained in healthy individuals, and no study has investigated the effects of sleep deprivation on respiratory function in critically ill patients. If the physiologic alterations seen in healthy individuals also occur in critically ill patients, they may adversely affect weaning from assisted ventilation.

Neuropsychological and Behavioral Effects of Sleep Alterations

Sleep deprivation affects cognitive functions. Many experiments have shown that specific neurocognitive domains, including executive attention, working memory, and concentration, are particularly vulnerable to sleep loss, the result being cognitive slowing and response perseveration.[86] Prolonged sleep deprivation over several days have been shown to trigger perceptual distortions and hallucinations in healthy individuals.[87] All these effects may play a role in the occurrence of delirium in ICU patients.[88]

SUMMARY

ICU patients experience severe sleep alterations with reductions in several sleep stages, marked sleep fragmentation, low sleep continuity, and circadian rhythm disorganization. The numerous sources of these sleep alterations are associated with disruptions of sleep neurobiological processes and sleep dynamics that could alter sleep restorative functions. A crucial issue is how to objectively quantity this particular sleep, which is the step before imaging sleep protection strategies. Understanding the neurobiology of sleep in the ICU is a major challenge for future sleep studies in critically ill patients.

REFERENCES

1. Drouot X, Cabello B, d'Ortho MP, et al. Sleep in the intensive care unit. Sleep Med Rev 2008;12: 391–403.
2. Parthasarathy S, Tobin MJ. Sleep in the intensive care unit. Intensive Care Med 2004;30:197–206.
3. Pisani MA, Friese RS, Gehlbach BK, et al. Sleep in the intensive care unit. Am J Respir Crit Care Med 2015;191:731–8.
4. Elliott R, McKinley S, Cistulli P. The quality and duration of sleep in the intensive care setting: an integrative review. Int J Nurs Stud 2011;48:384–400.
5. Rechtschaffen A, Kales A. A manual for standardized terminology, techniques and scoring system for sleep stages of human subjects. Washington, DC: Public Health Service, US Government Printing Office; 1968. p. 1–12.
6. Iber C, Ancoli-Israel S, Chesson A, et al. The AASM manual for the scoring of sleep and associated events: rules, terminology and technical specifications. 1st edition. Westchester (IL): American Academy of Sleep Medicine; 2007.
7. Bourne RS, Minelli C, Mills GH, et al. Clinical review: sleep measurement in critical care patients: research and clinical implications. Crit Care 2007; 11:226.
8. Cooper AB, Thornley KS, Young GB, et al. Sleep in critically ill patients requiring mechanical ventilation. Chest 2000;117:809–18.
9. Freedman NS, Gazendam J, Levan L, et al. Abnormal sleep/wake cycles and the effect of environmental noise on sleep disruption in the intensive care unit. Am J Respir Crit Care Med 2001;163: 451–7.
10. Watson PL. Measuring sleep in critically ill patients: beware the pitfalls. Crit Care 2007;11:159.
11. Drouot X, Roche-Campo F, Thille AW, et al. A new classification for sleep analysis in critically ill patients. Sleep Med 2012;13:7–14.
12. Watson PL, Ely EW, Malow B, et al. Scoring sleep in critically ill patients: limitations in standard methodology and the need for revised criteria. Crit Care Med 2006;34:A83.
13. Watson PL, Pandharipande P, Gehlbach BK, et al. Atypical sleep in ventilated patients: empirical electroencephalography findings and the path toward revised ICU sleep scoring criteria. Crit Care Med 2013;41(8):1958–67.
14. Young GB, McLachlan RS, Kreeft JH, et al. An electroencephalographic classification for coma. Can J Neurol Sci 1997;24:320–5.
15. Brochard L, Isabey D, Harf A, et al. Non-invasive ventilation in acute respiratory insufficiency in chronic obstructive bronchopneumopathy. Rev Mal Respir 1995;12:111–7 [in French].
16. Demedts M, Clement J, Schepers R, et al. Respiratory failure: correlation between encephalopathy, blood gases and blood ammonia. Respiration 1976;33:199–210.
17. Kilburn KH. Neurologic manifestations of respiratory failure. Arch Intern Med 1965;116:409–15.
18. Scala R, Naldi M, Archinucci I, et al. Noninvasive positive pressure ventilation in patients with acute exacerbations of COPD and varying levels of consciousness. Chest 2005;128:1657–66.
19. Halpern P, Neufeld MY, Sade K, et al. Middle cerebral artery flow velocity decreases and electroencephalogram (EEG) changes occur as acute hypercapnia reverses. Intensive Care Med 2003; 29:1650–5.
20. Bonnet MH. Acute sleep deprivation. In: Kryger MH, Roth T, Dement WC, editors. Principles and practice of sleep medicine. Philadelphia: Elsevier Saunders; 2005. p. 51–66.
21. Naitoh P, Kales A, Kollar EJ, et al. Electroencephalographic activity after prolonged sleep loss. Electroencephalogr Clin Neurophysiol 1969;27:2–11.
22. Rodin EA, Luby ED, Gottlieb JS. The electroencephalogram during prolonged experimental sleep deprivation. Electroencephalogr Clin Neurophysiol 1962; 14:544–51.
23. De Gennaro L, Ferrara M, Bertini M. Effect of slow-wave sleep deprivation on topographical distribution of spindles. Behav Brain Res 2000;116:55–9.
24. Sforza E, Chapotot F, Pigeau R, et al. Effects of sleep deprivation on spontaneous arousals in humans. Sleep 2004;27:1068–75.
25. Gabor JY, Cooper AB, Hanly PJ. Sleep disruption in the intensive care unit. Curr Opin Crit Care 2001;7: 21–7.
26. Weinhouse GL, Schwab RJ. Sleep in the critically ill patient. Sleep 2006;29:707–16.
27. Quentin S, Thille A, Roche-Campo F, et al. Atypical sleep in ICU: role of hypercapnia and sleep deprivation. Am J Resp Crit Care Med 2014;189:A3615.
28. Wang D, Piper AJ, Wong KK, et al. Slow wave sleep in patients with respiratory failure. Sleep Med 2011; 12:378–83.
29. Schenck CH, Mahowald MW. Injurious sleep behavior disorders (parasomnias) affecting patients on intensive care units. Intensive Care Med 1991;17: 219–24.
30. Cochen V, Arnulf I, Demeret S, et al. Vivid dreams, hallucinations, psychosis and REM sleep in Guillain-Barre syndrome. Brain 2005;128:2535–45.

31. Roche-Campo F, Drouot X, Thille AW, et al. Sleep quality for predicting noninvasive ventilation outcome in patients with acute hypercapnic respiratory failure. Crit Care Med 2010;38:705–6.

32. Ioffe S, Jansen AH, Chernick V. Hypercapnia alters sleep state pattern. Sleep 1984;7:219–22.

33. Aurell J, Elmqvist D. Sleep in the surgical intensive care unit: continuous polygraphic recording of sleep in nine patients receiving postoperative care. Br Med J (Clin Res Ed) 1985;290:1029–32.

34. Kavey NB, Ahshuler KZ. Sleep in herniorrhaphy patients. Am J Surg 1979;138:683–7.

35. Knill RL, Moote CA, Skinner MI, et al. Anesthesia with abdominal surgery leads to intense REM sleep during the first postoperative week. Anesthesiology 1990;73:52–61.

36. Orr WC, Stahl ML. Sleep disturbances after open heart surgery. Am J Cardiol 1977;39:196–201.

37. Hardin KA, Seyal M, Stewart T, et al. Sleep in critically ill chemically paralyzed patients requiring mechanical ventilation. Chest 2006;129:1468–77.

38. Fanfulla F, Ceriana P, D'Artavilla Lupo N, et al. Sleep disturbances in patients admitted to a step-down unit after ICU discharge: the role of mechanical ventilation. Sleep 2011;34:355–62.

39. Broughton R, Baron R. Sleep patterns in the intensive care unit and on the ward after acute myocardial infarction. Electroencephalogr Clin Neurophysiol 1978;45:348–60.

40. Elliott R, McKinley S, Cistulli P, et al. Characterisation of sleep in intensive care using 24-hour polysomnography: an observational study. Crit Care 2013;17:R46.

41. Johns MW, Large AA, Masterton JP, et al. Sleep and delirium after open heart surgery. Br J Surg 1974;61:377–81.

42. Parthasarathy S, Tobin MJ. Effect of ventilator mode on sleep quality in critically ill patients. Am J Respir Crit Care Med 2002;166:1423–9.

43. Bonnet MH. Performance and sleepiness as a function of frequency and placement of sleep disruption. Psychophysiology 1986;23:263–71.

44. Drouot X, Bridoux A, Thille AW, et al. Sleep continuity: a new metric to quantify disrupted hypnograms in non-sedated intensive care unit patients. Crit Care 2014;18:628.

45. Tweedie IE, Bell CF, Clegg A, et al. Retrospective study of temperature rhythms of intensive care patients. Crit Care Med 1989;17:1159–65.

46. Gazendam JA, Van Dongen HP, Grant DA, et al. Altered circadian rhythmicity in patients in the ICU. Chest 2013;144:483–9.

47. Nuttall GA, Kumar M, Murray MJ. No difference exists in the alteration of circadian rhythm between patients with and without intensive care unit psychosis. Crit Care Med 1998;26:1351–5.

48. Claustrat B, Brun J, Chazot G. The basic physiology and pathophysiology of melatonin. Sleep Med Rev 2005;9:11–24.

49. Shilo L, Dagan Y, Smorjik Y, et al. Patients in the intensive care unit suffer from severe lack of sleep associated with loss of normal melatonin secretion pattern. Am J Med Sci 1999;317:278–81.

50. Mundigler G, Delle-Karth G, Koreny M, et al. Impaired circadian rhythm of melatonin secretion in sedated critically ill patients with severe sepsis. Crit Care Med 2002;30:536–40.

51. Frisk U, Olsson J, Nylen P, et al. Low melatonin excretion during mechanical ventilation in the intensive care unit. Clin Sci (Lond) 2004;107:47–53.

52. Gehlbach BK, Chapotot F, Leproult R, et al. Temporal disorganization of circadian rhythmicity and sleep-wake regulation in mechanically ventilated patients receiving continuous intravenous sedation. Sleep 2012;35:1105–14.

53. Olofsson K, Alling C, Lundberg D, et al. Abolished circadian rhythm of melatonin secretion in sedated and artificially ventilated intensive care patients. Acta Anaesthesiol Scand 2004;48:679–84.

54. Bourne RS, Mills GH. Melatonin: possible implications for the postoperative and critically ill patient. Intensive Care Med 2006;32:371–9.

55. Elliott R, Rai T, McKinley S. Factors affecting sleep in the critically ill: an observational study. J Crit Care 2014;29:859–63.

56. Elliott RM, McKinley SM, Eager D. A pilot study of sound levels in an Australian adult general intensive care unit. Noise Health 2010;12:26–36.

57. Freedman NS, Kotzer N, Schwab RJ. Patient perception of sleep quality and etiology of sleep disruption in the intensive care unit. Am J Respir Crit Care Med 1999;159:1155–62.

58. Meyer TJ, Eveloff SE, Bauer MS, et al. Adverse environmental conditions in the respiratory and medical ICU settings. Chest 1994;105:1211–6.

59. Walder B, Francioli D, Meyer JJ, et al. Effects of guidelines implementation in a surgical intensive care unit to control nighttime light and noise levels. Crit Care Med 2000;28:2242–7.

60. Harma MI, Ilmarinen J, Yletyinen I. Circadian variation of physiological functions in physically average and very fit dayworkers. J Hum Ergol (Tokyo) 1982;11(Suppl):33–46.

61. Nakagawa Y. Continuous observation of EEG patterns at night and daytime of normal subjects under restrained conditions. I. Quiescent state when lying down. Electroencephalogr Clin Neurophysiol 1980;49:524–37.

62. Schweitzer P. Drugs that disturb sleep and wakefulness. In: Kryger MH, Roth T, Dement WC, editors. Principles and practices of sleep medicine. 4th edition. Philadelphia: Elsevier; 2005. p. 499.

63. Achermann P, Borbely AA. Dynamics of EEG slow wave activity during physiological sleep and after administration of benzodiazepine hypnotics. Hum Neurobiol 1987;6:203–10.

64. Borbely AA, Mattmann P, Loepfe M, et al. Effect of benzodiazepine hypnotics on all-night sleep EEG spectra. Hum Neurobiol 1985;4:189–94.

65. Wilson S, Argyropoulos S. Antidepressants and sleep: a qualitative review of the literature. Drugs 2005;65:927–47.

66. Winkelman JW, James L. Serotonergic antidepressants are associated with REM sleep without atonia. Sleep 2004;27:317–21.

67. Gimenez S, Clos S, Romero S, et al. Effects of olanzapine, risperidone and haloperidol on sleep after a single oral morning dose in healthy volunteers. Psychopharmacology (Berl) 2007;190:507–16.

68. Bourne RS, Mills GH. Sleep disruption in critically ill patients–pharmacological considerations. Anaesthesia 2004;59:374–84.

69. Legros B, Bazil CW. Effects of antiepileptic drugs on sleep architecture: a pilot study. Sleep Med 2003;4:51–5.

70. Placidi F, Scalise A, Marciani MG, et al. Effect of antiepileptic drugs on sleep. Clin Neurophysiol 2000;111(Suppl 2):S115–9.

71. Cronin AJ, Keifer JC, Davies MF, et al. Postoperative sleep disturbance: influences of opioids and pain in humans. Sleep 2001;24:39–44.

72. Cammarano WB, Pittet JF, Weitz S, et al. Acute withdrawal syndrome related to the administration of analgesic and sedative medications in adult intensive care unit patients. Crit Care Med 1998;26:676–84.

73. Tung A, Lynch JP, Mendelson WB. Prolonged sedation with propofol in the rat does not result in sleep deprivation. Anesth Analg 2001;92:1232–6.

74. Tung A, Bergmann BM, Herrera S, et al. Recovery from sleep deprivation occurs during propofol anesthesia. Anesthesiology 2004;100:1419–26.

75. Kondili E, Alexopoulou C, Xirouchaki N, et al. Effects of propofol on sleep quality in mechanically ventilated critically ill patients: a physiological study. Intensive Care Med 2012;38:1640–6.

76. Van Dongen HP, Maislin G, Mullington JM, et al. The cumulative cost of additional wakefulness: dose-response effects on neurobehavioral functions and sleep physiology from chronic sleep restriction and total sleep deprivation. Sleep 2003;26:117–26.

77. Bryant PA, Trinder J, Curtis N. Sick and tired: does sleep have a vital role in the immune system? Nat Rev Immunol 2004;4:457–67.

78. Dinges DF, Douglas SD, Zaugg L, et al. Leukocytosis and natural killer cell function parallel neurobehavioral fatigue induced by 64 hours of sleep deprivation. J Clin Invest 1994;93:1930–9.

79. Born J, Lange T, Hansen K, et al. Effects of sleep and circadian rhythm on human circulating immune cells. J Immunol 1997;158:4454–64.

80. Spiegel K, Sheridan JF, Van Cauter E. Effect of sleep deprivation on response to immunization. JAMA 2002;288:1471–2.

81. Friese RS, Bruns B, Sinton CM. Sleep deprivation after septic insult increases mortality independent of age. J Trauma 2009;66:50–4.

82. Cooper KR, Phillips BA. Effect of short-term sleep loss on breathing. J Appl Physiol Respir Environ Exerc Physiol 1982;53:855–8.

83. Schiffman PL, Trontell MC, Mazar MF, et al. Sleep deprivation decreases ventilatory response to CO_2 but not load compensation. Chest 1983;84:695–8.

84. White DP, Douglas NJ, Pickett CK, et al. Sleep deprivation and the control of ventilation. Am Rev Respir Dis 1983;128:984–6.

85. Chen HI, Tang YR. Sleep loss impairs inspiratory muscle endurance. Am Rev Respir Dis 1989;140:907–9.

86. Durmer JS, Dinges DF. Neurocognitive consequences of sleep deprivation. Semin Neurol 2005;25:117–29.

87. Babkoff H, Sing HC, Thorne DR, et al. Perceptual distortions and hallucinations reported during the course of sleep deprivation. Percept Mot Skills 1989;68:787–98.

88. Watson PL, Ceriana P, Fanfulla F. Delirium: is sleep important? Best Pract Res Clin Anaesthesiol 2012;26:355–66.

Sleep and the Endocrine System

Dionne Morgan, MBBS[a], Sheila C. Tsai, MD[a,b],*

KEYWORDS

- Circadian rhythms • Sleep apnea • Endocrine abnormalities • Hormonal regulation
- Sleep disorders • Sleep deprivation • Critical illness • Critical care

KEY POINTS

- The endocrine system is influenced by both circadian rhythms and sleep-wake state.
- Hormonal abnormalities can contribute to sleep disruption and disorders.
- Sleep disorders can lead to hormonal dysregulation, resulting in endocrine abnormalities.
- Sleep fragmentation and deprivation are common in critically ill patients and may be associated with various hormonal disturbances.

INTRODUCTION

The endocrine system is a group of specialized organs or glands that secrete hormones directly into the circulation. These hormones are instrumental in growth, metabolism, and maintaining homeostasis. Similarly, sleep plays an important role in human homeostasis. Some hormonal secretion patterns are controlled mainly by the body's internal circadian pacemaker, located in the hypothalamus within the suprachiasmatic nucleus (SCN), whereas other hormones are primarily affected by the sleep-wake state. Sleep and the endocrine system are closely intertwined, with many hormonal secretions influenced by sleep. In addition, sleep quality and duration affect hormonal function such that sleep disorders and sleep fragmentation can contribute to endocrine abnormalities. Conversely, endocrine dysfunction can significantly affect sleep. In this article, the effect of sleep and sleep disorders on endocrine function and the influence of endocrine abnormalities on sleep are discussed. Sleep disruption and its associated endocrine consequences in the critically ill patient are also reviewed.

CIRCADIAN RHYTHM AND SLEEP-WAKE STATE CONTROL OF HORMONAL SECRETION

The primarily circadian-regulated hormones include those produced by the hypothalamic-pituitary axis, such as adrenocorticotropic hormone (ACTH) and cortisol, thyroid stimulating hormone, and melatonin. Growth hormone (GH), prolactin (PRL), and renin secretion are sleep related. Sleep, especially slow wave sleep (SWS), is associated with increased GH, growth hormone–releasing hormone (GHRH), and ghrelin levels.

Adrenocorticotropic Hormone and Cortisol

The hypothalamic-pituitary-adrenal axis (HPA) is primarily under circadian rhythm control. Cortisol and ACTH levels peak in the early morning and decline during the day. The primary circadian

This article originally appeared in Critical Care Clinics, Volume 31, Issue 3, July 2015.
Disclosure statement: The authors do not have any commercial or financial conflicts of interest pertaining to this article.
^a Department of Medicine, National Jewish Health, 1400 Jackson Street, A02, Denver, CO 80206, USA;
^b University of Colorado Denver, Aurora, CO 80045, USA
* Corresponding author.
E-mail address: tsais@njhealth.org

Sleep Med Clin 11 (2016) 115–126
http://dx.doi.org/10.1016/j.jsmc.2015.10.002

control is evidenced by the fact that daytime sleep does not significantly inhibit cortisol secretion. This diurnal variation in cortisol secretion persists even when sleep is altered and is not significantly affected by the absence of sleep or by sleep at an unusual time of day. The 24-hour periodicity of corticotropic activity is therefore primarily controlled by circadian rhythmicity.

However, secretion is also weakly modulated by the sleep-wake state. Sleep onset is normally associated with a decrease in cortisol secretion and nadir levels of cortisol and ACTH levels occur during the first part of sleep. Cortisol secretion is already low in the late evening, and sleep initiation results in prolongation of the low secretory state. At the end of sleep, morning awakening is associated with a burst of cortisol secretion. In sleep deprivation, the cortisol secretion pattern seems to be dampened such that the nadir of cortisol secretion is higher and the maximum morning cortisol level is lower than during nocturnal sleep.[1]

Melatonin

Melatonin release is controlled by the light-dark cycle and SCN through a series of complex polysynaptic pathways. It is produced and released from the pineal gland directly into the blood and cerebrospinal fluid. Melatonin levels start to increase in the evening and peak in the early morning. Melatonin is postulated to promote sleep by decreasing the firing rate of SCN neurons. Its production is suppressed by exposure to bright light.

Thyroid-Stimulating Hormone

Thyroid-stimulating hormone (TSH) is primarily under circadian control but is significantly influenced by the sleep-wake state. During daylight, TSH levels are low and stable. Starting in the early evening, TSH levels increase quickly and peak shortly before sleep onset. Sleep inhibits TSH levels from increasing further. Therefore, sleep has an inhibitory effect on TSH secretion, most notable during SWS. During the latter part of the sleep period, there is a progressive decline in TSH levels. The circadian effect on TSH secretion is predominant with some influence from sleep. For example, sleep deprivation results in higher TSH levels during the night because of the lack of sleep's inhibitory effect. But this inhibitory effect of sleep on TSH secretion seems to depend on time of day because daytime sleep does not seem to have this same suppressive effect on daytime TSH secretion.

Growth Hormone

GH secretion is largely influenced by sleep. The release of GH from the anterior pituitary gland is stimulated by hypothalamic GHRH and inhibited by somatostatin. In addition, ghrelin, a peptide produced by the stomach, acts as a potent endogenous stimulus for GH secretion by binding to the GH secretagogue receptor. GH secretion increases during sleep with less influence by the time of day. The sleep-onset GH pulse is the largest in men. Most GH secretion is associated with SWS (stage N3), although GH secretion also occurs in the absence of SWS. The amount of GH secretion closely correlates with the duration of stage N3 sleep. In older age, both N3 sleep and GH release decrease.

Prolactin

PRL secretion is strongly linked to sleep. Levels increase shortly after sleep, regardless of the time of day, although this stimulatory effect is greatest at night. During nocturnal sleep, the PRL levels peak around the middle of the sleep period. Awakenings associated with sleep disruption inhibit nocturnal PRL release. Therefore, the secretion of PRL is mainly sleep dependent.

In addition, a potential role of PRL in regulating rapid eye movement (REM) or SWS has been suggested because of a close temporal relationship between increased PRL secretion and SWS. However, this correlation is not as close as that seen with GH, and the normal secretory pattern of PRL does not decline with age despite a decline in SWS.

Gonadotropic Hormones

Gonadotropic hormone secretion seems to have both circadian rhythmicity and sleep influences. Gonadotropin-releasing hormone from the hypothalamus controls the secretion of luteinizing hormone (LH) and follicle-stimulating hormone (FSH) by the anterior pituitary. In men, LH is responsible for testosterone secretion, whereas FSH stimulates spermatogenesis. In women, the gonadotropins regulate the release of estrogen and progesterone and control the menstrual cycle.

The 24-hour patterns of gonadotropin release and gonadal steroid levels vary according to gender and the stage of life. There is a pulsatile increase in LH and FSH levels at sleep onset in children. As the child approaches puberty, the amplitude of the nocturnal pulses increases, which is one marker of puberty.

Testosterone production varies diurnally, but its production depends directly on sleep, with testosterone levels normally increasing at sleep onset. In young adult men, a notable diurnal rhythm in circulating testosterone levels exists, with minimal levels in the late evening and a clear nocturnal increase leading to maximal levels in the early morning. Approximately 3 hours of SWS is required, irrespective of whether it occurs during the day or at night, for peak testosterone production to occur, and levels remain stable thereafter while sleep is maintained. After waking, the plasma concentration of testosterone declines in proportion to the duration of time awake.[2] With sleep fragmentation experiments, the nocturnal increase in testosterone is attenuated, especially if no REM sleep is achieved.[3]

Renin-Angiotensin-Aldosterone System

Some circadian rhythmicity occurs in the renin-angiotensin-aldosterone system, with more urine flow and increased electrolyte excretion occurring during the day. Increased renin and aldosterone levels during sleep decrease urine output. In addition, plasma renin activity is synchronized with non-rapid eye movement (NREM)-REM cycles: higher levels occur during NREM sleep, and the lowest levels occur during REM sleep. Therefore, decreased urine flow and increased urine osmolality occurs during REM sleep. However, sleep deprivation decreases the usual elevation in aldosterone levels occurring during sleep, which results in increased sodium excretion.

Leptin and Ghrelin

Sleep plays an important role in energy balance. Both sleep and circadian rhythms control leptin secretion. Leptin is a hormone primarily secreted by adipocytes that promotes satiety and increases metabolism. Higher levels are noted in obese versus lean individuals suggesting possible leptin resistance. Levels fluctuate in response to caloric balance and increase at night. Leptin levels peak at night (around 2:30 AM) and nadir in the early afternoon (around 1 PM).[4] This nocturnal elevation of leptin level is thought to suppress hunger during sleep and may increase SWS.[5] When controlling for nutrition and activity, a shift in nighttime to daytime sleep results in leptin peaks during both day and night.[5,6]

Ghrelin is released primarily from the stomach, stimulates appetite, and promotes weight gain. Its release is controlled more by sleep-wake state than by circadian influences.[7] Ghrelin levels typically increase during the first half of the night and decrease in the second half, even when fasting. Ghrelin also enhances GH secretion and may stimulate SWS.[8]

Insulin and Glucose

A complex relationship between sleep, insulin, and glucose control also exists. Decreased glucose tolerance is noted during sleep, whether sleep occurs during the daytime or nighttime. This occurrence is thought to be related to decreased brain glucose use, decreased muscle use and tone, and anti-insulin effects of GH. Although decreased glucose metabolism occurs during NREM sleep, increased glucose metabolism occurs during REM sleep and wakefulness.[9]

Improved insulin sensitivity seems to occur at the end of sleep.[10] The improved glucose control at the end of the night is thought to be due to multiple factors, including increased metabolism during REM and wake time, greater body activity, augmented noninsulin-mediated glucose removal, and action by previously secreted insulin.[11,12]

EFFECTS OF ENDOCRINE ABNORMALITIES ON SLEEP

The previous section discussed normal hormonal secretion and the influence of sleep on hormonal balance. This section discusses endocrine disorders and their effect on sleep.

Acromegaly and Sleep Apnea

Acromegaly results from excessive GH production. In addition to notable physical findings, such as elongated digits and coarsening of features, several of other morphologic abnormalities can predispose to sleep apnea. These features include soft-tissue changes such as macroglossia, elongation and thickening of the soft palate, swelling and thickening of the pharyngeal walls, and thickening of the true and false vocal cords, which result in pharyngeal airway narrowing and an increased tendency of the airway to collapse.[13] Bony changes also contribute to this increased risk of obstructive sleep apnea (OSA): more vertical bony growth of the face results in posterior placement of the tongue, thus narrowing of the pharyngeal airspace. In addition, a more inferior position of the hyoid bone may contribute to upper airway instability.[14]

The relationship between sleep-disordered breathing and excessive GH production dates back to the late 1800s when Roxburgh and Collis linked acromegaly, snoring, and excessive daytime sleepiness.[15] More recent studies have demonstrated a high prevalence of sleep-disordered breathing in patients with acromegaly. An Australian study found a high prevalence of sleep apnea in acromegalic patients with approximately 60% of the patients with acromegaly having sleep apnea.[16] The same research group found that 33% of patients with acromegaly had central sleep apnea possibly due to increased hypercapnic ventilatory response.[17]

The prevalence of sleep apnea in those already treated for their acromegaly has been investigated. Although this percentage is lower than in untreated acromegalic patients, the prevalence remains high at more than 20%.[18] Surgical treatment of acromegaly may improve sleep-disordered breathing. Improvement in obstructive sleep apnea syndrome (OSAS) has been noted after transphenoidal hypophysectomy alone or transphenoidal hypophysectomy and radiation. However, uvulopalatopharyngoplasty has not been shown to improve OSA in these patients.[19] Treatment with octreotide has also been demonstrated to improve sleep-disordered breathing in patients with acromegaly. After 6 months of octreotide treatment, up to a 50% decline in respiratory events has been reported.[20,21] However, other studies have found that treatment of acromegaly does not result in resolution of the sleep-disordered breathing.[22,23] Furthermore, central sleep apnea seems to persist despite intracranial resection with or without radiation therapy.[23]

Thyroid Hormone and Sleep Disorders

Both hypothyroidism and hyperthyroidism can cause or exacerbate sleep disorders, such as OSAS, insomnia, and hypersomnia.

Symptoms of hypothyroidism overlap with those of OSA and may be difficult to distinguish. OSA may be a consequence of hypothyroidism. Up to 50% of hypothyroid patients have some degree of sleep-disordered breathing compared with 29% in the euthyroid control group.[24] Hypothyroidism can potentially cause or exacerbate OSAS for several reasons, including excess weight gain, reduction in ventilatory drive, thyroid myopathy, and abnormal mucopolysaccharide content in upper airway tissue. In addition, the presence of a goiter, independent of any concurrent hypothyroidism or hyperthyroidism, has occasionally been reported as a cause of OSAS due to mechanical constriction of the upper airway.

Evidence varies and is conflicting as to whether thyroid hormone supplementation improves sleep-disordered breathing. In some studies, thyroid hormone replacement has been shown to improve sleep-disordered breathing in hypothyroid patients with OSA.[25] In patients with sleep apnea and hypothyroidism, treatment of sleep apnea is recommended until thyroid replacement has been achieved because of reports of angina in patients initiated on thyroid replacement before management of sleep apnea. This angina resolves with initiation of continuous positive airway pressure (CPAP) therapy.[26] Fatigue and lack of energy are prominent features of hypothyroidism. In addition,

the symptom of sleepiness has been noted quite commonly.[27]

Sleep propensity is increased even in patients with subclinical hypothyroidism.[28] Thyroid replacement therapy has been used with success in the management of sleepiness in patients diagnosed with idiopathic hypersomnia who were treated for subclinical hypothyroidism.[29] As such, patients with symptoms of hypersomnia should be evaluated for thyroid abnormalities.

Both hyperthyroidism and overdose of thyroid supplements have been associated with insomnia complaints.[30] Hyperthyroidism has been more typically associated with difficulty falling asleep rather than maintenance insomnia.[31] Thyroid excess may also contribute to restlessness with a higher prevalence of restless legs syndrome,[32] which in turn may exacerbate insomnia complaints.

Hypothalamic-Pituitary-Adrenal-Cortisol Axis Disorders and Sleep

Adrenal insufficiency, primarily due to deficient cortisol secretion, results in severe fatigue, sleepiness, and poor-quality sleep. These symptoms may persist even in patients who are on treatment.[33] Sleep-wake disorders have also been attributed to elevated cortisol levels. Furthermore, there has been a link between cortisol levels and chronic insomnia: higher nighttime levels are noted in patients with insomnia.[34,35] This relationship may be bidirectional but suggests that elevated cortisol levels may contribute to chronic insomnia.

There is limited information concerning a possible link between Cushing syndrome and an increased risk of OSAS. One study found that 18% of 22 subjects demonstrated an Respiratory Disturbance Index (RDI) of greater than or equal to 17.5.[36] In addition, there has been a link between exogenous corticosteroid therapy and sleep apnea.[37] Furthermore, well-known complications of corticosteroid therapy include issues with insomnia, in addition to other neuropsychiatric issues.[38]

Sex Hormones and Sleep Disturbances

Testosterone

Patients with low testosterone levels often note a lack of energy or fatigue. There is also a decline in sleep quality after middle age and with increasing age in men. This decline may be due in part to reduced testosterone levels in aging men.[39] Decreased testosterone may lead to increased fat mass, and there may be poorer sleep quality associated with obesity.[40,41] Weight loss may improve plasma testosterone levels in obese men.[42]

Although based largely on anecdotal evidence, exogenous testosterone has been considered to have a deleterious effect in OSA. Current guidelines suggest that it is contraindicated in the presence of untreated OSA.[43] In one study involving obese men with severe OSA and low plasma testosterone levels, testosterone supplementation, irrespective of baseline testosterone level, resulted in worsening of the oxygen desaturation index and nocturnal hypoxemia at 7 weeks but not at 18 weeks.[44] Testosterone supplementation may affect sleep in other ways. In one study of young men engaging in resistance exercises and taking anabolic steroids, there was a reduction in sleep efficiency and alteration of sleep architecture.[45]

Estrogen and progesterone
Several issues can potentially affect sleep in postmenopausal women such as alterations in mood, hot flashes, insomnia, and an increased prevalence of upper airway instability. The Wisconsin Sleep Cohort Study demonstrated that postmenopausal women are more frequently affected by respiratory instability. Postmenopausal women were more likely to manifest OSAS, even when corrected for body mass index (BMI) and age.[46] Hormonal therapy is often used to assist with insomnia associated with hot flashes in perimenopausal and postmenopausal women. Evidence suggests that administration of hormones can improve sleep quality in women. In one study, women who did not use hormone therapy reported more sleep difficulties than those on hormonal therapy.[47] The Sleep Heart Health Study examined the prevalence of an RDI greater or equal to 15 in women without and with hormonal therapy and found that there was 50% reduction in the elevated RDI rate in the hormone users.[48] Overall, these data suggest that hormonal therapy may be a useful adjunct, although not a replacement for therapies such as CPAP, in treating OSAS in postmenopausal women.

Melatonin Effects on Sleep
Melatonin plays a role in the regulation of human sleep. In addition to its direct sleep-facilitating effect, melatonin may improve sleep through a chronobiotic effect by entraining the circadian system to a desired sleep-wake cycle.[49,50] Exogenous melatonin decreases sleep latency, and the sustained release and transdermal formulations can increase total sleep time and sleep maintenance.[51–53] Exogenous melatonin, in 0.3-mg up to 5-mg doses, has also been shown to improve sleep efficiency in healthy people during the daytime when endogenous melatonin production is absent.[54] These results are consistent with the hypothesis that both exogenous and endogenous melatonin promote sleep by opposing the wake-promoting signal from the circadian clock. The intake of either low-dose (0.3 mg) or high-dose (5 mg) melatonin has a similar effect on sleep efficiency, indicating no additional benefit of exogenous melatonin concentrations more than the endogenous nighttime levels.[55] These findings also suggest that daytime melatonin intake may be useful for individuals, such as rotating shift workers, who need to obtain sleep during the daytime.

THE EFFECT OF SLEEP DISORDERS ON HORMONAL REGULATION
Sleep Deprivation

Sleep deprivation is common in industrialized countries. Insufficient sleep may occur as a result of voluntary sleep restriction, insomnia, or shift work. Decreased sleep is associated with increased risk for obesity, diabetes, and hypertension.

Adrenocorticotropic hormone and cortisol
Studies have shown that partial or complete sleep deprivation results in elevations of evening cortisol levels.[56] Conversely, sleep deprivation also results in a significant reduction of cortisol secretion the next day. This reduction in cortisol secretion seems to be related to an increase in SWS during the recovery night, which exerts an inhibitory effect on the HPA axis.[57] The impact of restricted sleep on the HPA axis seems to depend on the time of day. In addition, the amplitude of normal circadian rhythm decline in cortisol levels is reduced with insufficient sleep.[58]

Insulin and glucose metabolism
The interactions between sleep, circadian function, and glucose metabolism have also been evaluated.[59] Both sleep insufficiency and sleep fragmentation have been linked to abnormal glucose metabolism. It has been shown that sleep restriction affects glucose tolerance through a direct effect on insulin sensitivity. There is decreased insulin sensitivity associated with loss of sleep that is not compensated for by an increase in insulin release.[60] Subsequent studies in healthy human subjects involving sleep restriction and assessments of glucose metabolism have confirmed an approximately 20% reduction in insulin sensitivity without simultaneous increases in insulin levels, resulting in reduced glucose tolerance and, subsequently, an increased risk of diabetes.[61] In

addition, the association of short sleep duration, usually less than 6 hours per night, with an increased risk of diabetes has been shown in multiple cross-sectional epidemiologic studies.[62]

Leptin, ghrelin, and appetite regulation

The duration of sleep plays an important role in the regulation of leptin and ghrelin levels in humans. Sleep loss may affect energy expenditure due its impact on the levels of leptin and ghrelin. Leptin and ghrelin exert opposing effects on appetite: leptin promotes satiety, whereas ghrelin promotes increased food intake and reduced fat metabolism. Several studies have shown that partial sleep deprivation is associated with significant decreases in leptin levels and conversely increases in levels of ghrelin. Although there is an increase in ghrelin levels after partial sleep restriction, the nocturnal increase in ghrelin levels is modestly reduced during acute total sleep deprivation.[7] Leptin levels decline with sleep restriction, although the nocturnal peak in leptin persists.[63] In a study of sleep deprivation in healthy adult men, while rigorously controlling diet and activity, the decline in leptin levels was observed.[64] This decline in leptin levels correlates with increases in sympathetic nervous system activity, which suggests that increased autonomic activity might reduce leptin secretion. The association between sleep duration and leptin and ghrelin levels was observed in the Wisconsin Sleep Cohort Study. Limited total sleep time was associated with higher ghrelin and reduced leptin levels.[65] These findings would support the postulate that sleep deprivation may alter the ability of leptin and ghrelin to accurately signal caloric need and so lead to increased food intake due to an internal misperception of insufficient energy availability.

It is likely that the increased hunger and food intake are potential mechanisms by which sleep deprivation contributes to weight gain and obesity. In a study of healthy young male subjects, limiting sleep opportunity to only 4 hours versus 10 hours resulted in elevated daytime ghrelin and decreased daytime leptin levels. These changes were associated with both increased hunger and appetite.[64] In another trial, when subjects underwent 5 nights of insufficient sleep of only 5 hours per night, they had increased food intake and total daily energy expenditure. The increased food intake during the insufficient sleep schedule exceeded energy expenditure and so contributed to weight gain.[66]

Insomnia

Adrenocorticotropic hormone and cortisol

Investigators have studied the effect of chronic insomnia on the HPA axis and associated clinical consequences. In insomnia, higher nighttime cortisol levels have been noted. With chronic insomnia, there is an overall and sustained increase in ACTH and cortisol secretion, although maintaining the normal circadian pattern. It is possible that the chronic activation of the HPA axis places patients with insomnia at risk of significant medical morbidity.[67] Therapy for patients with insomnia may include sleep restriction combined with cognitive behavioral therapy. Lower cortisol levels occur during treatment, which confirms part of the proposed physiologic mechanisms behind insomnia. These data support the benefit of sleep restriction in contributing to a decrease in hyperarousal insomnia.[68]

Insulin and glucose metabolism

Studies in healthy volunteers have demonstrated that sleep fragmentation results in abnormal glucose metabolism, especially if there is associated suppression of SWS.[69] In addition, prospective population-based studies have linked poor sleep quality to incident diabetes. In one study, the risk of type 2 diabetes was found to be almost 3 times higher in subjects with insomnia, defined by a sleep duration less than 5 hours versus those with a longer sleep duration.[70,71]

Obstructive Sleep Apnea

Sleep-disordered breathing may have several adverse effects on the endocrine hormonal axes, especially with regard to glucose metabolism and insulin resistance.[72,73]

Insulin and glucose metabolism

The link between OSA and impaired glucose metabolism due to insulin resistance seems to occur independently of obesity. Patients with OSA have been shown to have higher fasting serum glucose and insulin resistance index, independent of adiposity. The severity of OSA is associated with increased insulin resistance.[74] Similarly, an increased apnea-hypopnea index has been associated with worsened glucose tolerance and insulin resistance independent of obesity.[75] It is postulated that the primary mechanism linking OSA to impaired glucose metabolism and diabetes may be a consequence of sleep fragmentation with diminished SWS. Sleep fragmentation is associated with elevated sympathetic nervous activity, which could lead to alterations in glucose metabolism.[69] It is possible that through mechanisms such as enhanced sympathetic activity, endothelial dysfunction, and impairment of peripheral vasodilation, insulin resistance may contribute to the metabolic syndrome.

The metabolic syndrome

The metabolic syndrome is a complex of metabolic disturbances diagnosed when 3 of the following 5 characteristics are present: abdominal obesity, increased serum triglyceride levels, low high-density lipoprotein (HDL) levels, elevated blood pressure, and elevated plasma glucose levels. Patients with OSA seem to be at higher risk of developing certain features of metabolic syndrome, specifically hypertension, insulin resistance, and type 2 diabetes. OSA has been independently associated with an increased prevalence of the metabolic syndrome.[76]

Even after adjusting for obesity, OSA has been associated with increased systolic and diastolic blood pressure, higher fasting insulin and triglyceride concentrations, decreased levels of HDL cholesterol, and increased cholesterol to HDL ratio. Therefore, it has been concluded that metabolic syndrome is more likely to be present in patients with OSA.[77] It is also likely that OSA and metabolic syndrome share similar pathophysiologic mechanisms. Patients with sleep apnea are often obese and have a heightened sympathetic drive, endothelial dysfunction, systemic inflammation, insulin resistance, hypercoagulability, and high plasma leptin levels, which are also secondary factors associated with metabolic syndrome.

Circadian Rhythm Disorders

Circadian misalignment occurs when the internal circadian clock is not properly aligned with the external environment, including light-dark, sleep-wake, and fasting-feeding cycles. This condition can occur acutely with jet lag or on a chronic basis with shift work, delayed sleep phase, or advanced sleep phase disorders. With nearly 20% of the working population in industrialized countries being shift workers,[78] the impact of shift work disorder can be quite significant. Night-shift work is an example of severe circadian misalignment, as workers are awake, active, and eating during their biological night and trying to sleep and fast during their biological day. Several studies have examined the effects of circadian misalignment on sleep and related hormones.

Adrenocorticotropic hormone, cortisol, and thyroid-stimulating hormone

The impact of delayed sleep phase syndrome (DSPS) on cortisol and TSH release has been investigated. One study showed that the hormonal rhythms were delayed in patients with DSPS, although there was no difference in total 24-hour secretions of TSH and cortisol when compared with controls. Based on these results, it would seem that the hormonal delay in DSPS is due

more to the phase delay of the circadian clock rather than any overt hormonal dysfunction.[79]

Abnormally high cortisol levels have also been noted at the end of wake and start of sleep. Therefore, it has been postulated that the high cortisol secretion seen in circadian misalignment could contribute to insulin resistance and hyperglycemia.[80]

Insulin, glucose metabolism, and appetite regulation

Investigators have tested the different effects of phase advance and phase delay, compared with a daily 24-hour cycle, on sleep, energy expenditure, substrate oxidation, appetite, and related hormones in energy balance. They found that the primary effect of a phase shift, whether phase advanced or phase delayed, was a combined disturbance of glucose-insulin metabolism. Glucose concentrations were higher without any concomitant change in insulin concentrations.[81]

Acute circadian misalignment results in an increase in postprandial glucose and insulin levels with a concurrent decline in leptin levels. Similarly, low leptin levels are associated with appetite stimulation. An increase in appetite coupled with decreased energy expenditure could account for the increased risk of obesity noted in shift workers.[80]

There is considerable epidemiologic evidence that shift work is associated with increased risk for obesity, diabetes, and cardiovascular disease. Shift workers suffering from chronic sleep deprivation and circadian rhythm misalignment seem to be at an increased risk of type 2 diabetes.[82,83] Prospective studies have demonstrated this association. For example, in the Nurses' Health Study, researchers found that subjects who worked rotating night shifts had an increased risk for diabetes, even after adjusting for traditional diabetic risk factors, including BMI.[82] The risk was also noted to be higher in those with longer duration of shift work as compared with no shift work.

Evidence suggests that increased insulin resistance may be an intrinsic adverse effect of circadian rhythm misalignment on glucose metabolism, independent of sleep loss.[84] However, further prospective and interventional studies are needed to evaluate the role of circadian rhythm misalignment in the development and severity of type 2 diabetes.

Melatonin, gonadotropin, and oncogenic effect

Melatonin rhythms are also delayed in patients with DSPS, although the total 24-hour secretion of melatonin is similar to controls.[79] Shift workers may exhibit altered nighttime melatonin secretion and reproductive hormone profiles that could increase their risk of hormone-dependent cancers. Several studies have been conducted to investigate the effect of circadian rhythm disruption on reproductive hormone production and nocturnal production of melatonin as a possible cause for breast cancer.[85] Melatonin is known to affect regulation of gonadal function because decreased concentrations, as seen in circadian rhythm misalignment, result in increased pituitary gonadotropin release, leading to testosterone or estrogen production.

Melatonin also has been found to have tumor suppressive properties. For example, in rodent models, pinealectomy was found to enhance tumor growth,[86] whereas exogenous melatonin administration has demonstrated anticancer activity.[87] Overall, the antitumor effect of melatonin may be due to its direct effect on hormone-dependent proliferation through interaction with nuclear receptors, an effect on cell cycle control, and possible increase in p53 tumor-suppressor gene expression.[85]

Disorders of Hypersomnia

Limited data exist regarding hypersomnia disorders and associated endocrine abnormalities. However, patients with narcolepsy are often obese and have been reported to be at increased risk of diabetes. Yet, there is a paucity of studies looking at the endocrine consequences of narcolepsy. In a case-control study, investigators studied glucose metabolism using the oral glucose tolerance test and assessed dynamic function of the HPA axis with the dexamethasone suppression test in narcoleptic patients.[88] The study showed that, independent of obesity, narcolepsy is not associated with impaired glucose metabolism. In addition, there was no alteration in dynamic HPA function, although the negative feedback response to dexamethasone was mildly enhanced in narcolepsy cases. Similarly, other studies using BMI-matched controls have not shown any increased risk of type 2 diabetes or impaired glucose metabolism, independent of BMI, in narcoleptic patients.[89,90]

SLEEP AND ENDOCRINE ABNORMALITIES IN CRITICALLY ILL PATIENTS

Sleep fragmentation and deprivation are common in critically ill patients and may be associated with various hormonal disturbances. Patients experience poor sleep quality characterized by frequent disruptions and loss of circadian rhythms because of factors such as environmental noise; light; patient care activities, such as vital signs checks, drug administration, and diagnostic testing; patient-ventilator dyssynchrony; and pain or discomfort. Although the total number of hours of sleep in a 24-hour period may be normal (7–9 hours), approximately 50% of the sleep time occurs as short periods of light sleep during the day.[91] In patients in the intensive care unit (ICU), there is an increased percentage of wakefulness and stage N1 sleep (40%–60%) with decreased amounts of N2 (20%–40%), N3 (10%), and REM sleep (10%).[92] Thus, there is a significant reduction in the total time spent in restorative N3 and REM sleep stages.

It has been shown that there is loss of the normal circadian secretion of melatonin in critical illness, especially in sepsis, which seems to occur independently of light exposure.[93,94] In one study of patients with sepsis, investigators found that despite the exclusion of exposure to ambient light in the ICU, there was loss of periodic excretion of the melatonin urinary metabolite 6-sulfatoxymelatonin.[95] In addition, this noncircadian release of melatonin seems to persist for several weeks after recovery from sepsis that may contribute to continued sleep disturbances after ICU discharge.

The disruption of sleep, particularly restriction of SWS, as is seen in critically ill patients, negatively affects glucose metabolism and results in blunted insulin secretion with decreased insulin sensitivity.[60,69] ICU-related sleep disruption could therefore contribute to and exacerbate glucose abnormalities in critical illness; this is of particular importance in the critically ill patient, who is susceptible to episodes of hyperglycemia and the adverse outcomes associated with inadequate glucose control.

Exogenous corticosteroid administration may exacerbate the poor sleep and sleep disruption that is seen in these critically ill patients. Similarly, cortisol and catecholamine levels along with indices of energy expenditure, such as oxygen consumption (V_{O_2}) and carbon dioxide production (V_{CO_2}), tend to increase in sleep deprivation. The persistent sleep disruption that occurs in the critically ill patient, especially in the setting of sepsis, intensifies this stress response.[56,60]

Furthermore, in the acute phase of critical illness, increased levels of GH and PRL are initially noted. This increase seems to occur regardless of sleep onset and is likely due to increased pituitary activity.[96] However, with prolonged critical illness, the normal pulsatile secretion of GH and PRL is impaired, which may be a consequence of the potent inhibitory effect of sleep deprivation on GH and PRL release.[96,97] This decrease in GH and PRL levels may play a role in critical illness muscle wasting and impaired immunity.

SUMMARY

This article discusses the interactions between sleep and endocrine function. The authors have demonstrated the importance of sleep quality and quantity on maintaining hormonal balance. Disrupting this balance can have significant health consequences. Abnormalities in the endocrine system, such as excess GH secretion or thyroid hormone production, can lead to significant sleep disruption, such as sleep apnea and insomnia, respectively. Treating these hormonal abnormalities can improve sleep. Similarly, poor-quality or insufficient sleep can have a major impact on hormonal balance. Considerable research supports the effect of poor sleep on insulin and glucose metabolism, as well as on appetite regulation. Growing evidence supports the adverse consequences of sleep restriction, insomnia, and circadian rhythm abnormalities on endocrine balance and overall health. Restoring sleep quantity and improving sleep quality may assist in hormonal regulation, which is of particular importance in the critically ill patient who experiences sleep fragmentation and deprivation with loss of circadian rhythms. Understanding the sleep disruption and endocrine imbalances that occur in critically ill patients supports the importance of sleep and the need to optimize sleep in this patient population.

REFERENCES

1. Van Cauter E, Blackman JD, Roland D, et al. Modulation of glucose regulation and insulin secretion by circadian rhythmicity and sleep. J Clin Invest 1991; 88:934–42.
2. Axelsson J, Ingre M, Akerstedt T, et al. Effects of acutely displaced sleep on testosterone. J Clin Endocrinol Metab 2005;90:4530–5.
3. Luboshitzky R, Herer P, Levi M, et al. Relationship between rapid eye movement sleep and testosterone secretion in normal men. J Androl 1999;20: 731–7.
4. Sinha MK, Ohannesion JP, Heiman ML, et al. Nocturnal rise of leptin in lean, obese, and non insulin-dependent diabetes mellitus subjects. J Clin Invest 1996;97:1344–7.
5. Simon C, Grofier C, Schlienger JL, et al. Circadian and ultradian variations of leptin in normal man under continuous enteral nutrition: relationship to sleep and body temperature. J Clin Endocrinol Metab 1998;83:1893–9.
6. Saad MF, Riad-Gabriel MG, Khan A, et al. Diurnal and ultradian rhythmicity of plasma leptin: effects of gender and adiposity. J Clin Endocrinol Metab 1998;83:453–9.
7. Dzaja A, Dalal MA, Himmerich H, et al. Sleep enhances nocturnal plasma ghrelin levels in healthy subjects. Am J Physiol Endocrinol Metab 2004; 286:E963–7.
8. Weikel JC, Wichniak A, Ising M, et al. Ghrelin promotes slow-wave sleep in humans. Am J Physiol Endocrinol Metab 2003;284:E407–15.
9. Kern W, Offenheuser S, Born J, et al. Entrainment of ultradian oscillations in the secretion of insulin and glucagons to the nonrapid eye movement/rapid eye movement sleep rhythm in humans. J Clin Endocrinol Metab 1996;81:1541–7.
10. Levy I, Recasens A, Casamitjana R, et al. Nocturnal insulin and C-peptide rhythms in normal subjects. Diabetes Care 1987;10:148–51.
11. Boyle PJ, Scott JC, Krentz AJ, et al. Diminished brain glucose metabolism is a significant determinant for falling rates of systemic glucose utilization during sleep in normal humans. J Clin Invest 1994; 93:529–35.
12. Van Cauter E, Polonsky KS, Scheen AJ. Roles of circadian rhythmicity and sleep in human glucose regulation. Endocr Rev 1997;18:716–38.
13. Colao A, Ferone D, Marzullo P, et al. Systemic complications of acromegaly: epidemiology, pathogenesis, and management. Endocr Rev 2004; 25:102–52.
14. Hochban W, Ehlenz K, Conradt R, et al. Obstructive sleep apnoea in acromegaly: the role of craniofacial changes. Eur Respir J 1999;14:196–202.
15. Roxburgh F, Collis AJ. Notes on a case of acromegaly. Br Med J 1896;2:63–5.
16. Grunstein RR, Ho KY, Sullivan CE. Sleep apnea in acromegaly. Ann Intern Med 1991;115:527–32.
17. Grunstein RR, Ho KY, Berthon-Jones M, et al. Central sleep apnea is associated with increased ventilatory response to carbon dioxide and hypersecretion of growth hormone in patients with acromegaly. Am J Respir Crit Care Med 1994;150:496–502.
18. Rosenow F, Reuter S, Deuss U, et al. Sleep apnoea in treated acromegaly: relative frequency and predisposing factors. Clin Endocrinol (Oxf) 1996;45: 563–9.
19. Mickelson SA, Rosenthal LD, Rock JP, et al. Obstructive sleep apnea syndrome and acromegaly. Otolaryngol Head Neck Surg 1994;111: 25–30.
20. Grunstein RR, Ho KKY, Sullivan CE. Effect of octreotide, a somatostatin analog, on sleep apnea in patients with acromegaly. Ann Intern Med 1994;121: 478–83.
21. Herrmann BL, Wessendorf TE, Ajaj W, et al. Effects of octreotide on sleep apnoea and tongue volume (magnetic resonance imaging) in patients with acromegaly. Eur J Endocrinol 2004;151:309–15.
22. Pekkarinen T, Partinen M, Pelkonen R, et al. Sleep apnoea and daytime sleepiness in acromegaly:

relationship to endocrinological factors. Clin Endocrinol (Oxf) 1987;27:649–54.

23. Pelttari L, Polo O, Rauhala E, et al. Nocturnal breathing abnormalities in acromegaly after adenomectomy. Clin Endocrinol (Oxf) 1995;43:175–82.

24. Pelttari L, Rauhala E, Polo O, et al. Upper airway obstruction in hypothyroidism. J Intern Med 1994;236:177–81.

25. Jha A, Sharma SK, Tandon N, et al. Thyroxine replacement therapy reverses sleep-disordered breathing in patients with primary hypothyroidism. Sleep Med 2006;7:55–61.

26. Grunstein RR, Sullivan CE. Sleep apnea and hypothyroidism: mechanisms and management. Am J Med 1988;85:775–9.

27. Krishnan PV, Vadivu AS, Alappatt A, et al. Prevalence of sleep abnormalities and their association among hypothyroid patients in an Indian population. Sleep Med 2012;13:1232–7.

28. Resta O, Carratù P, Carpagnano GE, et al. Influence of subclinical hypothyroidism and T4 treatment on the prevalence and severity of obstructive sleep apnoea syndrome (OSAS). J Endocrinol Invest 2005;28:893–8.

29. Shinno H, Inami Y, Inagaki T, et al. Successful treatment with levothyroxine for idiopathic hypersomnia patients with subclinical hypothyroidism. Gen Hosp Psychiatry 2009;31:190–3.

30. Lu CL, Lee YC, Tsai SJ, et al. Psychiatric disturbances associated with hyperthyroidism: an analysis report of 30 cases. Zhonghua Yi Xue Za Zhi (Taipei) 1995;56:393–8.

31. Sridhar GR, Putcha V, Lakshmi G. Sleep in thyrotoxicosis. Indian J Endocrinol Metab 2011;15:23–6.

32. Pereira JC Jr, Pradella-Hallinan M, Pessoa HL. Imbalance between thyroid hormones and the dopaminergic system might be central to the pathophysiology of restless legs syndrome: a hypothesis. Clinics 2010;65:547–54.

33. Aulinas A, Webb SM. Health-related quality of life in primary and secondary adrenal insufficiency. Expert Rev Pharmacoecon Outcomes Res 2014;14:873–88.

34. Seelig E, Keller U, Klarhöfer M, et al. Neuroendocrine regulation and metabolism of glucose and lipids in primary chronic insomnia: a prospective case-control study. PLoS One 2013;8:e61780.

35. Xia L, Chen GH, Li ZH, et al. Alterations in hypothalamus-pituitary-adrenal/thyroid axes and gonadotropin-releasing hormone in the patients with primary insomnia: a clinical research. PLoS One 2013;8:e71065.

36. Shipley JE, Schteingart DE, Tandon R, et al. Sleep architecture and sleep apnea in patients with Cushing's disease. Sleep 1992;15:514–8.

37. Berger G, Hardak E, Shaham B, et al. Preliminary prospective explanatory observation on the impact of 3-month steroid therapy on the objective measures of sleep-disordered breathing. Sleep Breath 2012;16:549–53.

38. Kenna HA, Poon AW, de los Angeles CP, et al. Psychiatric complications of treatment with corticosteroids: review with case report. Psychiatry Clin Neurosci 2011;65:549–60.

39. Miller CM, Rindflesch TC, Fiszman M, et al. A closed literature-based discovery technique finds a mechanistic link between hypogonadism and diminished sleep quality in aging men. Sleep 2012;35:279–85.

40. Shi Z, Araujo AB, Martin S, et al. Longitudinal changes in testosterone over five years in community-dwelling men. J Clin Endocrinol Metab 2013;98:3289–97.

41. Resta O, Foschino Barbaro MP, Bonfitto P, et al. Low sleep quality and daytime sleepiness in obese patients without obstructive sleep apnoea syndrome. J Intern Med 2003;253:536–43.

42. Grossmann M. Low testosterone in men with type 2 diabetes: significance and treatment. J Clin Endocrinol Metab 2011;96:2341–53.

43. Hanafy HM. Testosterone therapy and obstructive sleep apnea: is there a real connection? J Sex Med 2007;4:1241–6.

44. Hoyos CM, Killick R, Yee BJ, et al. Effects of testosterone therapy on sleep and breathing in obese men with severe obstructive sleep apnoea: a randomized placebo-controlled trial. Clin Endocrinol 2012;77:599–607.

45. Venancio DP, Tufik S, Garbuio SA, et al. Effects of anabolic androgenic steroids on sleep patterns of individuals practicing resistance exercise. Eur J Appl Physiol 2008;102:555–60.

46. Young T, Finn L, Austin D, et al. Menopausal status and sleep-disordered breathing in the Wisconsin Sleep Cohort Study. Am J Respir Crit Care Med 2003;167:1181–5.

47. Sarti CD, Chiantera A, Graziottin A, et al. Hormone therapy and sleep quality in women around menopause. Menopause 2005;12:545–51.

48. Cistulli PA, Barnes DJ, Grunstein RR, et al. Effect of short-term hormone replacement in the treatment of obstructive sleep apnoea in postmenopausal women. Thorax 1994;49:699–702.

49. Burgess HJ, Revell VL, Molina TA, et al. Human phase response curves to three days of daily melatonin: 0.5 mg versus 3.0 mg. J Clin Endocrinol Metab 2010;95:3325–31.

50. Sack RL, Brandes RW, Kendall AR, et al. Entrainment of free-running circadian rhythms by melatonin in blind people. N Engl J Med 2000;343:1070–7.

51. Sack RL, Hughes RJ, Edgar DM, et al. Sleep-promoting effects of melatonin: at what dose, in whom, under what conditions, and by what mechanisms? Sleep 1997;20:908–15.

52. Sharkey KM, Fogg LF, Eastman CI. Effects of melatonin administration on daytime sleep after

simulated night shift work. J Sleep Res 2001;10: 181–92.

53. Aeschbach D, Lockyer BJ, Dijk DJ, et al. Use of transdermal melatonin delivery to improve sleep maintenance during daytime. Clin Pharmacol Ther 2009;86:378–82.

54. Wyatt JK, Dijk DJ, Ritz-De Cecco A, et al. Sleep facilitating effect of exogenous melatonin in healthy young men and women is circadian-phase dependent. Sleep 2006;29:609–18.

55. Zhdanova IV, Wurtman RJ. Efficacy of melatonin as a sleep-promoting agent. J Biol Rhythms 1997;12: 644–50.

56. Leproult R, Copinschi G, Buxton O, et al. Sleep loss results in an elevation of cortisol levels the next evening. Sleep 1997;20:865–70.

57. Vgontzas AN, Mastorakos G, Bixler EO, et al. Sleep deprivation effects on the activity of the hypothalamic–pituitary–adrenal and growth axes: potential clinical implications. Clin Endocrinol 1999; 51:205–15.

58. Guyon A, Balbo M, Morselli LL, et al. Adverse effects of two nights of sleep restriction on the hypothalamic-pituitary-adrenal axis in healthy men. J Clin Endocrinol Metab 2014;99:2861–8.

59. Reutrakul S, Van Cauter E. Interactions between sleep, circadian function, and glucose metabolism: implications for risk and severity of diabetes. Ann N Y Acad Sci 2014;1311:151–73.

60. Spiegel K, Leproult R, Van Cauter E. Impact of sleep debt on metabolic and endocrine function. Lancet 1999;354:1435–9.

61. Buxton OM, Pavlova M, Reid EW, et al. Sleep restriction for 1 week reduces insulin sensitivity in healthy men. Diabetes 2010;59:2126–33.

62. Knutson KL, Van Cauter E. Associations between sleep loss and increased risk of obesity and diabetes. Ann N Y Acad Sci 2008;1129:287–304.

63. Mullington JM, Chan JL, Van Dongen HP, et al. Sleep loss reduces diurnal rhythm amplitude of leptin in healthy men. J Neuroendocrinol 2003;15:851–4.

64. Spiegel K, Leproult R, L'Hermite-Baleriaux M, et al. Leptin levels are dependent on sleep duration: relationships with sympathovagal balance, carbohydrate regulation, cortisol, and thyrotropin. J Clin Endocrinol Metab 2004;89:5762–71.

65. Taheri S, Lin L, Austin D, et al. Short sleep duration is associated with reduced leptin, elevated ghrelin, and increased body mass index. PLoS Med 2004; 1(3):e62.

66. Markwald RR, Melanson EL, Smith MR, et al. Impact of insufficient sleep on total daily energy expenditure, food intake, and weight gain. Proc Natl Acad Sci U S A 2013;110(4):5695–700.

67. Vgontzas A, Bixler EO, Lin HM, et al. Chronic insomnia is associated with nyctohemeral activation of the hypothalamic-pituitary-adrenal axis: clinical implications. J Clin Endocrinol Metab 2001;86(8): 3787–94.

68. Vallières A, Ceklic T, Bastein CH, et al. A preliminary evaluation of the physiological mechanisms of action for sleep restriction therapy. Sleep Disord 2013;2013:726372.

69. Tasali E, Leproult R, Ehrmann DA, et al. Slow-wave sleep and the risk of type 2 diabetes in humans. Proc Natl Acad Sci U S A 2008;105:1044–9.

70. Vgontzas AN, Liao D, Pejovic S, et al. Insomnia with short sleep duration and mortality: the Penn State cohort. Sleep 2010;33:1159–64.

71. Vgontzas AN, Liao D, Pejovic S, et al. Insomnia with objective short sleep duration is associated with type 2 diabetes: a population-based study. Diabetes Care 2009;32:1980–5.

72. Attal P, Chanson P. Endocrine aspects of obstructive sleep apnea. J Clin Endocrinol Metab 2010; 95:483–95.

73. Yee B, Liu P, Phillips C, et al. Neuroendocrine changes in sleep apnea. Curr Opin Pulm Med 2004;10:475–81.

74. Ip MS, Lam B, Ng MM, et al. Obstructive sleep apnea is independently associated with insulin resistance. Am J Respir Crit Care Med 2002;165:670–6.

75. Punjabi NM, Sorkin JD, Katzel LI, et al. Sleep-disordered breathing and insulin resistance in middle-aged and overweight men. Am J Respir Crit Care Med 2002;165:677–82.

76. Svatikova A, Wolk R, Gami AS, et al. Interactions between obstructive sleep apnea and the metabolic syndrome. Curr Diab Rep 2005;5:53–8.

77. Coughlin SR, Mawdsley L, Mugarza JA, et al. Obstructive sleep apnoea is independently associated with an increased prevalence of metabolic syndrome. Eur Heart J 2004;25:735–41.

78. McMenamin T. A time to work: recent trends in shift work and flexible schedules. Mon Labor Rev 2007;3–15.

79. Shibui K, Uchiyama M, Kim K, et al. Melatonin, cortisol and thyroid-stimulating hormone rhythms are delayed in patients with delayed sleep phase syndrome. Sleep Biol Rhythms 2003;1:209–14.

80. Scheer F, Hilton M, Mantzoros C, et al. Adverse metabolic and cardiovascular consequences of circadian misalignment. Proc Natl Acad Sci U S A 2009;106:4453–8.

81. Gonnissen H, Rutters F, Mazuy C, et al. Effect of a phase advance and phase delay of the 24-h cycle on energy metabolism, appetite, and related hormones. Am J Clin Nutr 2012;96:689–97.

82. Pan A, Schernhammer ES, Sun Q, et al. Rotating night shift work and risk of type 2 diabetes: two prospective cohort studies in women. PLoS Med 2011; 8(12):e1001141.

83. Monk TH, Buysse DJ. Exposure to shift work as a risk factor for diabetes. J Biol Rhythms 2013;28: 356–9.

84. Leproult R, Holmbäck U, Van Cauter E. Circadian misalignment augments markers of insulin resistance and inflammation, independently of sleep loss. Diabetes 2014;63:1860–9.

85. Davis S, Mirick DK. Circadian disruption, shift work and the risk of cancer: a summary of the evidence and studies in Seattle. Cancer Causes Control 2006;17:539–45.

86. Tamarkin L, Cohen M, Roselle D, et al. Melatonin inhibition and pinealectomy enhancement of 7,12-dimethylbenz(a)anthracene-induced mammary tumors in the rat. Cancer Res 1981;41:4432–6.

87. Mocchegiani E, Perissin L, Santarelli L, et al. Melatonin administration in tumor-bearing mice (intact and pinealectomized) in relation to stress, zinc, thymulin and IL-2. Int J Immunopharmacol 1999;21:27–46.

88. Maurovich-Horvat E, Keckeis M, Zuzana Lattov Z, et al. Hypothalamo–pituitary–adrenal axis, glucose metabolism and TNF-alpha in narcolepsy. J Sleep Res 2014;23:425–31.

89. Beitinger PA, Fulda S, Dalal MA, et al. Glucose tolerance in patients with narcolepsy. Sleep 2012;35:231–6.

90. Engel A, Helfrich J, Manderscheid N, et al. Investigation of insulin resistance in narcoleptic patients: dependent or independent of body mass index? Neuropsychiatr Dis Treat 2011;7:351–6.

91. Cooper AB, Thornley KS, Young GB, et al. Sleep in critically ill patients requiring mechanical ventilation. Chest 2000;117:809–18.

92. Freedman NS, Gazendam J, Levan L, et al. Abnormal sleep/wake cycles and the effect of environmental noise on sleep disruption in the intensive care unit. Am J Respir Crit Care Med 2001;163:451–7.

93. Shilo L, Dagan Y, Smorjik Y, et al. Patients in the intensive care unit suffer from severe lack of sleep associated with loss of normal melatonin secretion pattern. Am J Med Sci 1999;317:278–81.

94. Perras B, Meier M, Dodt C. Light and darkness fail to regulate melatonin release in critically ill humans. Intensive Care Med 2007;33:1954–8.

95. Mundigler G, Delle-Karth G, Koreny M, et al. Impaired circadian rhythm of melatonin secretion in sedated critically ill patients with severe sepsis. Crit Care Med 2002;30:536–40.

96. Van den Berghe G. Novel insights into the neuroendocrinology of critical illness. Eur J Endocrinol 2000;143:1–13.

97. Vanhorebeek I, Langouche L, Van den Berghe G. Endocrine aspects of acute and prolonged critical illness. Nat Clin Pract Endocrinol Metab 2006;1:20–31.

Congestive Heart Failure and Central Sleep Apnea

Scott A. Sands, PhD[a,b], Robert L. Owens, MD[c,]*

KEYWORDS

- Congestive heart failure • Central sleep apnea • Cheyne stokes respiration • Loop gain

KEY POINTS

- Congestive heart failure (CHF) is a common clinical syndrome among patients in the intensive care unit (ICU), who frequently require noninvasive or mechanical ventilation.
- CHF affects breathing control by increasing chemosensitivity and circulatory delay, predisposing to central sleep apnea, classically in a crescendo–decrescendo pattern of respiration known as Cheyne–Stokes respiration (CSR).
- Few data are available to determine prevalence of CSR in the ICU, or how CSR might affect clinical management and weaning from mechanical ventilation.

CLINICAL CONSIDERATIONS

Historical Perspective

An abnormal respiratory pattern has long been recognized as an ominous sign of congestive heart failure (CHF). The observations of 3 physicians who have lent their names to the pattern remain informative:

> His breathing was very particular: he would cease breathing for twenty or thirty seconds, and then begin to breathe softly, which increased until he breathed extremely strong, or rather with violent strength, which gradually died away till we could not observe that he breathed at all. He could not lie down without running the risk of being suffocated, therefore he was obliged to sit up in his chair.
> —John Hunter, 1781[1]

The patient suddenly developed palpitations and displayed signs of severe congestive heart failure. The only particularity in the last period of his illness, which lasted eight or nine days, was in the state of respiration. For several days his breathing was irregular; it would entirely cease for a quarter of a minute, then it would become perceptible, though very low, then by degrees it became heaving and quick, and then it would gradually cease again. This revolution in the state of his breathing occupied about a minute, during which there were about thirty acts of respiration.
> —John Cheyne, 1818

> This symptom [periodic breathing], as occurring in its highest degree, I have only seen

This article originally appeared in Critical Care Clinics, Volume 31, Issue 3, July 2015.

Disclosure Statement: Dr S.A. Sands is supported by a National Health and Medical Research Council of Australia Early Career Fellowship and R.G. Menzies award (1053201). Dr R.L. Owens is supported by the National Institutes of Health K23 HL105542. He has previously consulted for Philips Respironics.

[a] Division of Sleep Medicine, Brigham and Women's Hospital and Harvard Medical School, 221 Longwood Avenue, Boston, MA 02115, USA; [b] Department of Allergy, Immunology and Respiratory Medicine and Central Clinical School, Alfred Hospital and Monash University, 55 Commercial Rd, Melbourne, VIC 3004, Australia; [c] Division of Pulmonary and Critical Care Medicine, University of California San Diego, 9300 Campus Point Drive, #7381, La Jolla, CA 92037, USA

* Corresponding author.

E-mail address: rowens@ucsd.edu

http://dx.doi.org/10.1016/j.jsmc.2015.10.003
1556-407X/16/$ – see front matter © 2016 Elsevier Inc. All rights reserved.

during a few weeks previous to the death of the patient.

—*William Stokes, 1854*

The initial observations by Hunter, Cheyne, and Stokes were made in patients close to death. They were the first to note the characteristic waxing and waning respiratory pattern of "Cheyne–Stokes respiration" (CSR), a common pattern of central sleep apnea in patients with CHF. CSR is characterized by complete cessation of respiratory effort and airflow (apnea phase) alternating with profound hyperventilation (hyperventilation phase). Such patterns occur during wakefulness, but are typically more prominent during sleep (**Fig. 1**). The apnea phase of CSR causes arterial hypoxemia, and the hyperventilation phase produces surges in blood pressure, arousal from sleep, and dyspnea (**Fig. 2**).[2–5] Typically, CSR has a periodicity of 45 to 90 seconds, and occurs during non–rapid eye movement (REM) sleep stages 1 and 2. CSR severity is typically measured by quantifying the percent of total sleep time in CSR, and by the number of apneas and central hypopneas per hour of sleep (apnea–hypopnea index).[6] Despite advances in the treatment of CHF (eg, β-blockade, spironolactone), untreated CSR remains highly prevalent during sleep and retains its association with increased morbidity and mortality independent of the severity of heart failure (**Boxes 1–4**).[7–10]

Epidemiology in Stable Congestive Heart Failure

One of the first rigorous studies to use polysomnography by Javaheri and colleagues[11] found a

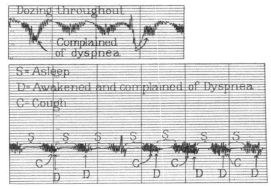

Fig. 2. Increased ventilatory drive during the hyperventilation phase of Cheyne–Stokes respiration results in dyspnea in a patient with heart failure. (*Adapted from* Harrison TR, King CE, Calhoun JA, et al. Congestive heart failure: Xx. Cheyne-Stokes respiration as the cause of paroxysmal dyspnea at the onset of sleep. Arch Intern Med 1934;53(6):897; with permission.)

high prevalence (40%) of CSR in patients with systolic heart failure. This prevalence has been a relatively consistent finding depending on the population studied (with increased prevalence with worsening heart failure) and the threshold and technology used to diagnosis sleep disordered breathing.[12–15] Although early epidemiologic studies predated the widespread use of advanced heart failure therapies, even the most recent studies continue to show a consistently high prevalence of CSR.[14,16] CSR is not limited to systolic heart failure; CSR is common in patients with symptomatic heart failure with preserved

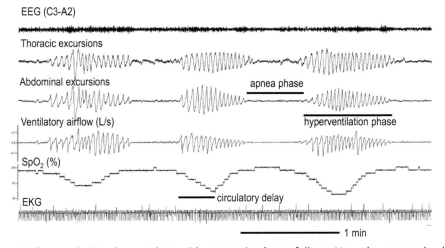

Fig. 1. Cheyne–Stokes respiration in a patient with congestive heart failure. Note the crescendo–decrescendo pattern of respiratory effort and airflow. The lung-to-ear circulatory delay can be approximated by the time from resumption of airflow to the start of the increase in oxygen saturation. EEG, electroencephalogram; EKG, electrocardiogram; SpO2, oxygen saturation.

Box 1
Features of Cheyne–Stokes respiration

- Waxing and waning respiratory pattern
- Baseline hyperventilation and hypocapnia is typical
- Periodicity of 45–90 seconds
- Improved in REM and slow-wave sleep

Abbreviation: REM, rapid eye movement.

Box 3
Pathophysiology/mechanisms of Cheyne–Stokes respiration in congestive heart failure

- Increased chemosensitivity owing to
  - Increased left atrial pressure
  - Hypoxemia
- Increased circulatory delay
- Low lung volumes

ejection fraction[17] (diastolic dysfunction), and is also common in patients with asymptomatic systolic dysfunction.[18] Additional risk factors for CSR include male gender, older age, the presence of atrial fibrillation, nocturnal ventricular arrhythmias, low arterial partial pressure of CO_2 ($Paco_2$), dyspnea with minimal exertion (New York Heart Association class $\geq$II), nocturnal dyspnea, very low ejection fraction (<20%), left atrial enlargement, and high N-terminal of the prohormone brain natriuretic peptide (NT-proBNP).[5,10,12,14,15,19,20]

Congestive Heart Failure in the Intensive Care Unit

CHF is among the most common causes of admission to hospitals in the United States, especially in those over 65 years of age, with more than 1 million hospital admissions per year.[21] Approximately 10% of these patients will require admission to the intensive care unit (ICU).[22] Despite the high number of hospital/ICU admissions, there are few data regarding the prevalence of CSR among hospitalized patients. Hoffman and colleagues[23] noted CSR in 44% of CHF patients after weaning from mechanical ventilation for cardiogenic pulmonary edema. More recently, Padeletti and colleagues[24] found moderate to severe CSR (apnea–hypopnea index of >15) in 75% of patients admitted for an acute exacerbation of systolic CHF, with an average of 51% of total sleep time spent exhibiting CSR. Thus, CSR seems to be more prevalent (~75%) in decompensated CHF in inpatients than in stable CHF outpatients (~40%).

Unfortunately, data on the prevalence of CSR in the ICU and effects on outcomes are lacking. Given the pathophysiologic changes that occur in severe heart failure (that requires ICU admission for management), we might expect a very high rate of CSR. However, the most acutely ill patients may be on mechanical ventilation and sedated, often with narcotics. Mechanical ventilation also provides ventilatory and cardiac support for the patient in heart failure, because both cardiac preload and afterload are reduced while on positive end-expiratory pressure (PEEP).[25,26] Thus, CSR is likely to be most relevant during the process of ventilator weaning[23] when such support is removed. It is during the process of moving

Box 2
Types/causes of central sleep apnea in the intensive care unit

- Cheyne–Stokes respiration
- Stroke/neurologic disease
- Narcotic induced

Box 4
Treatment of Cheyne–Stokes respiration

- Treat congestive heart failure
  - Improve cardiac function, left atrial pressure, and pulmonary congestion to decrease circulatory delay and decrease chemosensitivity
- Position patient to improve lung volumes
  - Lateral
  - Bed elevation
- PAP therapy
  - Continuous positive airway pressure
  - Bilevel positive airway pressure with backup rate
  - Adaptive servoventilation
- Supplemental oxygen therapy to reduce chemosensitivity
- Medication
  - Respiratory stimulants to lower CO_2
  - Sedatives to facilitate stable sleep
  - Low-dose opioids to reduce chemosensitivity

toward liberation from mechanical ventilation that sedatives are decreased, PEEP and supplemental oxygen levels are lowered, and patients are placed on spontaneous modes (ie, patient triggered) of ventilation.

PATHOPHYSIOLOGIC CONSIDERATIONS
Control of Breathing

The physiologic control of breathing is maintained by a negative feedback system that acts to regulate acid–base status and the partial pressure of arterial carbon dioxide ($Paco_2$), and ensure adequate oxygenation. The primary components of the ventilatory control system are chemoreceptor inputs located in the medulla that respond to changes in acid–base status and the peripheral chemoreceptors in the carotid bodies that are sensitive to both changes in Pao_2 and $Paco_2$. Central and peripheral chemoreceptor inputs are integrated in the medulla and act to modulate breath amplitude (and timing to a lesser extent), ultimately resulting in a level of ventilation conducive to survival. Importantly, there are other sensors in the lungs and circulation whose inputs modify the behavior of the respiratory control system, including pulmonary stretch receptors, irritant receptors, and the "J" (juxtacapillary) receptors, which may become important in disease states and are discussed elsewhere in this article.[27–31]

The Concept of Loop Gain

The stability of the respiratory feedback loop has been quantified using the engineering criterion, loop gain. Briefly, loop gain is the magnitude of the ventilatory response of the respiratory control system to a sinusoidal respiratory disturbance (at the frequency of CSR). Feedback loops with a value of loop gain that exceeds 1.0 (response is greater than the disturbance) are intrinsically unstable and periodic oscillations in breathing inevitably occur (**Fig. 3**). When loop gain is less than 1 (response < disturbance), transient oscillations are attenuated and thereby temporary. Detailed descriptions of loop gain have been given previously.[32–34] Consider a period of hyperventilation (disturbance) that causes a reduction in $Paco_2$. This reduction in $Paco_2$ is sensed by chemoreceptors after a circulatory delay, which in turn elicit a later reduction in ventilatory drive (response). In an unstable system, the decrease in ventilatory drive causes a greater degree of hypoventilation than the original hyperventilatory disturbance. Oscillations re amplified and self-sustained with no specific initiating factor required. The concept of loop gain has been applied successfully to predict

the occurrence of CSR (**Fig. 4**)[35] and the resistance to its suppression with treatment.[36,37]

Detailed analyses of the control system consistently reveal 4 primary factors that contribute to loop gain,[32,35,36,38–40] according to the relationship:

$$\text{Loop gain} = G \frac{Paco_2}{\text{Lung Volume}} T \qquad (1)$$

where G is the chemosensitivity, defined as the change in ventilation in response to a change in $Paco_2$; $Paco_2$ is the arterial partial pressure of CO_2 (with the assumption here that inspired $Pco_2 = 0$); lung volume is the end-expiratory lung volume (eg, functional residual capacity); and T is a timing factor that incorporates the lung–chemoreceptor circulatory delay. A similar equation can be written for the ventilatory feedback control of arterial Po_2.

How Congestive Heart Failure Predisposes to Cheyne–Stokes respiration

Equation 1 provides the framework for identifying the factors that predispose an individual to CSR. Indeed, there is evidence that each of these factors plays a role in the development or effective treatment of CSR.

Circulatory Delay

Classically, an increased lung-to-chemoreceptor circulatory delay (T) has been implicated as the cause of CSR. Patients with heart failure can have elevated circulatory delay as a result of decreased cardiac output. CHF patients with a lower left ventricular ejection fraction, lower cardiac output, and elongated circulatory delays are at elevated risk of CSR.[11,19,41,42] Further evidence includes the observation that the lung-to-ear circulation delay (approximating the lung-to-chemoreceptor delay) is equal to the delay between the nadir CO_2 level and apnea during CSR.[43] Raising cardiac output with exercise, pharmacologic intervention, or cardiac resynchronization can also reduce the ventilatory oscillations in CHF.[44–46] However, such interventions may also effect other factors (Equation 1) contributing to stabilization. Moreover, many CHF patients with low LVEF and increased circulatory delays do not have CSR.[35] Thus, the other factors identified in Equation 1 are likely important as well.

Chemosensitivity

Increased chemosensitivity (G) is the most powerful determinant of CSR.[35,47–49] Specifically, CHF–CSR severity is strongly associated with the

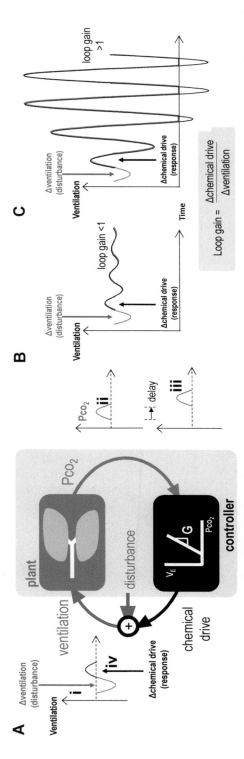

Fig. 3. Loop gain provides a framework to understand the pathophysiology of Cheyne–Stokes respiration. (*A*) Simplified conceptual block diagram of the respiratory control system. A disturbance to this system (*i*, hypoventilation) temporarily increases alveolar and arterial CO_2 (P_{CO_2}) at the lungs (*ii*) as determined by the "plant." After a circulatory delay (*iii*), the controller perceives the blood gas change and increases its output to oppose the original disturbance (*iv*). Whether or not this oscillation grows and manifests CSR depends on the loop gain of the system. (*B*) If loop gain is less than 1.0, each response is smaller than the prior disturbance and transient disturbances are damped away. (*C*) If loop gain exceeds 1.0, each response is greater than the prior disturbance, and oscillations grow until Cheyne–Stokes respiration is established. P_{CO_2}, partial pressure of CO_2; V_E, minute ventilation during exercise.

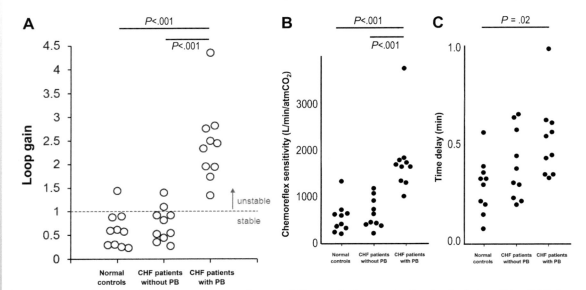

Fig. 4. Loop gain determines the presence or absence of Cheyne–Stokes respiration (periodic breathing [PB]) during wakefulness. (*A*) Congestive heart failure (CHF) patients with PB had higher loop gain compared with CHF patients without PB and healthy controls. Increased loop gain in CHFPB was owing to elevated chemosensitivity (*B*) and increased circulatory delay (*C*). (*Data from* Francis DP, Willson K, Davies LC, et al. Quantitative general theory for periodic breathing in chronic heart failure and its clinical implications. Circulation 2000;102(18):2218; and Kee K, Sands SA, Edwards BA, et al. Positive airway pressure in congestive heart failure. Sleep Med Clin 2010;5:398.)

dynamic ventilatory response to CO_2,[49] suggesting an essential role for elevated peripheral chemoreceptor (carotid bodies) activity in CSR. Increased chemosensitivity is thought to be owing to increased left atrial pressure (**Fig. 5**).[50] Additional evidence includes:

i. Increased pulmonary capillary wedge pressure (PCWP) is common in patients with CSR and is correlated with CSR severity.[42,46,50]

ii. CSR is associated with increased NT-proBNP levels,[10,51] a biomarker of left ventricular stretch and increased PCWP.[52–55]

iii. Left atrial size is associated with CSR and chemosensitivity.[56]

iv. PCWP is associated with hypocapnia,[57] a marker of increased chemosensitivity[58] and predictor of CSR.[12]

v. Raising left atrial pressure acutely increases chemosensitivity in dogs.[59]

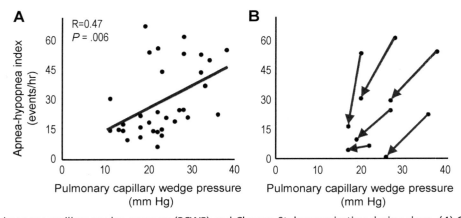

Fig. 5. Pulmonary capillary wedge pressure (PCWP) and Cheyne–Stokes respiration during sleep. (*A*) Correlation between the PCWP and Cheyne–Stokes respiration severity (apnea–hypopnea index). (*B*) Reducing PCWP with medical intervention for heart failure improves Cheyne–Stokes respiration. (*Adapted from* Solin P, Bergin P, Richardson M, et al. Influence of pulmonary capillary wedge pressure on central apnea in heart failure. Circulation 1999;99(12):1578; with permission.)

vi. CSR is associated with cardiogenic pulmonary edema in the form of reduced pulmonary diffusing capacity,[60] presumably via increased pulmonary capillary pressure.

vii. CSR is linked with fluid status, including the degree of overnight rostral fluid shift.[61]

viii. The reduction in PCWP with vasodilator (nitroprusside) is linearly associated with the reduction in CSR.[46]

Increased left atrial pressure is believed to increase chemosensitivity directly via stretch receptors in the left atrium or pulmonary vein[31,62,63] and indirectly through pulmonary edema via juxtapulmonary capillary receptors (J receptors, pulmonary C fibers). It is important to note, however, that such vagal afferents may not explain entirely hypersensitive chemoreflexes in CHF–CSR, given that CSR has been seen to persist despite lung transplantation (and hence vagal denervation).[64] Other factors that may increase chemosensitivity include reduced cardiac output via reduced carotid arterial blood flow[65] and hypoxemia (via pulmonary congestion). Hypoxemia increases chemosensitivity both acutely and over time.[60,66] Indeed, recent evidence in rabbits suggests that afferent activity from carotid body glomus cells is increased in CHF, an effect which is unlikely to be related directly to cardiac pressures.[67]

Lung Volume

Reduced end-expiratory lung volume is another factor that can increase loop gain, destabilize breathing, and promote CSR.[35,36,68] End-expiratory lung volume is decreased in CHF as a result of lung edema and/or pleural effusions, cardiomegaly. Lowered lung volume acts to increase loop gain by lowering the lung gas volume for buffering ventilation-induced fluctuations in P_{CO_2} and P_{O_2}.[36,68] Lowered end-expiratory lung volume, however, does not seem to differentiate between CHF patients and without CSR at baseline.[35] Nonetheless, manipulating lung volume can have an important effect on improving CSR.[36,68] Szollosi and colleagues[69] found that the lateral sleeping position attenuated the CSR severity (apnea–hypopnea index) by approximately 60% compared with the supine position. Importantly, the lateral position attenuates apnea-associated oxygen desaturation without affecting event duration. The decreased desaturation speed in lateral versus supine positions is consistent with the known increase in lung volume in the lateral position,[70] and provides indirect evidence that lung volume might be of major importance in the pathogenesis of CSR. Whether the lateral position affects other factors, including cardiac output or

chemosensitivity in CHF patients, is currently unknown.

Behavioral State Effects

Behavioral state can also have a major effect on CSR severity. Although CSR can be observed during wakefulness, it is greatly exacerbated by the transition to sleep,[71] which may seem counterintuitive given the reduced chemosensitivity during sleep.[72–74] However, accompanying the transition from wake to sleep is an abrupt reduction in ventilatory drive (for any given P_{aCO_2}); likewise, accompanying the transition from sleep to wake (arousal) is an abrupt increase in ventilatory drive. Thus, any oscillation in ventilatory drive that is accompanied by transitions in state[75] is enhanced and hence ventilation is destabilized further.[76] CSR is most common in light non-REM sleep (stage 1) and is suppressed most powerfully in deep non-REM sleep (slow-wave sleep).[69,77] Deeper sleep presumably promotes stable breathing via increased arousal threshold (fewer arousals/awakenings) and reduced chemosensitivity compared with lighter sleep.[72–74] The observation that a sedative (zolpidem) can greatly improve CSR in patients without CHF[78] further highlights the importance of behavioral state on ventilatory instability. CSR is also reduced but not always absent in REM sleep,[36,69,77] whereas chemosensitivity is reduced in REM,[79] the arousal threshold is similar in REM to stage 1[80] and profound (non–CO_2-related) disturbances to ventilatory control are characteristic of this state. A final consideration is that sleep may promote CSR via the lowered end-expiratory lung volume that occurs with sleep onset.[81]

TREATMENT OF CHEYNE–STOKES RESPIRATION

In patients with CHF, untreated but not treated CSR is associated with increased mortality,[8,82,83] leading to the view that improving severe ventilatory oscillations of CSR may promote survival. Ongoing clinical trials are assessing whether CSR treatment improves mortality. In the meantime, clinicians treat symptomatic CSR to achieve improvements in quality of life, as well as nocturnal hypoxemia, sympathoexcitation, ventricular irritability, and for small improvements in cardiac function.[82,84–90] Although no such data exist for CSR in the ICU, we review the general treatment strategies in this article.

Treatment of Heart Failure

Based on the discussion so far, therapies for the treatment of CSR first focus on improving CHF. It is expected that treatments that improve cardiac output, decrease left atrial pressure, and improve lung volume should improve CSR. For example, intensive medical therapy that included diuretics and afterload reduction can successfully lower PCWP and improve CSR (see **Fig. 5**).[50] Similarly, β-blockers,[91–93] cardiac resynchronization therapy,[44,94] left ventricular assist devices[95] and transplantation[96–98] have been associated with improvements in CSR over time. Rapid changes in cardiac function, as might happen in the ICU, can quickly affect CSR severity. Kara and colleagues[99] have shown that there are acute improvements/worsening in the CSR with acute administration/withdrawal of cardiac resynchronization. Although CHF treatment can be effective at resolving CSR, in many patients CSR can persist despite the most aggressive therapies, including cardiac resynchronization therapy,[100] left ventricular assist devices,[101] and even heart transplantation.[96] Thus, additional treatments are needed for CSR.

Positive Airway Pressure

Positive airway pressure, whether applied as PEEP from a mechanical ventilator or in noninvasive form as continuous positive airway pressure (CPAP), has the potential to improve CSR acutely via multiple mechanisms:

i. Acutely increasing lung volume, which increases the gas volume for buffering ventilation-induced changes in P_{CO_2} and P_{O_2}.[36,68,102]
ii. Stabilization of the upper airway, which may play a covert role in CSR in some patients.[103]
iii. Improved hypoxemia that in turn reduces chemosensitivity, both acutely and further over time.[104,105] CPAP may improve oxygenation by improving microatelectasis in cardiogenic pulmonary edema.[106] CPAP also improves CSR-related desaturation independent of CSR resolution,[36] presumably via increased lung volume.
iv. Improved cardiac function by lowering cardiac preload and afterload. Such effects could theoretically increase cardiac output, decrease circulatory time, and lower PCWP (and chemosensitivity).[107] However, despite improvements in afterload, cardiac output and circulatory time do not typically change with CPAP.[26,84] Long-term CPAP can improve chemosensitivity over time.[84,89,104]

Although variability in the mechanism of action may help to explain the variable effect size of CPAP in CSR,[82,85] it is those with the most unstable breathing pattern (the greatest loop gain) that tend to respond insufficiently to CPAP.[36] The majority of CPAP-related suppression of CSR is immediate,[36,88] consistent with major effects of CPAP acting via increased lung volume[36,68,102] and relief of hypoxemia. Smaller additional suppression of CSR can be observed over time,[104] and are presumably via improvements in cardiac function. Such improvements in cardiac function are seen exclusively in those in whom CPAP improves CSR, and not in those in whom CPAP fails to resolve CSR nor in those with CHF but without CSR.[82,108] Given that CPAP is associated only with beneficial outcomes when CSR is suppressed, the early use of more aggressive therapy for CSR may be warranted.

Given the variable CSR response to CPAP, there has been increasing interested in bilevel positive airway pressure (PAP) and more advanced ventilation algorithms, such as adaptive-servo ventilation (ASV). Bilevel PAP offers the advantages of CPAP but, when used in a spontaneous/timed mode, can provide ventilation during periods of apnea. Importantly, bilevel PAP without any backup rate during periods of apnea may destabilize respiration further by augmenting hyperventilation (effectively raising chemosensitivity "G" in Equation 1), and can worsen central apneas during sleep.[109] When applied to patients with CSR, bilevel PAP (with a backup rate) can show small further improvements in the CSR severity over CPAP.[110] ASV also provides PEEP; however, the amount of inspiratory pressure varies dynamically to prevent hypopneas and maintain a constant minute ventilation. Inspiratory pressure increases as the patient's inspiratory effort decreases, but decreases as the patient augments their inspiratory effort. Preliminary data have been promising[83,100,111–119] and long-term outcome data are pending (NCT01128816 and NCT00733343).

Oxygen

Supplemental inspired oxygen therapy maintains arterial oxygenation during CSR, but can also resolve CSR effectively in many patients.[117,120–122] Relief of hypoxemia is expected to reduce chemosensitivity ("G" in Equation 1) and thereby reduce loop gain.[105] However, the effect of supplemental oxygen on CSR is heterogeneous (unlike the uniform resolution of CSR when oxygen is used for altitude-induced central sleep apnea), demonstrating that hypoxemia alone is not sufficient to explain CSR.

Medications

Ventilatory stimulants have also been used to improve CSR in CHF patients, including acetazolamide[71,87] and theophylline.[123] Stimulants act to lower Pa_{CO_2} (see Equation 1), which lowers plant gain and acts to stabilize breathing.[124] The administration of supplemental CO_2 has a similar effect on plant gain,[37] and can suppress CSR powerfully.[43,125] As yet, a long-term therapeutic benefit of stimulants for CHF–CSR has not yet been proven. Alternatively, the use of sedatives/hypnotics can improve CSR in patients without CHF[78]; the efficacy of this approach in heart failure patients is unknown. A mild dose of an opiate analgesic (eg, dihydrocodeine), as routinely administered in the ICU, can lower chemosensitivity and improve CSR and dyspnea during wakefulness[126,127]; however, improvements in CSR during sleep and long-term benefits have not been established. Judicious administration of medications on a case-by-case basis may be warranted to treat symptomatic CSR and associated sequelae in those who do not tolerate mask-pressure–based therapies.

Lung Volume Manipulation

One of the simplest yet underrecognized means to improve CSR is the manipulation of body position. Positional therapy via lateral positioning[69,77,128] and bed elevation[129] have potent effects on CSR severity. Given the low likelihood of "side effects," manipulating body position to treat CSR may yield improved outcomes (**Fig. 6**).

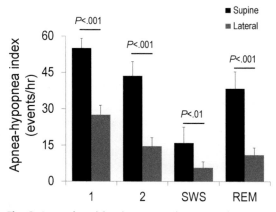

Fig. 6. Lateral position improves Cheyne–Stokes respiration in patients with heart failure in all sleep stages. Note also that Cheyne–Stokes respiration severity is mild in slow wave sleep (SWS) and most severe in stage 1 non-REM sleep. REM, rapid eye movement. (*Adapted from* Szollosi I, Roebuck T, Thompson B, et al. Lateral sleeping position reduces severity of central sleep apnea/Cheyne-Stokes respiration. Sleep 2006;29(8):1045–51; with permission.)

Novel and Future Therapies

Several new therapies are emerging for the treatment of CSR. Phrenic nerve stimulation, applied during the hypopnea phase of CSR, can resolve central events.[130,131] Dynamic CO_2 therapy, applied during the hyperventilation phase of CSR to prevent hypocapnia, can resolve CSR during wakefulness without considerably raising mean ventilation.[132,133] Finally, denervation of the carotid body chemoreceptors has been shown in animal studies to improve survival in CHF, and a case patient with CHF improved sleep disordered breathing, exercise capacity and quality of life.[134,135]

INTENSIVE CARE UNIT MANAGEMENT
General Considerations

Although data are not available, CSR is most likely to occur during the period of ventilator weaning. When sufficient clinical progress provides for reduced sedation, and a switch to a spontaneous mode of breathing, the underlying respiratory pattern will be revealed. Additionally, PEEP is frequently decreased as patients move toward liberation from mechanical ventilation. As PEEP is decreased, preload and afterload increase, which may tend to exacerbate CHF and CSR.

Recognition

The first step in the ICU management of CSR is recognition. Although apneas may be noted, especially by ventilator alarms, the initial management may be focused on (1) changing alarm settings to decrease alerts, or (2) changing ventilator modes from a spontaneous mode to an assist/control mode of ventilation. (An assist/control mode assists all spontaneous respiratory efforts, but in the absence of patient effort and apnea the ventilator controls minute ventilation by delivering a breath from the ventilator.) Alternatively, depending on the ventilator and alarm settings, some ventilators primarily alarm for a low minute ventilation (rather than apnea) when in a spontaneous mode of ventilation. The response may be to increase the amount of pressure support provided. As explained, this may paradoxically increase hyperventilation and further destabilize breathing.[136] Only with proper recognition can appropriate steps be taken to treat underlying heart failure, and manage the patient correctly. Respiratory therapists as well as physicians need to be familiar with the recognition of CSR.

Differential Diagnosis

For the patient not on mechanical ventilation, the differential for apnea includes obstructive sleep apnea. Although endotracheal intubation stents the upper airway open, patients on noninvasive positive pressure ventilation may still have upper airway obstruction if the airway pressure (expiratory positive airway pressure) is inadequate to hold open the upper airway. Obstructive sleep apnea is extremely common, and is likely as prevalent in patients with CHF as CSR. It too, may even more likely in the acutely decompensated patient as a result of excess edema fluid and narrowing of the pharyngeal airway.[137] Bedside evaluation of the sleeping patient should focus on signs of flow limitation, such as snoring, as well as evidence of ongoing respiratory effort during the apnea, such as paradoxic movement of the thorax and abdomen. CHF patients may have both obstructive and central sleep apnea, such that both upper airway and ventilator control require interventions.

Another important consideration is central sleep apnea owing to opioids, which are commonly used both for sedation while on mechanical ventilation, and for treatment of dyspnea in CHF.[138] Central sleep apnea owing to narcotics is generally believed to exhibit an ataxic, irregular pattern with reduced respiratory rate and occasional missed breaths.[139] However, many patients with narcotic-induced apneas exhibit a quasiperiodic or crescendo–decrescendo pattern similar to CSR (see **Fig. 6**).[140] The presence of CSR in the absence of hypocapnia may suggest opioid involvement.

Stroke (cerebral vascular accident) is another consideration. In fact, the patient described by Dr John Cheyne had both CHF and stroke.[141] CSR is seen in approximately 20% to 50% of patients recovering from recent stroke.[142–145] CSR is more common in patients with severe stroke, in those with concurrent CHF (low ejection fraction), and in those with longer hospital admissions.[143–145] The mechanisms of stroke-related CSR are not well-studied. Studies from more than 50 years ago illustrated that stroke, even in the absence of CHF, can cause an increase in chemosensitivity and CSR.[146,147] Likewise, more recent evidence suggests that CSR in stroke is caused by an increase in chemosensitivity (as indicated by observations of lower carbon dioxide) in stroke patients with CSR versus those without CSR.[143] The role of high chemosensitivity (and high loop gain) is confirmed further by the case observation that medical agents that stabilize breathing can ameliorate CSR.[148] Whether treating CSR has a beneficial effect on stroke outcomes remains unclear, but available observation data illustrate that stroke-related CSR and associated sleepiness can be managed effectively with ASV.[149] Thus, the new appearance of central

sleep apnea in a patient with improving CHF should prompt a neurologic evaluation.

Treatment

As discussed, if possible, the best treatment includes further efforts at heart failure treatment, especially therapies designed to lower the left atrial/PCWP. Other medical therapies with respiratory stimulants may or may not be practical in critically ill patients.

Patient Positioning

Given the effects of lung volume on loop gain, proper patient positioning to maximize lung volumes may have an important clinical impact. Lung volumes are greater when sitting or lying lateral than when lying supine.[150] If possible, supine patients with CSR could be moved to a different position to improve lung volumes.

Ventilator Management

For patients with CSR manifest on a pressure support mode, it is worthwhile both diagnostically and therapeutically to decrease pressure support as much as possible to assess the underlying respiratory pattern. Again, a decrement in support may decrease apneic periods, which may be sufficiently brief (and without substantial oxygen desaturation) to consider moving toward liberation from the ventilator. The most robust stress test would be to monitor the patient in the absence of pressure support and PEEP, because this mimics the additional stress that the heart is under once liberated from mechanical ventilation. If prolonged apneas are noted, a spontaneous mode with a backup rate (eg, synchronized intermittent mandatory ventilation). Most modern ventilators can also provide ASV.

Noninvasive Positive Pressure Ventilation Management

Once extubated, the treatment algorithm may not be substantially different than the list in the discussion of Cheyne–Stokes respiration. Noninvasive positive pressure ventilation can be used to provide mechanical support to the left ventricle and limit CSR, especially during sleep. Again, CPAP, bilevel PAP with a backup rate, and ASV could all be tried. Such therapy may be necessary not only in the ICU but during the remainder of hospitalization and after discharge.

SUMMARY

There are few data about the prevalence of CSR owing to CHF in the ICU. Nevertheless, CSR is expected to be highly prevalent among those with CHF, and treatment should focus on the underlying mechanisms by which CHF increases loop gain and promotes unstable breathing. Several important questions await further study: Does earlier recognition of CSR facilitate ventilator management and ultimately hasten weaning from mechanical ventilation? Does treatment of CSR during acute illness facilitate faster recovery? The answers to these questions could substantially impact a large number of ICU patients.

REFERENCES

1. Ward M. Periodic respiration. A short historical note. Ann R Coll Surg Engl 1973;52(5):330–4.

2. van de Borne P, Oren R, Abouassally C, et al. Effect of Cheyne-Stokes respiration on muscle sympathetic nerve activity in severe congestive heart failure secondary to ischemic or idiopathic dilated cardiomyopathy. Am J Cardiol 1998;81(4):432–6.

3. Trinder J, Merson R, Rosenberg JI, et al. Pathophysiological interactions of ventilation, arousals, and blood pressure oscillations during Cheyne-Stokes respiration in patients with heart failure. Am J Respir Crit Care Med 2000;162(3 Pt 1): 808–13.

4. Harrison TR, King CE, Calhoun JA, et al. Congestive heart failure: Xx. Cheyne-Stokes respiration as the cause of paroxysmal dyspnea at the onset of sleep. Arch Intern Med 1934;53(6):891–910.

5. Rees PJ, Clark TJ. Paroxysmal nocturnal dyspnoea and periodic respiration. Lancet 1979;2(8156–8157):1315–7.

6. Berry RB, Budhiraja R, Gottlieb DJ, et al. Rules for scoring respiratory events in sleep: update of the 2007 AASM manual for the scoring of sleep and associated events. Deliberations of the sleep apnea definitions task force of the American Academy of Sleep Medicine. J Clin Sleep Med 2012; 8(5):597–619.

7. Lanfranchi PA, Braghiroli A, Bosimini E, et al. Prognostic value of nocturnal Cheyne-Stokes respiration in chronic heart failure. Circulation 1999; 99(11):1435–40.

8. Jilek C, Krenn M, Sebah D, et al. Prognostic impact of sleep disordered breathing and its treatment in heart failure: an observational study. Eur J Heart Fail 2010;13:68–75.

9. Yumino D, Wang H, Floras JS, et al. Relationship between sleep apnea and mortality in patients with ischemic heart failure. Heart 2009;95(10):819–24.

10. Amir O, Reisfeld D, Sberro H, et al. Implications of Cheyne-Stokes breathing in advanced systolic heart failure. Clin Cardiol 2010;33(3):E8–12.

11. Javaheri S, Parker TJ, Liming JD, et al. Sleep apnea in 81 ambulatory male patients with stable heart failure. Types and their prevalences, consequences, and presentations. Circulation 1998; 97(21):2154–9.

12. Sin DD, Fitzgerald F, Parker JD, et al. Risk factors for central and obstructive sleep apnea in 450 men and women with congestive heart failure. Am J Respir Crit Care Med 1999;160(4):1101–6.

13. Tremel F, Pepin JL, Veale D, et al. High prevalence and persistence of sleep apnoea in patients referred for acute left ventricular failure and medically treated over 2 months. Eur Heart J 1999; 20(16):1201–9.

14. Yumino D, Wang H, Floras JS, et al. Prevalence and physiological predictors of sleep apnea in patients with heart failure and systolic dysfunction. J Card Fail 2009;15(4):279–85.

15. Javaheri S. Sleep disorders in systolic heart failure: a prospective study of 100 male patients. The final report. Int J Cardiol 2006;106(1):21–8.

16. MacDonald M, Fang J, Pittman SD, et al. The current prevalence of sleep disordered breathing in congestive heart failure patients treated with beta-blockers. J Clin Sleep Med 2008;4(1):38–42.

17. Chan J, Sanderson J, Chan W, et al. Prevalence of sleep-disordered breathing in diastolic heart failure. Chest 1997;111(6):1488–93.

18. Lanfranchi PA, Somers VK, Braghiroli A, et al. Central sleep apnea in left ventricular dysfunction: prevalence and implications for arrhythmic risk. Circulation 2003;107(5):727–32.

19. Oldenburg O, Lamp B, Faber L, et al. Sleep-disordered breathing in patients with symptomatic heart failure: a contemporary study of prevalence in and characteristics of 700 patients. Eur J Heart Fail 2007;9(3):251–7.

20. Blackshear JL, Kaplan J, Thompson RC, et al. Nocturnal dyspnea and atrial fibrillation predict Cheyne-Stokes respirations in patients with congestive heart failure. Arch Intern Med 1995; 155(12):1297–302.

21. Fang J, Mensah GA, Croft JB, et al. Heart failure-related hospitalization in the U.S., 1979 to 2004. J Am Coll Cardiol 2008;52(6):428–34.

22. Safavi KC, Dharmarajan K, Kim N, et al. Variation exists in rates of admission to intensive care units for heart failure patients across hospitals in the United States. Circulation 2013;127(8):923–9.

23. Hoffman R, Agatston A, Krieger B. Cheyne-Stokes respiration in patients recovering from acute cardiogenic pulmonary edema. Chest 1990;97(2): 410–2.

24. Padeletti M, Green P, Mooney AM, et al. Sleep disordered breathing in patients with acutely decompensated heart failure. Sleep Med 2009; 10(3):353–60.

25. Malhotra A, Owens RL. What is central sleep apnea? Respir Care 2010;55(9):1168–78.

26. Naughton MT, Rahman MA, Hara K, et al. Effect of continuous positive airway pressure on intrathoracic and left ventricular transmural pressures in patients with congestive heart failure. Circulation 1995;91(6):1725–31.

27. Adrian ED. Afferent impulses in the vagus and their effect on respiration. J Physiol 1933;79(3):332–58.

28. Hamilton RD, Winning AJ, Horner RL, et al. The effect of lung inflation on breathing in man during wakefulness and sleep. Respir Physiol 1988; 73(2):145–54.

29. Hatridge J, Haji A, Perez-Padilla JR, et al. Rapid shallow breathing caused by pulmonary vascular congestion in cats. J Appl Physiol 1989;67(6): 2257–64.

30. Lalani S, Remmers JE, MacKinnon Y, et al. Hypoxemia and low Crs in vagally denervated lambs result from reduced lung volume and not pulmonary edema. J Appl Physiol 2002;93(2):601–10.

31. Paintal AS. Mechanism of stimulation of type J pulmonary receptors. J Physiol 1969;203(3): 511–32.

32. Khoo MC, Kronauer RE, Strohl KP, et al. Factors inducing periodic breathing in humans: a general model. J Appl Physiol 1982;53(3):644–59.

33. Edwards BA, Sands SA, Skuza EM, et al. Increased peripheral chemosensitivity via dopaminergic manipulation promotes respiratory instability in lambs. Respir Physiol Neurobiol 2008;164(3):419–28.

34. Wellman A, Jordan AS, Malhotra A, et al. Ventilatory control and airway anatomy in obstructive sleep apnea. Am J Respir Crit Care Med 2004;170(11): 1225–32.

35. Francis DP, Willson K, Davies LC, et al. Quantitative general theory for periodic breathing in chronic heart failure and its clinical implications. Circulation 2000;102(18):2214–21.

36. Sands SA, Edwards BA, Kee K, et al. Loop gain as a means to predict a positive airway pressure suppression of Cheyne-Stokes respiration in patients with heart failure. Am J Respir Crit Care Med 2011;184(9):1067–75.

37. Sands SA, Edwards BA, Kee K, et al. Loop gain explains the resolution of Cheyne-Stokes respiration using inspired CO_2 in patients with heart failure [abstract]. Am J Respir Crit Care Med 2012;185: A6697.

38. Nugent ST, Finley JP. Periodic breathing in infants: a model study. IEEE Trans Biomed Eng 1987;34: 482–5.

39. Wilkinson MH, Sia KL, Skuza EM, et al. Impact of changes in inspired oxygen and carbon dioxide on respiratory instability in the lamb. J Appl Physiol 2005;98(2):437–46.

40. Carley DW, Shannon DC. A minimal mathematical model of human periodic breathing. J Appl Physiol 1988;65(3):1400–9.

41. Mortara A, Sleight P, Pinna GD, et al. Association between hemodynamic impairment and Cheyne-Stokes respiration and periodic breathing in chronic stable congestive heart failure secondary to ischemic or idiopathic dilated cardiomyopathy. Am J Cardiol 1999;84(8):900–4.

42. Oldenburg O, Bitter T, Wiemer M, et al. Pulmonary capillary wedge pressure and pulmonary arterial pressure in heart failure patients with sleep-disordered breathing. Sleep Med 2009;10(7):726–30.

43. Lorenzi-Filho G, Rankin F, Bies I, et al. Effects of inhaled carbon dioxide and oxygen on Cheyne-Stokes respiration in patients with heart failure. Am J Respir Crit Care Med 1999;159(5 Pt 1): 1490–8.

44. Sinha AM, Skobel EC, Breithardt OA, et al. Cardiac resynchronization therapy improves central sleep apnea and Cheyne-Stokes respiration in patients with chronic heart failure. J Am Coll Cardiol 2004; 44(1):68–71.

45. Murphy RM, Shah RV, Malhotra R, et al. Exercise oscillatory ventilation in systolic heart failure: an indicator of impaired hemodynamic response to exercise. Circulation 2011;124(13):1442–51.

46. Olson TP, Frantz RP, Snyder EM, et al. Effects of acute changes in pulmonary wedge pressure on periodic breathing at rest in heart failure patients. Am Heart J 2007;153(1):104.e1–7.

47. Topor ZL, Johannson L, Kasprzyk J, et al. Dynamic ventilatory response to CO(2) in congestive heart failure patients with and without central sleep apnea. J Appl Physiol 2001;91(1):408–16.

48. Javaheri S. A mechanism of central sleep apnea in patients with heart failure. N Engl J Med 1999; 341(13):949–54.

49. Solin P, Roebuck T, Johns DP, et al. Peripheral and central ventilatory responses in central sleep apnea with and without congestive heart failure. Am J Respir Crit Care Med 2000;162(6):2194–200.

50. Solin P, Bergin P, Richardson M, et al. Influence of pulmonary capillary wedge pressure on central apnea in heart failure. Circulation 1999;99(12): 1574–9.

51. Poletti R, Passino C, Giannoni A, et al. Risk factors and prognostic value of daytime Cheyne-Stokes respiration in chronic heart failure patients. Int J Cardiol 2009;137(1):47–53.

52. Speksnijder L, Rutten JH, van den Meiracker AH, et al. Amino-terminal pro-brain natriuretic peptide (NT-proBNP) is a biomarker of cardiac filling pressures in pre-eclampsia. Eur J Obstet Gynecol Reprod Biol 2010;153(1):12–5.

53. Tschope C, Kasner M, Westermann D, et al. Elevated NT-ProBNP levels in patients with increased left ventricular filling pressure during exercise despite preserved systolic function. J Card Fail 2005;11(5 Suppl):S28–33.

54. Knebel F, Schimke I, Pliet K, et al. NT-ProBNP in acute heart failure: correlation with invasively measured hemodynamic parameters during recompensation. J Card Fail 2005;11(5 Suppl): S38–41.

55. Pudil R, Tichy M, Praus R, et al. NT-proBNP and echocardiographic parameters in patients with acute heart failure. Acta Med 2007;50(1):51–6.

56. Calvin AD, Somers VK, Johnson BD, et al. Left atrial size, chemosensitivity, and central sleep apnea in heart failure. Chest 2014;146(1):96–103.

57. Lorenzi-Filho G, Azevedo ER, Parker JD, et al. Relationship of carbon dioxide tension in arterial blood to pulmonary wedge pressure in heart failure. Eur Respir J 2002;19(1):37–40.

58. Manisty CH, Willson K, Wensel R, et al. Development of respiratory control instability in heart failure: a novel approach to dissect the pathophysiological mechanisms. J Physiol 2006;577(Pt 1): 387–401.

59. Chenuel BJ, Smith CA, Skatrud JB, et al. Increased propensity for apnea in response to acute elevations in left atrial pressure during sleep in the dog. J Appl Physiol 2006;101(1):76–83.

60. Szollosi I, Thompson BR, Krum H, et al. Impaired pulmonary diffusing capacity and hypoxia in heart failure correlates with central sleep apnea severity. Chest 2008;134(1):67–72.

61. Yumino D, Redolfi S, Ruttanaumpawan P, et al. Nocturnal rostral fluid shift: a unifying concept for the pathogenesis of obstructive and central sleep apnea in men with heart failure. Circulation 2010; 121(14):1598–605.

62. Lloyd TC Jr. Breathing response to lung congestion with and without left heart distension. J Appl Physiol (1985) 1988;65(1):131–6.

63. Kappagoda CT, Ravi K. The rapidly adapting receptors in mammalian airways and their responses to changes in extravascular fluid volume. Exp Physiol 2006;91(4):647–54.

64. Solin P, Snell GI, Williams TJ, et al. Central sleep apnoea in congestive heart failure despite vagal denervation after bilateral lung transplantation. Eur Respir J 1998;12(2):495–8.

65. Ding Y, Li YL, Schultz HD. Role of blood flow in carotid body chemoreflex function in heart failure. J Physiol 2011;589(Pt 1):245–58.

66. Dempsey JA, Smith CA, Blain GM, et al. Role of central/peripheral chemoreceptors and their interdependence in the pathophysiology of sleep apnea. Adv Exp Med Biol 2012;758:343–9.

67. Schultz HD, Marcus NJ, Del Rio R. Mechanisms of carotid body chemoreflex dysfunction during heart failure. Exp Physiol 2015;100:124–9.

68. Edwards BA, Sands SA, Feeney C, et al. Continuous positive airway pressure reduces loop gain and resolves periodic central apneas in the lamb. Respir Physiol Neurobiol 2009;168(3): 239–49.

69. Szollosi I, Roebuck T, Thompson B, et al. Lateral sleeping position reduces severity of central sleep apnea/Cheyne-Stokes respiration. Sleep 2006; 29(8):1045–51.

70. Hurewitz AN, Susskind H, Harold WH. Obesity alters regional ventilation in lateral decubitus position. J Appl Physiol 1985;59(3):774–83.

71. Fontana M, Emdin M, Giannoni A, et al. Effect of acetazolamide on chemosensitivity, Cheyne-Stokes respiration, and response to effort in patients with heart failure. Am J Cardiol 2011; 107(11):1675–80.

72. Douglas NJ, White DP, Weil JV, et al. Hypoxic ventilatory response decreases during sleep in normal men. Am Rev Respir Dis 1982;125(3):286–9.

73. Douglas NJ, White DP, Weil JV, et al. Hypercapnic ventilatory response in sleeping adults. Am Rev Respir Dis 1982;126(5):758–62.

74. White DP, Douglas NJ, Pickett CK, et al. Hypoxic ventilatory response during sleep in normal premenopausal women. Am Rev Respir Dis 1982; 126(3):530–3.

75. Domenico Pinna G, Robbi E, Pizza F, et al. Sleep-wake fluctuations and respiratory events during Cheyne-Stokes respiration in patients with heart failure. J Sleep Res 2014;23(3):347–57.

76. Khoo MC, Berry RB. Modeling the interaction between arousal and chemical drive in sleep-disordered breathing. Sleep 1996;19(10 Suppl): S167–9.

77. Sahlin C, Svanborg E, Stenlund H, et al. Cheyne-Stokes respiration and supine dependency. Eur Respir J 2005;25(5):829–33.

78. Quadri S, Drake C, Hudgel DW. Improvement of idiopathic central sleep apnea with zolpidem. J Clin Sleep Med 2009;5(2):122–9.

79. Hudgel DW, Martin RJ, Johnson B, et al. Mechanics of the respiratory system and breathing pattern during sleep in normal humans. J Appl Physiol 1984;56(1):133–7.

80. Edwards BA, Eckert DJ, McSharry DG, et al. Clinical predictors of the respiratory arousal threshold in patients with obstructive sleep apnea. Am J Respir Crit Care Med 2014;190(11):1293–300.

81. Ballard RD, Irvin CG, Martin RJ, et al. Influence of sleep on lung volume in asthmatic patients and normal subjects. J Appl Physiol 1990;68(5): 2034–41.

82. Arzt M, Floras JS, Logan AG, et al. Suppression of central sleep apnea by continuous positive airway pressure and transplant-free survival in heart failure: a post hoc analysis of the Canadian Continuous Positive Airway Pressure for Patients with Central Sleep Apnea and Heart Failure Trial (CANPAP). Circulation 2007;115(25):3173–80.

83. Oldenburg O, Bitter T, Wellmann B, et al. Reduced mortality in heart failure patients with nocturnal Cheyne-Stokes respiration receiving adaptive servoventilation therapy. J Am Coll Cardiol 2013; 61(10_S).

84. Naughton MT, Benard DC, Rutherford R, et al. Effect of continuous positive airway pressure on central sleep apnea and nocturnal PCO2 in heart failure. Am J Respir Crit Care Med 1994;150(6 Pt 1):1598–604.

85. Naughton MT, Liu PP, Bernard DC, et al. Treatment of congestive heart failure and Cheyne-Stokes respiration during sleep by continuous positive airway pressure. Am J Respir Crit Care Med 1995;151(1):92–7.

86. Bradley TD, Logan AG, Kimoff RJ, et al. Continuous positive airway pressure for central sleep apnea and heart failure. N Engl J Med 2005;353(19): 2025–33.

87. Javaheri S. Acetazolamide improves central sleep apnea in heart failure: a double-blind, prospective study. Am J Respir Crit Care Med 2006;173(2): 234–7.

88. Javaheri S. Effects of continuous positive airway pressure on sleep apnea and ventricular irritability in patients with heart failure. Circulation 2000; 101(4):392–7.

89. Arzt M, Schulz M, Wensel R, et al. Nocturnal continuous positive airway pressure improves ventilatory efficiency during exercise in patients with chronic heart failure. Chest 2005;127(3):794–802.

90. Sharma BK, Bakker JP, McSharry DG, et al. Adaptive servoventilation for treatment of sleep-disordered breathing in heart failure: a systematic review and meta-analysis. Chest 2012;142(5): 1211–21.

91. Tamura A, Kawano Y, Naono S, et al. Relationship between beta-blocker treatment and the severity of central sleep apnea in chronic heart failure. Chest 2007;131(1):130–5.

92. Kohnlein T, Welte T. Does beta-blocker treatment influence central sleep apnoea? Respir Med 2007;101(4):850–3.

93. Silva CP, Lorenzi-Filho G, Marcondes B, et al. Reduction of central sleep apnea in heart failure patients with beta-blockers therapy. Arq Bras Cardiol 2010;94(2):223–9, 39–45, 6–32. [in Portuguese, Spanish].

94. Skobel EC, Sinha AM, Norra C, et al. Effect of cardiac resynchronization therapy on sleep quality, quality of life, and symptomatic depression in patients with chronic heart failure and Cheyne-Stokes respiration. Sleep Breath 2005;9(4):159–66.

95. Vazir A, Hastings PC, Morrell MJ, et al. Resolution of central sleep apnoea following implantation of a left ventricular assist device. Int J Cardiol 2010; 138(3):317–9.

96. Mansfield DR, Solin P, Roebuck T, et al. The effect of successful heart transplant treatment of heart failure on central sleep apnea. Chest 2003; 124(5):1675–81.

97. Braver HM, Brandes WC, Kubiet MA, et al. Effect of cardiac transplantation on Cheyne-Stokes respiration occurring during sleep. Am J Cardiol 1995; 76(8):632–4.

98. Thalhofer SA, Kiwus U, Dorow P. Influence of orthotopic heart transplantation on breathing pattern disorders in patients with dilated cardiomyopathy. Sleep Breath 2000;4(3):121–6.

99. Kara T, Novak M, Nykodym J, et al. Short-term effects of cardiac resynchronization therapy on sleep-disordered breathing in patients with systolic heart failure. Chest 2008;134(1):87–93.

100. Miyata M, Yoshihisa A, Suzuki S, et al. Adaptive servo ventilation improves Cheyne-Stokes respiration, cardiac function, and prognosis in chronic heart failure patients with cardiac resynchronization therapy. J Cardiol 2012;60(3):222–7.

101. Padeletti M, Henriquez A, Mancini DM, et al. Persistence of Cheyne-Stokes breathing after left ventricular assist device implantation in patients with acutely decompensated end-stage heart failure. J Heart Lung Transpl 2007;26(7): 742–4.

102. Krachman SL, Crocetti J, Berger TJ, et al. Effects of nasal continuous positive airway pressure on oxygen body stores in patients with Cheyne-Stokes respiration and congestive heart failure. Chest 2003;123(1):59–66.

103. Jobin V, Rigau J, Beauregard J, et al. Evaluation of upper airway patency during Cheyne-Stokes breathing in heart failure patients. Eur Respir J 2012;40(6):1523–30.

104. Arzt M, Schulz M, Schroll S, et al. Time course of continuous positive airway pressure effects on central sleep apnoea in patients with chronic heart failure. J Sleep Res 2009;18(1):20–5.

105. Lloyd BB, Jukes MG, Cunningham DJ. The relation between alveolar oxygen pressure and the respiratory response to carbon dioxide in man. Q J Exp Physiol Cogn Med Sci 1958;43(2):214–27.

106. Lenique F, Habis M, Lofaso F, et al. Ventilatory and hemodynamic effects of continuous positive airway pressure in left heart failure. Am J Respir Crit Care Med 1997;155(2):500–5.

107. Bradley TD, Holloway RM, McLaughlin PR, et al. Cardiac output response to continuous positive airway pressure in congestive heart failure. Am Rev Respir Dis 1992;145(2 Pt 1):377–82.

108. Sin DD, Logan AG, Fitzgerald FS, et al. Effects of continuous positive airway pressure on cardiovascular outcomes in heart failure patients with and without Cheyne-Stokes respiration. Circulation 2000;102(1):61–6.

109. Johnson KG, Johnson DC. Bilevel positive airway pressure worsens central apneas during sleep. Chest 2005;128(4):2141–50.

110. Kohnlein T, Welte T, Tan LB, et al. Assisted ventilation for heart failure patients with Cheyne-Stokes respiration. Eur Respir J 2002;20(4):934–41.

111. Oldenburg O, Schmidt A, Lamp B, et al. Adaptive servoventilation improves cardiac function in patients with chronic heart failure and Cheyne-Stokes respiration. Eur J Heart Fail 2008;10(6):581–6.

112. Pepperell JC, Maskell NA, Jones DR, et al. A randomized controlled trial of adaptive ventilation for Cheyne-Stokes breathing in heart failure. Am J Respir Crit Care Med 2003;168(9):1109–14.

113. Philippe C, Stoica-Herman M, Drouot X, et al. Compliance with and effectiveness of adaptive servoventilation versus continuous positive airway pressure in the treatment of Cheyne-Stokes respiration in heart failure over a six month period. Heart 2006;92(3):337–42.

114. Szollosi I, O'Driscoll DM, Dayer MJ, et al. Adaptive servo-ventilation and dead space: effects on central sleep apnoea. J Sleep Res 2006;15(2):199–205.

115. Teschler H, Dohring J, Wang YM, et al. Adaptive pressure support servo-ventilation: a novel treatment for Cheyne-Stokes respiration in heart failure. Am J Respir Crit Care Med 2001;164(4):614–9.

116. Owada T, Yoshihisa A, Yamauchi H, et al. Adaptive servoventilation improves cardiorenal function and prognosis in heart failure patients with chronic kidney disease and sleep-disordered breathing. J Card Fail 2013;19(4):225–32.

117. Yoshihisa A, Suzuki S, Miyata M, et al. A single night' beneficial effects of adaptive servo-ventilation on cardiac overload, sympathetic nervous activity, and myocardial damage in patients with chronic heart failure and sleep-disordered breathing. Circ J 2012;76(9):2153–8.

118. Haruki N, Takeuchi M, Kaku K, et al. Comparison of acute and chronic impact of adaptive servo-ventilation on left chamber geometry and function in patients with chronic heart failure. Eur J Heart Fail 2011;13(10):1140–6.

119. Kasai T, Usui Y, Yoshioka T, et al. Effect of flow-triggered adaptive servo-ventilation compared with continuous positive airway pressure in patients with chronic heart failure with coexisting obstructive sleep apnea and Cheyne-Stokes respiration. Circ Heart Fail 2010;3(1):140–8.

120. Javaheri S, Ahmed M, Parker TJ, et al. Effects of nasal O2 on sleep-related disordered breathing in ambulatory patients with stable heart failure. Sleep 1999;22(8):1101–6.

121. Hanly PJ, Millar TW, Steljes DG, et al. The effect of oxygen on respiration and sleep in patients with congestive heart failure. Ann Intern Med 1989;111(10):777–82.

122. Krachman SL, D'Alonzo GE, Berger TJ, et al. Comparison of oxygen therapy with nasal continuous positive airway pressure on Cheyne-Stokes respiration during sleep in congestive heart failure. Chest 1999;116(6):1550–7.

123. Javaheri S, Parker TJ, Wexler L, et al. Effect of theophylline on sleep-disordered breathing in heart failure. N Engl J Med 1996;335(8):562–7.

124. Edwards BA, Sands SA, Eckert DJ, et al. Acetazolamide improves loop gain but not the other physiological traits causing obstructive sleep apnoea. J Physiol 2012;590(Pt 5):1199–211.

125. Leung RS, Diep TM, Bowman ME, et al. Provocation of ventricular ectopy by Cheyne-Stokes respiration in patients with heart failure. Sleep 2004;27(7):1337–43.

126. Ponikowski P, Anker SD, Chua TP, et al. Oscillatory breathing patterns during wakefulness in patients with chronic heart failure: clinical implications and role of augmented peripheral chemosensitivity. Circulation 1999;100(24):2418–24.

127. Chua TP, Harrington D, Ponikowski P, et al. Effects of dihydrocodeine on chemosensitivity and exercise tolerance in patients with chronic heart failure. J Am Coll Cardiol 1997;29(1):147–52.

128. Zaharna M, Rama A, Chan R, et al. A case of positional central sleep apnea. J Clin Sleep Med 2013;9(3):265–8.

129. Soll BA, Yeo KK, Davis JW, et al. The effect of posture on Cheyne-Stokes respirations and hemodynamics in patients with heart failure. Sleep 2009;32(11):1499–506.

130. Zhang XL, Ding N, Wang H, et al. Transvenous phrenic nerve stimulation in patients with Cheyne-Stokes respiration and congestive heart failure: a safety and proof-of-concept study. Chest 2012;142(4):927–34.

131. Ponikowski P, Javaheri S, Michalkiewicz D, et al. Transvenous phrenic nerve stimulation for the treatment of central sleep apnoea in heart failure. Eur Heart J 2012;33(7):889–94.

132. Giannoni A, Baruah R, Willson K, et al. Real-time dynamic carbon dioxide administration: a novel treatment strategy for stabilization of periodic breathing with potential application to central sleep apnea. J Am Coll Cardiol 2010;56(22):1832–7.

133. Mebrate Y, Willson K, Manisty CH, et al. Dynamic CO2 therapy in periodic breathing: a modeling study to determine optimal timing and dosage regimes. J Appl Physiol 2009;107(3):696–706.

134. Marcus NJ, Del Rio R, Schultz EP, et al. Carotid body denervation improves autonomic and cardiac function and attenuates disordered breathing in congestive heart failure. J Physiol 2014;592(Pt 2):391–408.

135. Niewinski P, Janczak D, Rucinski A, et al. Carotid body removal for treatment of chronic systolic heart failure. Int J Cardiol 2013;168(3):2506–9.

136. Meza S, Mendez M, Ostrowski M, et al. Susceptibility to periodic breathing with assisted ventilation during sleep in normal subjects. J Appl Physiol 1998;85(5):1929–40.

137. White LH, Bradley TD. Role of nocturnal rostral fluid shift in the pathogenesis of obstructive and central sleep apnoea. J Physiol 2013;591(Pt 5):1179–93.

138. Mogri M, Khan MI, Grant BJ, et al. Central sleep apnea induced by acute ingestion of opioids. Chest 2008;133(6):1484–8.

139. Walker JM, Farney RJ, Rhondeau SM, et al. Chronic opioid use is a risk factor for the development of central sleep apnea and ataxic breathing. J Clin Sleep Med 2007;3(5):455–61.

140. Wang D, Teichtahl H, Drummer O, et al. Central sleep apnea in stable methadone maintenance treatment patients. Chest 2005;128(3):1348–56.

141. Cheyne J. A case of apoplexy, in which the fleshy part of the heart was converted into fat. Dublin Hosp Rep 1818;12:216–22. Cardiac Classics 1941. p. 317–20 [reprint].

142. Nachtmann A, Siebler M, Rose G, et al. Cheyne-Stokes respiration in ischemic stroke. Neurology 1995;45(4):820–1.

143. Nopmaneejumruslers C, Kaneko Y, Hajek V, et al. Cheyne-Stokes respiration in stroke: relationship to hypocapnia and occult cardiac dysfunction. Am J Respir Crit Care Med 2005;171(9):1048–52.

144. Bonnin-Vilaplana M, Arboix A, Parra O, et al. Cheyne-Stokes respiration in patients with first-ever lacunar stroke. Sleep Disord 2012;2012: 257890.

145. Siccoli MM, Valko PO, Hermann DM, et al. Central periodic breathing during sleep in 74 patients with acute ischemic stroke - neurogenic and cardiogenic factors. J Neurol 2008;255(11):1687–92.

146. Brown HW, Plum F. The neurologic basis of Cheyne-Stokes respiration. Am J Med 1961;30(6): 849–60.

147. Heyman A, Birchfield RI, Sieker HO. Effects of bilateral cerebral infarction on respiratory center sensitivity. Neurology 1958;8(9):694–700.

148. Garcia-Pachon E. Severe Cheyne-Stokes respiration in an awake patient after stroke. Internet J Pulm Med 2006;7(1).

149. Brill AK, Rosti R, Hefti JP, et al. Adaptive servo-ventilation as treatment of persistent central sleep apnea in post-acute ischemic stroke patients. Sleep Med 2014;15(11):1309–13.

150. Watson RA, Pride NB. Postural changes in lung volumes and respiratory resistance in subjects with obesity. J Appl Physiol 2005;98(2):512–7.

Moving?

Make sure your subscription moves with you!

To notify us of your new address, find your **Clinics Account Number** (located on your mailing label above your name), and contact customer service at:

Email: journalscustomerservice-usa@elsevier.com

800-654-2452 (subscribers in the U.S. & Canada)
314-447-8871 (subscribers outside of the U.S. & Canada)

Fax number: 314-447-8029

Elsevier Health Sciences Division
Subscription Customer Service
3251 Riverport Lane
Maryland Heights, MO 63043

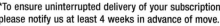

*To ensure uninterrupted delivery of your subscription, please notify us at least 4 weeks in advance of move.

ELSEVIER